To Jean and Bob Swenson
with my warmest regards,

Martin Goldberg.

MIND-INFLUENCING DRUGS

Effective Management of Patients with Emotional Illness

Edited by
Martin Goldberg, M.D. and Gerald Egelston

PSG Publishing Company, Inc.
Littleton, Massachusetts

Library of Congress Cataloging in Publication Data

Main entry under title:

Mind-influencing drugs.

    1. Psychopharmacology—Addresses, essays, lectures.
2. Mental illness—Diagnosis—Addresses, essays, lectures. 3. Diagnosis, Differential—Addresses, essays,
lectures. I. Egelston, Gerald. II. Goldberg, Martin,
1924-
RC483.M56   615'.78   76-19659
ISBN 0-88416-179-X

Printed in the United States of America.

International Standard Book Number: 0-88416-179-X

Library of Congress Catalog Card Number: 76-19659

CONTRIBUTORS

Walter C. Alvarez, M.D.
Professor of Medicine Emeritus
Mayo Foundation Graduate
   School
University of Minnesota Medical
   School
San Francisco, California

Doris Berlin, M.D., M.P.H.
Chief of Service for Education
   and Training
Hudson River Psychiatric Center
Poughkeepsie, New York
Clinical Associate Professor of
   Psychiatry
Albany Medical College
Albany, New York

Dean T. Collins, M.D.
Section Chief
C. F. Menninger Memorial
   Hospital
The Menninger Foundation
Topeka, Kansas

Gerald Egelston
Consultant, Professional
   Relations
New City, New York

Dana L. Farnsworth, M.D.
Henry K. Oliver Professor of
   Hygiene Emeritus
Harvard University
Cambridge, Massachusetts

Martin Goldberg, M.D.
Senior Attending Psychiatrist
Director of Marital Therapy
   Training and Research
The Institute of the Pennsylvania
   Hospital
Philadelphia, Pennsylvania

Burton J. Goldstein, M.D.
Professor of Psychiatry
Associate Professor of
   Pharmacology
Vice Chairman, Department of
   Psychiatry
University of Miami School of
   Medicine
Miami, Florida

Arthur A. Greenfield, D.O.
Associate Clinical Professor of
   Psychiatry
Ohio University College of
   Osteopathic Medicine
Dayton, Ohio

Harvey A. Horowitz, M.D.
Associate Psychiatrist
The Institute of the Pennsylvania
   Hospital
Philadelphia, Pennsylvania

Myer Mendelson, M.D.
Senior Attending Psychiatrist
The Institute of the Pennsylvania
   Hospital
Philadelphia, Pennsylvania

Alan Jay Ominsky, M.D.
Associate Professor of
   Anesthesiology
Assistant Professor of Psychiatry
School of Medicine
University of Pennsylvania
Philadelphia, Pennsylvania

Harcharan S. Sehdev, M.D.
Director, Children's Division
The Menninger Foundation
Topeka, Kansas

iv

Edward Stainbrook, M.D., Ph.D.
Professor and Chairman
Department of Human Behavior
University of Southern
    California School of Medicine
Professor of Human Behavior
University of Southern
    California Schools of Dentistry,
    Pharmacy, and Social Work
Los Angeles, California

Henry H. Swain, M.D.
Professor of Pharmacology
University of Michigan Medical
    School
Ann Arbor, Michigan

Raymond Waggoner, M.D.
Senior Clinical Consultant
State of Michigan Department of
    Mental Health
Lansing, Michigan

Allan B. Wells, M.D.
Associate Psychiatrist
The Institute of the Pennsylvania
    Hospital
Philadelphia, Pennsylvania

Harry Zall, M.D.
Attending Psychiatrist
The Institute of the Pennsylvania
    Hospital
Philadelphia, Pennsylvania

CONTENTS

FOREWORD

This interesting book can be of great help to all those medical specialists who have learned that a considerable percentage of the patients who consult them for "heart disease" or "stomach disease" really haven't what they think they have; they have a neurosis or minor psychosis, a great worry or great annoyance, attacks of migraine, or the end-result of a little stroke.

I, who for years was a gastroenterologist, President of the Society, and Editor of the Journal, later became largely a psychiatrist because I had learned that almost half of the patients who came to or were referred to me because of an uncomfortable "stomach" were suffering from a neurosis or minor psychosis, due often to an inherited hypersensitivity of their nervous system, or to some great annoyance, or worry, or unhappiness.

Most patients I saw suffering from a duodenal ulcer got the ulcer because of some great worry or unhappiness.

Another phenomenon which led me into much study of neurosis was that many of the patients who in a great clinic had been thoroughly examined were told that there "was nothing the matter with them" and they could go home. When some of these patients begged for more information and some help, or cure, some of my doctor friends got into the habit of asking me to see if I could find out what was wrong.

Often I made the diagnosis in two minutes by using the technique which dear old Dr. Charlie Mayo taught me, which was to ask the spouse what was wrong. To illustrate: a pleasant farmer was turned over to me after a thorough examination had failed to show why he was having spells of nausea and vomiting. I just asked his wife, "What caused the spells?" and she said, with some annoyance, "He gets into trouble when he goes on a binge of chewing tobacco and swallowing the juice." The man then grinned, and admitted that his wife was correct.

Also, I found it very important, when an able roentgenologist had reported the finding of gallstones, to keep my assistant from immediately telling a surgeon to operate. In many such cases, a few questions showed that the gallstones had never caused any trouble, and what was really bothering the patient was a syndrome that had come suddenly one day, obviously due to a little stroke.

Early in my long life-time of medical practice, I learned the unwisdom of trying to get some diagnoses made with the help of only a physical examination, some laboratory tests, and some X-ray studies. In thousands of cases, I found that in order to make a correct diagnosis, I had to look carefully at the patient; I had to make friends with him/her; I had to take a careful and thorough history, and sometimes a most careful family history; and sometimes I had to have electroencephalograms made. To show how helpful the electric brain records can be, one afternoon a big man of 55 came in and begged me to cure his impotence, which was so bad that he had never been able to have sexual intercourse, and he so wanted it. He told me that with three doctors in succession he had had nine years of mental treatment without result! Noting that he had tremendous knee jerks, such as sometimes are due to epilepsy, I sent him to my good friend, Dr. Frederic Gibbs, for the making of electroencephalograms, and in an hour, I had the report of "typical epilepsy." I gave the man Dilantin, and next morning, over the phone, he shouted with joy, telling me that his impotence was cured!

Some sixty years ago, I learned the great value, in many cases, of a good, honest family history. One day, a fine, sensible man, 40 years old, came in and begged me to cure the awful pains in his head that for years had made his life hardly worth living. Noting his stiff, brownish facial skin, such as one sees in a few elderly epileptics, I asked if he had ever had a convulsion, and he said, "No." Then I asked, "Have you any epileptic relatives?" and he said, "Yes, I have a brother who falls down every day. He is in the State Colony." I gave the man Dilantin, and soon he reported that, at long last, he was free from pain.

The need for looking carefully at many a patient was shown me years ago when the president of a big company begged me to find out what had gone wrong with his once very able vice-president, who, for several months, had not been getting much work done. The Chief had sent him, in succession, to four eminent doctors, and all had reported that they could not find anything wrong, and so the poor fellow was being sent to me.

When next morning he walked into my office, I was distressed to realize that the four eminent physicians had failed to make what looked to me like a very easy diagnosis. First, the man did not look at all like an able vice-president. He looked like a poor ditch digger; his face showed definite signs of a minor brain damage, and he was leaning on his wife's arm!

I asked the man's wife, "Did this terrible change in your husband come suddenly one day?" and she said, "Yes, in the evening of January 2nd, while sitting reading, suddenly he fell out of his chair, and since then he has been so changed for the worse that I hardly know him. He must have had a little stroke!" And there was the correct diagnosis.

As most of us know, the wise physician who is a good diagnostician, while he is taking a history, will keep studying the patient's facial expression, and learning about his/her character. In thousands of cases, the wise doctor will become satisfied that the patient's illness was brought on by some distressing or frightening event.

To illustrate: I will never forget a woman who tried for two weeks to get me to call a surgeon and have her gallbladder removed. I refused because an X-ray study of her gallbladder had shown no disease, and the symptoms of her behavior strongly indicated a great nervous shock, annoyance, and worry.

After two weeks, in which she kept strongly denying that there was any shock just before her illness came, she gave in and told me that the evening before she fell ill, a woman came and said, "You are not Mrs. R.; I am; that bigamist that married you had not divorced me before he married you. Give me $5,000.00, or I will have your supposed husband in jail tomorrow." My patient said she was able to buy off the visitor.

That is the sort of "cause for an illness" that many of our patients will try hard not to tell us about. In thousands of such cases, I got the story, as I did in this case, by keeping the patient around for a week or two, taking a new history every day. Often, in this way, I have made a good friend out of the patient, and then he/she told me the truth, even about insane relatives!

Many patients have confessed that they were able to tell me the truth about their illness and their bad heredity only after they developed a friendship for me.

This book will be of great service to all doctors, and particularly those we now call primary care physicians. It deals with the many problems and guises of emotional illness, and the drugs available today which make it possible to keep our patients productive.

After seventy years of being a physician, my convictions are even stronger that a doctor's best diagnostic tool is his own keen observation. That is why this book is important. It teaches what to look for, and how to manage the problem. And, all of this is based on the many years of practical experience of the authors.

Walter C. Alvarez, M.D.
San Francisco, California

FOREWORD

I am very much impressed with the scope and purpose of this book. The majority of osteopathic physicians are in primary care medicine, and I am reminded daily by my colleagues of the need for an understanding of current mind-influencing drugs. Questions about when to use a drug, what drug to use, and drug interactions are the essence of many calls I receive from physicians.

The osteopathic concept of medicine has its roots in the inter-relationships of structure and function. It was only natural that early in the history of osteopathic medicine the importance of behavior and emotions were noted. A major underpinning of the osteopathic concept is total patient care.

This book deals with many psychophysiologic issues in total patient care. It can be very valuable in enhancing the primary care physician's confidence in dealing with psychopharmacologic agents.

The need for a rational approach to psychotropic drug therapy is of paramount importance. Which drug to use, under what conditions, and side effects and contraindications are primary concerns, but they do not encompass all that must be considered in developing a drug regimen. Social and economic factors about the patient must be known and taken into account. A rational approach to drug therapy must be more than pharmacologically correct—it must be humane and reasonable. The scope and purpose of this book underscore the clinical and practical aspects of using mind-influencing drugs.

Masked depressions, anxieties expressed through somatic channels, "ambulatory schizophrenia," and "street drug" abuses are but a few of the problems that are prevalent in today's society. Can drugs be of value in the treatment of these problems? How? Which drug is appropriate for each particular problem?

We no longer tuck emotionally disturbed people away into institutions. Today, the emphasis is on treatment within the community. This imposes increased responsibility on those involved with primary health care. Not many years ago, drugs related to the treatment of emotional disturbances were nonexistent. Today, we are confronted with a formidable array of such drugs. Although choices provide a welcome freedom, they also impose dilemmas. In order to answer pressing issues related to drug use, a plethora of material has become available. Unfortunately, much of it is based on laboratory findings that do not translate this information into practical and clinical usage. It is understandable that many primary care physicians and allied health care people have shied away from attempting to become familiar with these drugs.

This book was conceived in the field; that is, the authors have become acquainted with the needs of primary care physicians through scientific seminars, presentations, and panel discussions. These programs were shared by primary care physicians and allied health professionals throughout the country. What is pertinent and important to the clinical workers has been made known to the authors, and they in turn have emphasized the practical and clinical aspects of the use of mind-influencing drugs.

This monograph should be a welcome addition to the armamentarium of those professionals who deal with the growing mass of emotionally stricken humanity.

Arthur A. Greenfield, D.O.
Dayton, Ohio

Perhaps among the most fortunate of all people are those who are encouraged to read and to enjoy reading. As children, they are helped to discover the excitement and adventure of reading, and they are exposed to the joys of reading. Books become their good friends.

All of this is certainly good for publishers. It enhances the marketplace. It is equally good for the child, for it takes a lot of pain out of learning. Most of all, it is good for all of us who would like to share our ideas, and that is what this book is all about, an opportunity for a group of practicing physicians and teachers to share their ideas, experience, and information about how to be of better service to the patient with emotional illness.

Unlike many books, this is not the recitation of one man's experience. It might be called a compilation, a collection, an anthology, or any of the many names we use to explain cooperative literary effort. But in its truest sense, this book is better called a distillation. Each chapter reflects the quintessential result of erudition, broad clinical experience, and all that was learned in teaching others.

Like all books, it began with a small idea that was given the opportunity to grow. One of the authors, whose primary job is the organizing and presenting of courses in postgraduate medical education for a major pharmaceutical company, read the newspaper reports of Medicare and Medicaid scandals in New York. Many of the stories referred to what was alleged to be the indiscriminate use of a number of the popular mind-influencing drugs. Most often mentioned were tranquilizing agents. If one were to believe the stories as reported, most of these drugs were not needed, were overprescribed, were not used by the patients even though prescribed, and, because they were considered to be safe, could be written for many people in large quantities. The scandal became worse in the minds of the public, because they were convinced none of the drugs were prescribed for need but rather to increase the flow of money from the public coffers into the pockets of the greedy.

The stories stirred the imagination and provoked enough curiosity to encourage a bit of investigation. Like most stories, it contained both fact and fancy. Scandal about fraud has become so common in our newspapers that a day or two later the stories were off the front page, but enough curiosity stayed on to at least prompt the asking of some questions.

From a variety of sources, including friends in medicine who would have good advice, bits and pieces of the stories were confirmed. Tranquilizers were among the most commonly prescribed drugs, and one led all prescribed drugs in numbers of prescriptions. For the most part they were relatively safe. They were usually prescribed at low dosage levels and, even if overused, were seldom good suicide tools. They often helped symptoms without helping the underlying cause of disease. Many primary care physicians used them because of convenience, but, often as a result of being very busy or even overworked, they had had too little opportunity to learn as much about the drugs and their uses as they should.

Some pharmacologists suggested that the potential for drug interaction was great enough to be a problem. Most felt that there was insufficient history taking before the drugs were prescribed.

Now the idea began to grow. "Mind-Influencing Drugs" was suggested to a number of program committees as a theme for some medical symposia. The committees were usually composed of busy primary care physicians. As each committee discussed plans for its meeting, it became apparent the idea was a good one. More and more subject material was suggested for papers to be given within the meetings, and all of it identified the needs of the several medical communities as reflected in the clinical experiences of the committee members.

It was time to try the idea. The first three programs were tried in Minneapolis, Denver, and Napa. In every instance they drew the largest audience the sponsoring medical society had had since the early days of sex programming.

Because of the newness of the theme, the meetings were taped for review. Each meeting varied slightly, as each committee had determined its own program, but certain basic ingredients were constant. The committees did not want another meeting about drug abuse. They were generally turned off by more information about how to care for the experimenter with illegal drugs. They *did* want to know how they could make better use of the huge armamentarium of legal drugs available to them to manage patients with emotional illness.

They wanted more information about diagnosis. They wanted the different states of disorder better identified. They wanted to know what drugs to use and when to use them, and in the tradition of all concerned physicians, they wanted to know what they should not do.

The first three meetings were so successful the news spread, and many additional medical communities wanted the same kind of program. More programs were held in centers both large and small, and even as this is being written, plans for some twenty additional programs are in final form. These will also be in large and small centers, one even in Alaska.

So far you have read of an idea that became a series of successful medical symposia. This same idea finally became this book. After each meeting, request after request was received for one paper or another, but the lectures had been spontaneously given, informal talks. They were not available in print. Finally it dawned on the authors that getting the information into one cover was really needed, and over a late pair of nightcaps, the little idea became a concept for a book.

Getting started was not very difficult. From the consensus of the many program committees and speakers, we had good guidelines as to what was needed. Most of the speakers had spoken at one or more of the programs. We had tapes of their talks which could become the basis of chapters.

Equally important for our purposes, we had a record of all the questions asked by the audiences after the lectures. And, we had taped their answers and the discussions the questions generated. The panelists were not always in complete accord. This led to discussion, and even argument; all of which was good, for every speaker was wiser for it.

Most of the speakers on the several programs were friends of many years. We all knew each other, liked each other, and believed in what we planned to do.

A few ideas for chapters were added to the outline of the book to give it a wider scope. We went to additional friends whose knowledge and talents were needed, and the book got underway.

Practical clinical experience is the basis for each chapter. The test of the material against audiences of busy practicing physicians gave each contributor a feel for what was needed. Add to these the ingredients of erudition, experience, communication, and the desire to help patients, and you have the chapters of our book.

There is sometimes redundancy and there are some varying opinions. Each writer has spoken his piece. All of which adds up to his best shot.

We assume this book will be read not cover-to-cover, but selectively as the reader is curious.

Each contributor tested and retested, tried and improved, fined and refined. He separated the fine ore of practical information from the dross of untried theory. All of this went into the minds of audiences and was played back as questions. It was finally processed as this book, a distillation of ideas, concepts, information, cooperation, and goodwill.

This is our book. We hope it will be one more useful weapon to attack the disorders of the patient with emotional illness.

Gerald Egelston
New City, New York

1 Mind-Influencing Drugs: Nature's Gifts from the Gods

Gerald Egelston

Canst thou not minister to a mind diseas'd;
Pluck from the memory a rooted sorrow;
Raze out the written troubles of the brain;
And with some sweet oblivious antidote
Cleanse the stuff'd bosom of that perilous
    stuff
Which weighs upon the heart?
Macbeth, Act V, Scene 3

INTRODUCTION

It has been a condition of man since his earliest day that he has sought to enlarge his life. He has searched out the greener pasture. He has won greater territory. Shelter and clothing were developed, and as his skills and accumulated knowledge increased, he lived more and more comfortably, until today most men live secure from climate and most natural disaster. He no longer falls asleep fearful of being killed and eaten by some huge beast of prey.

At the same time, we have substituted fear of things abstract for fear of things physical. We fear loss of income, loss of respect, loss of status, loss of love. As we have progressed to these fears generated in our imaginations, our dreams, and our own psyches, we have tried to find some protection from these worries, which are as troublesome to us as was the saber-toothed tiger to our caveman ancestors.

1

Seeking escape from reality is as important today as ever before. We are concerned with perpetuating life—not just life, but youth. Maintaining sexual drive is very important. We dream of some magic elixir that could make us irresistible to the opposite sex. We still fear and hate pain and look for better analgesics. Whether religiously or intellectually motivated, we should all like to enjoy some greater awareness, some experience greater than the reality that surrounds us.

Like our ancestors—caveman, bronze age, ancient, or even most recent—we are still concerned with these same elusive needs: escape from pain; extension of youthful feelings; escape from death; and at the same time, escape from life as circumscribed by our own intellect.

Today we avoid the mumbo-jumbo of the shaman, love philtres, dream potions, and all the other essences of magic. We now substitute an abundance of botanicals, pharmaceuticals, vaccines, and vitamins. With them we seek to escape illness, avoid pain, extend youth, avoid death, and just feel better. And, to complement all of these, we have today's psychotropics, the drugs that indeed influence our minds.

Mind-influencing drugs! When one considers all of the implications of this simple combination of three commonplace words, it is mind-boggling of itself. In the memories of many who will read this book, the concept of a drug that could in fact influence the mind was frightening. It brought to mind all manner of incantation, witchery, evil influences, and the occult. This was the stuff of medieval legends, of Iseult and her Tristan quaffing the cup that set their fate.

To be able to use a drug, a magic compound that would alter the mind or change a mood, has long been an aspiration of mankind. Probably through all history there have been men and women who have had special knowledge of naturally occurring substances that did in fact influence the mind. This was a secret knowledge of the witches, the shamans, the magicians, of the Merlins. But the ordinary people knew little of this; their dreams became the legends: Scheherazade spinning her tales, the fancies of the Brothers Grimm, or the folklore of our Appalachians.

Today, the use of psychotropics, the mind-influencing drugs, has become so commonplace that one of them (Valium) is probably the one drug prescribed more than any other in the United States.

Mind-influencing drugs seem to offer a quick cure for many

emotionally ill patients. Too often they correct the symptoms without curing the disease. This is not always bad; there can be a positive placebo effect. Too, the patient relieved of the urgency of his emotional problem may effectively arrive at his own cure. So, like all things in this world, there is a bit of both good and bad, and the mind-influencing drug becomes another tool which, used wisely and with compassion, can help many unhappy, unfortunate, and unproductive people.

Although today we have available for therapy elaborately contrived chemical compounds, mind-influencing drugs have been with us since our earliest ancestors. Knowledge of many of them is certainly prehistoric. It could be argued that the apple given to Eve influenced the mind; certainly it influenced Adam's approach to things. It might have paved the way for some of the early conjectures about glutamic acid (instant smart). In retrospect, though, the trouble in Eden was probably due less to the apple than to the pair on the ground.

CACTUS, MUSHROOMS, AND LOCO WEED

Were such things here as we do
Or have we eaten on the insane root
That takes the reason prisoner?
Macbeth, Act I, Scene 3

Prehistoric man was familiar with a number of the naturally occurring psychotropic agents, which were usually of botanical origin. There is legendary evidence that many were known and used by ancient peoples, often as part of their primitive religious observances.

Hallucination played a part in many early religious practices. It provided an experience that could not be explained other than as an extraordinary happening. Hallucinatory effect could be the explanation of the many legends about flying into the skies, communicating with powers of other worlds, witnessing the wheels of fire, and all the many experiences first handed down as recanted legends and later recorded as part of the histories of early cultures.

The seeming escape of the mind from earthly measure was sought out by many early societies. The early Israeli sought a communication with Divinity by fasting, and the phenomenon of hallucination induced by excessive fasting, today recognized and explained physiologically, may have played a contributing role in the genesis of some of the legends of the Old Testament.

Perhaps it was Krog—or Arg, or Mog, or whatever grunted name by which our early caveman ancestor was called—who first stumbled on a substance that took him to another dimension of consciousness. It may have been an unwitting intoxication with naturally fermented fruit, or it could have been the happenstance of picking up and eating some exotic mushroom, cactus bud, or some form of loco weed (*Datura inoxia*). Nature abounds in substances that, when ingested innocently or purposely, can affect our feelings, our emotions, and our level of consciousness.

There is no record of who first noted the cause and effect, but someone must have, for sooner or later, as societies developed, man sought substances that would, in a sense, take him out of his known world.

Since the effect was pleasurable, startling, frightening, or just unexplainable, it was a very human reaction to experiment with it. And, since there was no understandable reason for this unusual effect, it was equally human to ascribe it to some supernatural power. Of course, the next step was to tie it to a religious experience.

As man moved into history as it is recorded, he brought with him his accumulated knowledge and experience. Records of the use of some agents that did indeed affect the mind are mentioned in very early manuscripts. It is alleged that some references to the "Source of Happiness," or the "Laughter Maker" (hemp, *Cannabis sativa*), occur in Chinese writings on pharmacology from the third millennium BC. Other of the early Chinese sacred books (ca 1500 BC) refer to a marijuana-like plant. Indian and Persian writings refer to the effect of the hemp plant. Herodotus wrote of the Scythians' use of hemp in their vapor baths, and Homer spoke of the drug (probably marijuana) Helen brought to Troy from Egypt.

At the same time, cults based on the use of hallucinogens were growing up in the Western world. By the time of the conquistadores, the use of peyote and hallucinogenic mushrooms (*Psilocybe mexicana*) was part of the culture of the Aztecs, Mayans, and other early American societies. The mushroom stones of Guatemala give evidence of the existence of a very active use of the hallucinogenic mushroom. The Indians of eastern Brazil and the Indians of our own Southwest all were familiar with and used some kind of naturally occurring hallucinogen. Use was always related to religion and supernatural experience. The mushroom eaten by the Aztecs as a part of their worship was called "food of the gods," or "god's flesh" (teonanaxatl).

At one time it was thought that the peyote bud, which produces hallucination when ingested, might have been confused with a dried mushroom, but mushrooms found in Mexico today contain psilocybin, and in some areas of Mexico they continue to be used by Indian tribes in their ceremonies.

In his book *The Teachings of Don Juan*, Carlos Castaneda, an anthropologist from California, describes many of the rituals and effects of using peyote, *Datura inoxia*, and the mushroom *Psilocybe mexicana*. His book records his experiences while learning the ancient lore of hallucinatory experience from a Yaqui Indian sorcerer during the early 1960s.

Early American societies were familiar with many other hallucinogens they had discovered in nature, and cults grew up around them. To this day, Indians of South and Central America, of Mexico, and of the United States continue the cults of the *mescalito* (peyote), the *yerba del diablo* (*Datura inoxia*), and the sacred mushroom, or *humito (Psilocybe mexicana)*.

It is an interesting coincidence that as this was written there was shown on the New York educational television channel a special program about the Yanomamo Indians. The program was a filmed study of the Indians' culture. The Yanomamos live in an area of southern Venezuela. They use a hallucinogen to give them an experience in which they believe they can soar from their corporeal selves to other areas, where they can do damage to their enemies. The film showed the preparation of the material: it appeared to be scraped from the inner bark of some woody stem; it was not identified. The powdered material was packed into a long pipette that looked to be a hollow reed. It was then blown into the nostrils of the sorcerers by an apprentice or fellow sorcerer. The physiologic effect was prompt. It caused a large amount of mucous discharge from the nostrils and also had some emetic effect.

In a very short time, the sorcerers staggered into a kind of dance. Their movements were erratic, and they seemed to be jerked by invisible strings. Their grimacing, gesticulating, and prancing about seemed to be the movements of completely decerebrated creatures. It was during this period that they believed they escaped their bodies. Later, they slept.

So even today we have primitive societies using naturally

occurring drugs in rituals as old as time, and yet this is very little different from the "tripping" of hippies on LSD.

The peyote button is the crown of a small cactus which is relatively common in the desert areas of the Southwest. It is a cactus without spines, and it has a long, tapering root. Only the crown of the plant is used. It is cut from the plant and dried into a small, hard button sometimes called a mescal button. These buttons are softened in the mouth and swallowed.

The use of peyote goes back to pre-Columbian times. Its use spread from the Indians of what is now northern Mexico to the Indians of our Southwest. The Apaches were familiar with and used peyote. The use of peyote by the Mescalero Apaches gave its name to the drug mescaline.

The use of peyote became part of the ritual of the Native American Church, originally the First-Born Church of Christ. Some early Indian leaders encouraged its use in order to wean the Indian away from alcohol. During the early Spanish rule of Mexico, peyote was outlawed at the insistence of the clergy, but it was later legalized. In the United States, it has been in and out of legality, but today it is legalized for its ritual use in the Native American Church.

One of the nineteenth-century Indian leaders who advocated the use of peyote was Quanah Parker,* who was half Comanche and half white. He was first an important war chief; it is purported that his purpose in life was to collect more white scalps than any other Indian. But being an astute man, he could see that the spread of the whites throughout the West was inevitable. He saw that the contest for the land was too one-sided.

History has it that Parker went off to the wilderness to speak with the Great Spirit. There he was told that he should work to unite his Indian brothers and lead them to a freedom they'd never before known. Manitou, it is told, spoke to him of the peyote. He said it was of his own divine flesh, and that by its use Parker and his Indian brothers could communicate with the Great Spirit and could become one people and eventually reign again over the lands and the waters.

Another of the great Indian prophets was John Wilson, who was part Caddo and part Delaware. He too preached the cult of the peyote.

It is the consensus of anthropologists who have studied the

---

* Sometimes written Quanan Parker.

spread of the peyote cult that it has been of distinct advantage to the Indians. It has brought a common culture that spans tribal lines. It has cemented the relationships of the Indians and given them a solidarity they have never before enjoyed. The peyote cult requires complete abstinence from alcohol, which in itself is a blessing. Members of the Native American Church do seem to do better than other Indians. They are usually better adjusted, enjoy a fuller social and cultural life, and generally are better off economically. Using peyote as a replacement for alcohol (alcoholism is the major health problem of the urban American Indian) had most positive results.

Dr. Robert Bergman of the United States Public Health Service has written extensively of the peyote cult and its ritual use in the Native American Church. While serving as chief of the Mental Health Program of the United States Public Health Service for the Navajo Indians, he had the opportunity not only to observe the rituals but also to follow up on reported psychotic episodes related to the use of peyote. In his report presented to the American Psychiatric Association, Dr. Bergman recommended that a full-scale study be made of peyote as used successfully by the Indians, from whom he thought there was much to learn. This report was later published in the *American Journal of Psychiatry*.

It has been the privilege of the author to work with the Association of American Indian Physicians and to be banquet lecturer for them. In conversation with many Indian physicians, it was repeatedly told us that the ritual use of peyote was beneficial, and some of the physicians could tell us of their personal experiences with peyote.

As they related, if peyote were taken with the correct (ritual) preparation, it served to expand awareness and in some way helped one to think out his or her problems. The correct use of peyote requires a spiritual preparation as important as is the ritual preparation for the sacrament of communion in the Catholic Church. In describing the benefits of peyote, Quanah Parker is supposed to have said, "The white man goes into his church and talks about Jesus. The Indian goes into his tipi and talks with Jesus."

Peyote has been used by many drug experimenters, and for a while it was a fashionable drug in the hippie culture. In the 1960s it was supplanted by LSD and other newer drugs. Apparently those who regularly use drugs purely as an escape or merely as experimenters constantly turn to new drugs, hoping for a new and different experience.

HEMP

Give me an ounce of civet, good apothecary,
to sweeten my imagination.
    King Lear, Act IV, Scene 6

As noted earlier in this chapter, mention of hemp is made in some of the earliest records of the peoples of Asia and the Middle East. It was also known in Egypt and other areas of Africa. It was used for its fiber, for the oil from its seeds, and for medicinal reasons.

As medicine, it was used to ease the pangs of childbirth, to alleviate pain in general, and, although not a true energizer, it was used among laboring classes to help them accomodate to the rigors of their hard work.

Among African tribes, it was thrown onto smoldering campfires, and the tribal members could sit around the fire and inhale the fumes. The Scythians used hemp in their vapor baths (similar to the saunas of the Finnish and Scandinavian peoples) by throwing the stems and leaves on heated stones. The active ingredient of the hemp mixed with the other vapors of the bath and added an intoxicating effect that enhanced the feeling of well-being and relaxation of the bath itself.

Where the grape was readily available, alcohol was the intoxicant of choice. The Greeks used wine and introduced it to the Mediterranean areas they colonized. Wine was also in common use by the Israelites. However, hemp was also available to them and they knew of its uses. The use of hemp versus that of alcohol was a cultural choice.

The Celtic tribes also had knowledge of hemp. These tribes, which probably originated in the area that today is Bohemia or Czechoslovakia, spread all through western Europe and went south and east toward the Balkan peninsula. It was here that they made contact with the Greeks, who called them Keltoi; hence our name Celt. It was probably at this time that the Celts first became familiar with the many uses of hemp. Hemp seeds have been found in urns discovered in excavations in Germany that are believed to date back to at least the sixth century BC.

Hemp (marijuana, bhang) is probably the most ubiquitous mind-influencer we have, and its use continues in many forms in almost every culture. In India it is used as bhang: the stems, flowers, and leaves; as ganja: the flowering tops with the plant resin; and as charas: the highly potent resin referred to as hashish. In India and in other areas of the world, hemp is chewed, eaten, prepared in teas, and included in candies, sweetmeats, and even in some ice creams. It is often used for festive occasions, and usually it is used socially. Its use in this way might be compared to our festive use of champagne or a special holiday wine.

In the Western world, the pick-me-up of a cup of coffee or tea or the end-of-the-workday cocktail parallels the use of hemp in India and other societies of Asia. A few puffs of a pipe or a bit of bhang tea gives the same mild stimulation, helps ease fatigue, increases appetite, and just makes life a bit more pleasant. It is cheaper than alcohol or coffee and probably less likely to produce dependence.

In Africa, also, hemp has been used to alleviate fatigue. It has been used too as an intoxicant, as a painkiller during childbirth, and as a pacifier for babies and young children.

The use of hemp as an intoxicant and stimulant was common in the ancient world and into modern times. Apparently it caused an increased sense of bravado, of heroic effort, or even of evil intent. Its use by the Hashasheen is well documented, and it was also used by the Thuggees, whose infamous murdering sprees are part of the unhappier history of India. Seemingly, hemp in concentrated form releases inhibitions and enlarges upon prior intent.

In the history of the Old World, as in Western history, hemp has moved in and out of official favor. In the fourteenth century, its use was outlawed in large parts of the Arab world, and drastic punishments were decreed for users. Imprisonment was one of the milder penalties; under one emir of the time, the bastinado and other cruel physical punishments were meted out to convicted growers and users of hemp.

Unlike other plants that can produce mind-influencing effects, hemp is a very useful plant. It produces a high-quality fiber of great tensile strength. The seeds can be utilized as bird feed and they also produce an oil useful in the paint industry.

It is a small wonder that this plant of so many uses found its way around the world. It is easy to cultivate and grows well on marshy land as well as in fields with good drainage. Here we have a plant of many uses that also provides surcease from fatigue, a feeling of well-being, a supposed aphrodisiac response, and alleviation of pain. By many measures, it was a truly marvelous gift of nature, and it was thought of by many cultures as coming from the gods themselves. With so many things going for it, it is easy to understand why the use of hemp as a psychotropic agent has never been successfully suppressed in any society.

Hemp, or marijuana (its Spanish name), first came to the New World by way of the Spanish and Portuguese explorers. Slaves brought from Africa would have had familiarity with it and probably brought it with them as an intoxicant. The Spanish, seeking to exploit the new territories for agricultural opportunity as well as mineral wealth, brought it to South America as a crop plant.

Since the South American natives had the coca leaf and other energizer plants, it is likely that the use of marijuana as a mind-influencing agent spread rather slowly. But spread it did, and by the nineteenth century the use of marijuana was associated with the peoples of Mexico, Central America, and the islands and countries of the Caribbean. It reflected a kind of cultural snobbism to look down on the marijuana smoker when at the same time the United States had developed an urban subculture of hashish users.

In our South, poor laborers wise in the ways of hemp used it for all the many benefits their deprived counterparts in the Old World had found it to possess. Many slaves knew about hemp from their own African experience or by handed-down legend, and our coastal and border towns in the South had easy access to the cult of marijuana.

In North America, hemp was introduced by the first settlers from Europe. The use of hemp by the colonists was an extension of its use in Europe, where for many years it was used in the production of cloth. Hemp was grown in all the colonies and was an important export item. Kentucky was famous for its production of hemp, and the total hemp production of the colonies severely affected the economy of hemp-producing areas of Europe. It was commonly used in the cruder fabrics of the time and was important economically not only as a raw material but also as an end product in the many ropewalks of our Atlantic seaboard. Its use for fabric goes back to at least the twelfth century, when it was probably brought back from the Middle East by Crusaders. There is also evidence that hempen cloth and rope were brought to Europe even earlier, as trade items in the caravan trade.

Hemp as a fiber for cloth went out of fashion when cotton became more easily available, but its cultivation both for rope fiber and for the bird feed industry continued into this century.

During World War II, our government encouraged its cultivation to ensure a supply of rope fibers.

As a result of centuries of widespread cultivation, hemp grows wild over extensive areas of the United States, so it has never been a problem to find it. However, for most regular marijuana users, the native stuff is considered to be of poor quality because it has a lower concentration of cannabinols, which apparently are the active mind-influencing ingredients of the plant.

Most marijuana users seek out a supply of marijuana grown in Mexico, Hawaii, Asia, and other areas where a stronger "weed" seems to grow. There has been very little legal research done in the United States on the cultivation of marijuana for its drug properties. From the best information available, the quality of the "weed" seems to be more dependent on the strain of the hemp grown than on the area where it is grown. However, from a merchandising point of view, there is a lot to be said for Kona Gold, Maui Wowee, Thai Sticks, Acapulco Gold, Santa Marta (the Lafitte-Rothschild for the pot connoisseur), and Congolese Black.

The easy come-and-go across our border with Mexico, our readily accessible seaports, and the multiplicity of our cultural origins gave us many points of contact with the use of marijuana. It was very easy for the use of marijuana to become common in the United States, and of course, for many years marijuana was completely legal.

In the United States, as in every other society to date, suppression of the use of marijuana by legal action has been a dismal failure. In some states the penalties for possession have been as drastic as those for felonies such as assault. Many of the states are now taking a more realistic approach to the problem and enabling legislation has adjusted the laws downward for possession and use.

The history of marijuana in the United States has followed much the same pattern as the history of other natural psychotropic drugs. It has been legal: it has been available both over-the-counter and as a prescription drug prepared by reputable companies. Although its sale is now illegal in the United States, it is still legal in many countries, but its use as a pharmaceutical is not widespread. It has been underinvestigated as a useful therapeutic agent because it has suffered the stigma of being dangerous and illegal, and it remains so almost as an exercise in scientific blindness and legislative stupidity. The many legislative blunders relating to marijuana reflect the same obtuse thinking seen in the misguided steps that led to our Eighteenth Amendment and the excesses of the Volstead Act.

If anything, the use of marijuana has spread in the United States from limited use by segments of our society—such as jazz musicians in the 1930s and 1940s, the hippie communities, and certain ethnic groups—to all strata of our society. Youth is not influenced by the illogical arguments against its use. The Department of Health, Education, and Welfare points out that the many claims, pro and con, about marijuana have been neither proved nor disproved. Most influential to the spread of the use of marijuana has been its move out of the subcultures to acceptance by society generally. After many years of study, Dr. David Smith, a clinical pharmacologist and toxicologist at the University of California, observed that the use of marijuana in all strata of society in the San Francisco and Bay area was so common that it was completely acceptable. In fact, Dr. Smith speaks of marijuana as the "new social drug," a name he used as the title for the report on a symposium on marijuana held under the auspices of the Haight Ashbury Foundation.

Dr. Smith was one of the first of the "respectable" physicians who was moved to find ways of bringing good medical attention to the "hippies," a subculture of teenagers and young adults who tried to find a social bond in an undisciplined, loosely structured establishment that sought identity with peace and peaceful pursuits. Dr. Smith's famous Haight Ashbury Clinic was the prototype of the many storefront clinics that sprung up in the ghetto areas of our big cities. Dr. Smith's firsthand experience with the drug culture is probably more extensive than that of any other physician in the country. He has lectured extensively to both medical and lay audiences. He has served on the President's Commission on Drug Abuse, and he has long been in the vanguard of the fight for more realistic drug laws.

Most who read this will know more about the drug than is written here. It is also dealt with in a later chapter. Its history is interesting beyond that of most drugs by reason of its millenia of use, its very ubiquity, and its prevalence in our society today. In a recent series of articles in the *New York Daily News*, it was quoted that official estimates indicate the United States imports 20 tons of marijuana daily—a $6-billion-a-year industry—all of which is illegal. Like it or not, marijuana is here. It is easily obtained, and it is not too expensive. It has become part of our culture, and its use or possible misuse will bring problems to physicians. Marijuana is not considered to be addictive, although there is always the potential for psychologic dependence, and in some instances, it is considered a first step toward using dangerous, hard drugs. Despite any problems marijuana may pose, it is here!

The challenge, then, is ours. Shall we investigate marijuana thoroughly and seek out its pharmacologic properties? It has been used for the pain of childbirth and was thought to be mildly analgesic, if not a true anesthetic. It has been tried in the management of migraine; there has been conjecture that it has a use in ophthalmology. Research is needed, and it is long overdue.

We need no longer concern ourselves with the legends of the hashish eaters, and certainly the worries of marijuana dens, the old wives' tales of sexual psychopathy, should be put aside. Enlightened research, free of all our former misconceptions, is called for. If marijuana is indeed useful, let's find out. If it is at best a crutch, or another alcohol which can be used either positively or destructively, then we should know that, too. We can't deal with any problem successfully if we approach it with pejorative misconceptions.

We know that marijuana is not as destructive a drug as are the opium derivatives, the barbiturates, and the amphetamines. These have positive value when used judiciously, as is pointed out by contributors to this book. Apparently marijuana is less dangerous than either alcohol or nicotine, yet, since it does influence the mind, more knowledge about it is needed, and most importantly, more knowledge is needed by physicians.

THE EMPEROR'S MAGIC LEAF

One must compose a song of praise
to this magical substance.
    Attributed to Sigmund Freud

The Old World had hemp and, of course, the opium poppy, and their uses were well known before the discovery of the New World, whether we use 1492 and the coming of the Spanish as a baseline date, or whether we go back to the earlier contacts with the Western world made by the navigators of the North Atlantic in early Celtic times. Hemp readily found a new home in the West and joined the assortment of mind-influencing drugs already available to the inhabitants of the Americas. There were quite a few of these which were used commonly, as noted earlier: peyote, *Datura,* and *Psilocybe,* the latter two available in several forms. It was the coca leaf, however, that brought a new drug influence to the Old World.

As soon as the Spanish came into contact with the Incas, they learned about the coca leaf. Coca was as much a part of the Incan culture as the gold and silver the Spanish sought, and it was considered to be of greater value by the Incas. The coca leaf (*Erythroxylon coca*) is from a shrub of the Andes and contains a drug that was completely new to the Spanish. Chewed, it produced euphoria, a feeling of energy, of physical well-being, of mental comfort, and of loss of pain.

Under the Incas, the coca leaf became part of religious ritual. In this respect its history is much like that of the other drugs mentioned earlier. In all cultures, when something is not understood, it is often assigned religious significance. And if it is something which makes people feel better and creates its own demand, it isn't long before it becomes the prerogative of the priesthood to determine who might enjoy it. This was the case with the coca leaf among the Incas. Before the Spanish came, the emperor of the Incas, who controlled the priesthood and was considered by his subjects to be godlike, controlled all aspects of the use of the coca leaf. He controlled its production and disbursement; he decided who might use it, who might have it, and to whom it might be given as a reward. The right to chew the coca leaf was a reward worth more than gold or silver. Before the Spanish came, the emperor of the Incas controlled the coca leaf as popular stories today suggest the Godfather controls heroin.

After the Spanish arrived, however, this was changed. They were the conquerors, and they were the great exploiters of all they conquered. In no time at all the Incas were plundered of their treasures, and control of the coca leaf fell to the Spanish, who used it to more deeply enslave the conquered.

The control of the Indian by way of the drug was insidious and successful. No longer was the drug forbidden; instead, its use was encouraged. Enslaved by drug dependence, the Indians worked harder just for coca. Because of the effects of the drug, they could work harder, longer, and more willingly, and the "carrot-on-the-stick" was more coca leaf. Also, the Indians were dependent for food on their Spanish masters, who found out that this magical leaf suppressed appetite, so that the slave ate less.

Here was the perfect vicious circle. The slaves had to pay their taxes to the Spanish master in labor and in produce, and part of that produce had to be coca leaf. At best, the coca leaf helped them to alleviate some of their misery. When the slave died working for the Spanish, and he usually did, new slaves were constantly available, and they became slaves not only of the Spanish but also of the coca leaf. Later in history the British were to do much the same with opium in controlling China.

It is interesting to note that in the high Andes, where there was no Spanish contact, the coca leaf was used by the natives as a part of ordinary daily life with apparently no deleterious effects. In the rigorous life of the high mountain areas, where extreme cold and a rarified atmosphere make demands that only the Andean Indians can survive, the coca leaf is still in regular use, and among these people there is apparently no addiction. Many of these Indians who have chewed the coca leaf daily abandon the practice completely if they leave their high mountain homes and move to the lowlands.

The Spanish had taken the leaf home with them, but, as something to be chewed, its use did not become popular in Europe. Perhaps the Spanish, knowing the coca leaf had made possible their slave empire in the New World, were afraid of the drug. And besides, they had alcohol and, by midsixteenth century, nicotine.

There were attempts to make beverages of the coca leaf. The Spanish and Portuguese were quite familiar with the yerba maté (herb tea), but drinks made with coca leaf did not become popular. One concoction did have some vogue in nineteenth-century Europe. Mariani's wine was a red wine fortified with an elixir of coca leaf, but its popularity was not widespread or long-lived. Because it contained cocaine, it was a stimulant and kept one awake and also stilled hunger pangs. Perhaps it failed because it was ahead of its time. Were it available today, it would certainly be the most successful fad diet ever: just imagine a pleasant-tasting wine that combined pleasure for the palate, suppression of appetite, and a feeling of well-being and stimulation, all with sexual overtones.

It was not the coca leaf per se that influenced the Old World, but cocaine, an alkaloid and the active ingredient of the coca leaf. It was as cocaine that the coca leaf came into its own in modern times. Cocaine was first isolated in the 1840s, and shortly after, investigation of its uses began. It was tried as a stimulant for the military, and the reports were enthusiastic. Physicians tried it for all manner of illness.

The young Sigmund Freud tried it after reading of its effects on soldiers. He found it to have an antidepressive effect, and he was excited about its many possibilities. In some of his early considerations of the drug, he felt it would supplant morphine.

Freud also tried cocaine as a blocking agent for pain. He was not very successful in this, but in the hands of others, cocaine became the local anesthetic of choice of many physicians. Its use in this capacity continued well into the 1930s, when newer agents became available.

No matter where one reads of cocaine, one reads of Freud's many experiments with it and of his personal use of it. He was early to report on the incidence of cocaine psychosis. He believed cocaine to be a nonaddictive drug, but he was well aware of the dangers of its overuse.

There is still argument as to whether cocaine is truly addictive. Some users need to support their habit as terribly as do heroin addicts. Other users seem to be able to either enjoy it or leave it alone, and never develop a dependence.

The distinctions between addiction and dependence are subtle, and they vary in different people. Cocaine users suffer very little in the way of physical withdrawal symptoms, but they may suffer extreme psychologic symptoms. Chief among these is severe depression for which cocaine seems to provide the only relief. In some ways, this parallels the problems of the alcoholic. However, the cocaine user in withdrawal does not experience physical problems such as the delirium tremens (DTs) of the alcoholic or the horrible problems of the opiate addict who goes it "cold turkey."

Cocaine is a very active psychotropic drug, and in the United States its use as a street drug seems to be on the ascendance. It is illegal but has been relatively easy to get, and as there were more and more crackdowns by the law on amphetamines, the use of cocaine regained much of its popularity. Cocaine, like marijuana, was for many years completely uncontrolled and readily available. A whole cult grew up around its use. Many characters in real life (Freud, for example) were users and praised its benefits. In fiction, Sherlock Holmes led readers to believe that cocaine enhanced his renowned powers of deduction.

Because there were so many well-esteemed devotees of cocaine, its use had wide acceptance. Even though it was not always used as the pure drug, its inclusion in the patent medicines, tonics, and nostrums of the late nineteenth and early twentieth centuries made many people cocaine users. A patent medicine of 1885, French Wine Coca, advertised as a nerve and tonic stimulant, was the ancestor of Coca Cola.

The use of cocaine, snuffed into the nostrils in a finely powdered form, was very common. It produced an instant effect, a kind of "right-now" flash. It was and has again become popular in the subcultures of our society. Its use by members of the demimonde gave us many jingles, limericks, and songs. Some of these songs became very popular as swing and skat songs in the thirties: the very popular "Minnie The Moocher" had lyrics that spoke of cocaine.

In cocaine, or the coca leaf, we have found another tale of a naturally occurring mind-influencing drug. It takes its place in history as both boon and curse. It played its role in religion, in the conquering of the New World, and in the subjugation and exploitation of the Indian. It has had its day in medicine and has had its bad qualities discovered. It has been used wisely and carelessly in its time, but safer substitutes have replaced its use by most physicians. In most of the Western world today, it is associated with criminal activity, and it is purported to be used more illegally than legally.

THE DREAM FLOWER

Take thou this vial, being then in bed,
And this distilled liquor drink thou off;
When, presently, through all thy veins shall run
A cold and drowsy humour.
   Romeo and Juliet, Act IV, Scene 1

Although legend and history alike abound with stories of hemp, peyote, and the coca leaf, it is with opium that we find the lengthiest and most elaborate record of use. Anyone who has read the *Arabian Nights* or *Grimm's Fairytales,* or the exploits of Fu Manchu or Sherlock Holmes, knows about opium. Much of the lurid appeal of the yellow journalism of the early 1900s depended on the stories of the opium dens and the innocent girls sold into white slavery; the broken blossoms who ended their days escaping into their opium-induced dreams. There is no other mind-influencing drug in nature that has engendered so many happy stories or sordid tales nor has so woven itself into the fabric of our legends.

The opium poppy *(Papaver somniferum)* occurs naturally in many areas of Asia. No one is quite sure when its sleep-inducing properties were first discovered. Unlike other of nature's mind-influencing drugs, opium requires that something be done to the plant in order that its effects be experienced. Coca leaf can be chewed as is; hemp can be ingested as is; peyote, too, can be merely swallowed; but collecting the sap of the seed pod of the poppy required the development of a technique beyond that of just picking and eating. Yet this technique was discovered early, and the use of opium to produce narcosis was known to the shamans and magi of many pre-Christian societies. Because it induced sleep, alleviated pain, and could cause a happy lassitude, it came into use as a panacea.

In its early history, it was used in the draughts of the apothecaries and physickers. Many of its properties were kept privy to the knowing few who could use it to make their spells and incantations come true. It was the "knock-out drop" used by the shamans of the tribes of the high steppes, the healers of ancient China and India, the magi of Persia, and, of course, the many miraculous healers of the Dark and Middle Ages. By the time of the Renaissance, its properties were much better understood. Alchemists were working with it to refine it, and apothecaries were including it in many mixtures designed to alleviate pain. Shortly after opium reached the West, where alcohol was available, it was discovered these two readily formed a solution. Sleeping potions and possets to comfort pain and to quiet the restless, ill child all usually consisted of opium in wine. This was sometimes sweetened or combined with other ingredients, some of which were potentially lethal, and most of which, at best, produced no additional beneficial effects. The history and literature of witchcraft reveal that the concoctions of the Satanists followed very closely the formulae for the healing nostrums of the pre-Renaissance physician. Almost all of the witches' brews included the poppy (oh, a few two-tailed lizards, or some powdered frogs' eyes, or bits of blood or infant fat might be added). The physician, being more scientific, used henbane, nightshade, yew leaves, aconite, dissected and powdered animal tissue, or eggs. But the common denominator of all the mixtures that successfully alleviated pain and stilled the troubled breast was opium.

The medical sciences, limited as they were, were preserved with little change through the Dark Ages by the monks and scholars in the West. It was in the East and in the Arabic world that progress in the healing arts continued at this time. The Crusades, which brought the barely civilized Western world into close touch with the far more sophisticated Moslems, produced one very important benefit for the people of Europe: a resurgence of interest in the healing arts. With this came the knowledge of opium that the physicians of the East had been accumulating during the centuries when medical science in Europe was stagnating.

Now information about opium was organized. For diarrhea in infants, it was a specific, continued as such right into the twentieth century in the form of paregoric. It was used to alleviate pain, and it became a tool for the midwife and for the surgeon, that barber/butcher who practiced his greatest skills on the battlefields. Opium came into regular use by all of the healers of the Renaissance.

As with the coca leaf, opium became an object of investigation of the chemists. It was they who, in the nineteenth century, succeeded in extracting the active ingredient, an alkaloid, from opium. They promptly named it morphine, after Morpheus, the god of sleep. The chemists continued their work with opium and discovered another fraction, which they called codeine. They also went on to discover that heating morphine in the presence of acetic acid produced heroin. Their aims were laudable: they were trying to create purer, more active forms of opium that would give physicians better, controllable dosage forms. Since the use of opium was still legal and socially acceptable in the nineteenth century, there is little reason to believe that any of those experimenters could have known that they were opening the Pandora's box of the troubles and problems from which we suffer so much today. One wonders if they would have forgone their research had they guessed the potential for criminal activity deriving from heroin alone.

By the nineteenth century, opium, in one form or another, was the most commonly used drug we had. It was as readily accessible as aspirin is today and it had more regular users. Most of the over-the-counter products of the day contained opium. The use of opium in prescriptions was so common many physicians wrote it as "G.O.M." (God's own medicine). Even though there was suspicion that the opiates produced addiction, it was thought of by many to be less dangerous than alcohol.

Of course, the nature of addiction was less well understood. Physicians could observe the problems of addiction: withdrawal symptoms, both psychologic and physical, were noted and reported in many of the journals of the day; physicians were familiar with managing delirium tremens; and they could report on the gross appearance of the addict. The contrast of the unruly, aggressive, and destructive alcoholic and the tranquil, often sleeping, opium addict made opium appear preferable. A habit that could be supported within the home by simply taking a spoonful or so of some popular tonic was far more acceptable socially than a habit that was pursued in the public houses and saloons. The opium user sat smugly at home enjoying his own soporific glow; the alcoholic was the drunken wretch lying in the gutter or brawling in the streets. A sense of propriety and morality blinded the scientific mind from seeing the like dangers of the two forms of addiction.

By the time of our Civil War, opium, in one form or another, was used in all strata of society and all over the country. It didn't seem to matter if you bought your patent medicine for diarrhea or consumption, for menstrual cramps or a bad cough. The opium was in it. Godfrey's Cordial, Cherry Pectoral, McMunn's Elixir—concoction after concoction contained opium or morphine.

The opiates were legal, opium was imported legally, and the opium poppies were cultivated legally. Morphine was manufactured legally, and there was no limitation on its sale. It was not even necessary to go to a pharmacy to obtain them. They were available in the grocery store as well as the drug store. In the frontier and rural towns, the general store carried opiates along with horse liniment, barbed wire, calico for a sun bonnet, and all of the other necessities. If you couldn't get to the general store, you could get your opium or morphine from a mail-order house.

All of this was the outgrowth of the early cultivation of the opium poppy by the colonists. It was grown in Pennsylvania and New England, and later, opium poppies were grown throughout the eastern colonies, as well as in the newly won areas to the west. Eventually, poppy cultivation moved to Arizona and California, and both of these became big producers of opium. It is interesting to note that although the cultivation of the opium poppy was banned by some of the states, it was as late as 1942 before the ban became a federal law.

Use of opium became so widespread there were soon reports of opium- and morphine-eaters. Actually, they were usually drinkers, for the opiates were most readily available in elixirs, tonics, and wines. Laudanum, opium in alcohol, could be added to any beverage. Since the alcohol used was often of a proof low enough to be drunk without hurting the oral mucosa, laudanum was often drunk straight.

Many people of the times who were teetotalers and who morally abhorred the use of alcohol were morphine or opium users. It was not at all unusual for a physician to convert the alcoholic to the use of opium and believe he was effecting a cure.

More unfortunately, because of the easy availability of opium in proprietary medicines, many people became addicted to opium without realizing it. Pillars of church and community were often addicts. Most sadly, the statistics of the time included many addicted children. The numerous cures they were given for teething pain, running-off-the-bowels, colic, coughs, earache—any childhood pain or just fretfulness—all included opium. The mill worker who carried her baby with her to work quieted its crying with laudanum. The village mother, busy with her friends at a quilting bee, soothed the aching gums of her teething child with a syrup of molasses, sassafras, and opium. The cure-alls of the time were opiates. A century later, *opiate* remains in our language as a noun that describes anything that can give general satisfaction to the public or delude them into ignoring incipient danger.

At the same time, opium-eaters were increasing in number in Europe, particularly in countries such as England, where industrialization was moving more and more people from the land to the city. These poor and uneducated, with only their labor to provide them a livelihood, were easily wooed to opium. It was cheap, and it helped one forget the pain of the long day. For many it was better than gin, the panacea of an earlier London.

Addiction, though innocently acquired, became a social problem of consequence. It was observed that, if deprived of his supply of opium, an addict would lie, cheat, and steal to get his need filled. This was evidence of a weak will; it suggested decadence and moral impairment. No one thought of the addict as a poor, misbegotten creature who needed help. There was no pity for him, only scorn. The physicians of the day sat as judges and condemned the poor creatures for being viciously immoral. Neighbors, who witnessed the troubles brought to a family as father or mother, or often both, fell deeper into opium use, would also condemn them. Of course, these good people weren't likely to support a law that would control the sale of opiates and perhaps prohibit use of the tonic that kept grandma feeling so chipper or the syrup that was a sure cure for colic. Their attitude was that the addicts should spend their money for food instead of for supporting their habit. Didn't they have any gumption? In addition, it was considered good sense for a pharmacist or storekeeper to encourage the use of opiates: it was a sure way to increase one's business. It was silly to think that anyone would develop so fixed a habit for a drug that he would sacrifice his property and family to support it. They would not believe that anything which produced good business contributed to someone's moral degeneration. The addict was just weak willed.

The use of opium continued to be common well into this century. Many studies conducted in the several states suggested that opium and morphine were more likely to be the choices of women, whereas men preferred alcohol. Many professional men were regular users of morphine, but the smoking of opium was relatively less common among them. Many physicians used opium and morphine, often with the full sanction of society.

The late Dr. Windsor C. Cutting, former dean of Stanford University Medical School and later the first dean of the University of Hawaii Medical School, published an article in the 1942 *Stanford Medical Bulletin* about a physician who had become addicted to morphine as a medical student. This man had first used morphine as it was found in a then popular emulsion of cod liver oil. He had evidently used the cod liver oil emulsion when he was diagnosed as tubercular in 1878. He was apparently "cured" and lived an active, productive life. He soon noticed, however, that if he didn't take his medicine, he would experience a craving that could only be satisfied by morphine. He practiced medicine for many years, and although he would go off the drug for periods of time, he would eventually go back to it. He was once in some difficulty and was threatened with the loss of his license. This occasioned his taking the cure for a fourth time, but when he became ill some years later, he was administered some morphine and soon after he was again a regular user. He continued to be a user, and to practice medicine, until he was 81 years old.

Dr. Cutting told this author more about this physician in a conversation a few years ago in Hawaii. One of the interesting and amusing things Dr. Cutting related was that, at the age of 84, our morphine-using old gentleman confounded everyone by taking a series of psychologic tests in which he did better than many men 30 years his junior. Dr. Cutting said the only consistent problem the good doctor suffered as a result of regular morphine use was constipation. With case histories like this, one can readily understand the easy attitude of medicine of that time toward opium and morphine.

It was the opium smoker who was singled out in the public's mind as being dangerous, and this was probably the result of ethnic chauvinism. With the importation of cheap, coolie labor from the Orient to build railroads, work the crops, and generally do the menial work, there came the opium smokers. These were the frequenters of the opium dens, and in a time when there was fear of the Yellow Peril, the opium dens became the target first of the self-righteous and then of the politicians, who, scenting the spoils, soon made themselves heroes in the public eye by outlawing opium smoking.

San Francisco was first to pass a law prohibiting opium smoking, and soon other western cities with big Chinese communities followed suit. The journalists had a field day with lurid stories of white slavery. The Chinese were vilified and put upon at every turn, to the delight of men who had seen their jobs in jeopardy as a result of the burgeoning supply of cheap labor. It seemed that everyone was pleased except the poor men who sought surcease with the pipe-of-dreams.

Of course, the politicians revelled in the furor they had created, as they had made themselves heroes in the public eye and thus perpetuated themselves in their jobs. And, the dealers in opium were happy. The drug was now illegal, but the demand remained, and there could be only one result—illicit trade. The profits in opium on the black market increased twentyfold to fortyfold.

It is true that opium was used by prostitutes, but few of them smoked it; most of them used morphine. However, a few news stories and reviews in the magazines of the day, and the witch hunt for the poor devil who quietly smoked a pipe of opium, were reminiscent of an earlier period in Salem, when we hunted other witches.

The beneficial uses of opium and its derivatives spurred the creation of many synthetic compounds that resemble opiates in their effect. In the United States these synthetics have supplanted most of the opiates, and one of them, methadone, is being used in an attempt to salvage heroin addicts. (In this chapter, we are attempting to give some idea of the long history of experience mankind has had with mind-influencing agents. For this reason, we shall avoid discussion of the plethora of synthetics that are available today.)

Thus, opium provides another example of a useful, naturally occurring drug with infinite beneficial uses which becomes dangerous to society. The gifts of the gods, so generously provided, have been sullied by the stupidity of men. Hopefully, we shall some day exercise judgment, caution, and enlightenment in dealing with these rather miraculous gifts.

We have seen that peyote, as used positively, has been a boon to the Indian, and we are now beginning a new appraisal of hemp. Perhaps enlightened attitudes will lead to education about and to the employment of scientific values in making judgments on the nature and value of mind-influencing drugs.

NICOTINE

We just don't talk to each other until we've
had our morning cigarette, if we don't want to quarrel.
Many American couples

Unique, for many reasons, among the naturally occurring mind-influencing drugs is nicotine. It has one source, tobacco, and its history in the world, unlike that of hemp or opium, is relatively young. Tobacco first came to the attention of Europeans with Columbus' discovery of the New World, but in less than 50 years, its use had spread literally around the world. Columbus and his crew spoke of smoke drinkers. They had seen the Carib Indians smoking tobacco loosely rolled into a kind of cigar. To the Spanish sailors it appeared that the Indians, after firing the roll of leaves, would drink in the smoke. The Indians had also developed a crude pipe, in which they smoked the crumbled, dry leaves of tobacco.

The Indians were completely aware of the addictive power of tobacco. They knew of the craving they had for nicotine that could only be accommodated by smoking or chewing the leaves, or by breathing in the fumes from leaves thrown onto embers; and they knew they had the miseries without it.

When sea captains of the early 1500s persuaded some Indians to return to England with them, the Indians, knowing how much they were dependent on tobacco, would only make the trip if they could carry it along. It is reported that they did, and soon smoking was common in England.

The tobacco habit spread like wildfire. Sailors to the New World would try the smoke drinking and in a few days were caught up in the trap of nicotine addiction. Of course, this appetite had to be satisfied, so tobacco sailed with them wherever they went. They also carried the seeds, and wherever they touched shore, they would plant them to ensure future supplies of tobacco. It followed that the natives where the tobacco crops were started also became users and, of course, could then no longer do without nicotine.

Most regular smokers, particularly cigarette smokers, quarrel with the term *addict*. It sounds demeaning. They associate it with all the unpleasant stories they read about heroin, morphine, cocaine; they're not dope fiends! How they delude themselves. Nicotine is the most commonly used, and probably the most addictive, mind-influencing drug we have. Much research has gone into this, and there is much data to support that nicotine is more addictive than heroin. The confirmed nicotine user who quits smoking may have physiologic cravings for the drug for more than 18 months. It is true that the cured heroin addict may return to its use at a later time, but this is most often due to psychologic dependence.

When one considers how rapidly the use of nicotine spread over 400 years ago, it is unbelievable for its time. Today, dissemination of knowledge and technique takes only hours because of the speed of modern communication and transportation; one can span the Atlantic and return in less time than it took Columbus to sail 50 miles west. Just contemplate the implications of tobacco, commonly used by the Indians of the Americas, becoming known completely around the world in approximately 40 years. This coincided with the western hemisphere's finding its way into history and with the decades when Magellan, by sheer luck, was the first to circumnavigate the globe. Magellan's sailors carried tobacco and its seed to the Philippines, Malay, the Indonesian archipelago, and southern Asia. The use of tobacco became common all through Malay and also in Goa and the islands off China. By 1527, tobacco was a very important export of New Spain. Very early in the sixteenth century, the Dutch had introduced it to the Hottentots in Africa. It was soon used throughout the Arab world. By a fluke, tobacco reached Zipangu (Japan), that mysterious, cut-off-from-the-world land, by 1542. A few years later the smoking habit was well established there.

In Europe, the spread of its use was equally rapid. The seeds first brought to Spain and Portugal found their way to the other sea-bordering countries and from there to the interior of the continent. Since tobacco created its own, ever-demanding appetite, its use flourished.

The supplies were limited at first, but no price was too great to pay. At one time in England, tobacco traded ounce for ounce for silver. The principle still holds: no price is too high for the *hooked* smoker to pay. Cigarettes, the most commonly used form of nicotine, have gone from 5 to 65 to 75 cents (in nightclubs, often more than a dollar) for a pack of 20, and the demand continues.

When cigarette smoking was first definitively linked to lung cancer, it was opined that the tobacco companies might fall on hard times, and many of the companies diversified as a hedge against a flagging demand for cigarettes. It didn't happen. Cigarettes continue to be sold in ever-increasing amounts.

A greater price is paid in health. Smoking has been specifically identified as the principal cause of lung cancer. It is now also recognized as a causative factor in emphysema and eventual respiratory failure, heart disease, vascular disease, hypertension, gastric problems, and the gangrene-causing Buerger's disease. Almost everyone who reads this will have personally known cigarette smokers who were sure that their physical problems were not related to smoking. We have all seen them die, sometimes horribly painful deaths. We have all seen them crippled to half-existence. We know of survivors of dramatically extensive vascular surgery who continue to smoke. No matter where one looks, one sees total disregard of the definitive knowledge we now have about the deleterious effects of nicotine. Apparently, too few care! It is not unusual to see the concerned young mother-to-be puffing away, completely ignorant of, or completely ignoring, the proven potential of nicotine for teratogenicity. The learned physician Freud continued to smoke even though he underwent numerous surgical procedures for cancer. As a physician, he was well aware of the carcinogenic properties of nicotine for the oral mucosa, but he continued to smoke after undergoing an operation to remove a cancer of the lip. Nor did he stop smoking after the complete removal of his jaw. He lived with a prosthetic jaw and continued to smoke through horrible pain until his excruciating death from cancer. That a disciplined, knowledgeable giant such as Freud could not give up nicotine is testimony to its insidious power to addict.

Historically, nicotine as found in tobacco has played a greater role in world economy and politics than anything else but gold, and now oil. Socially, it established patterns of behavior that finally had to be codified in etiquette. Medically, it has also had an influence. It was used as a purgative, a stimulant, a tranquilizer, an emetic, a therapy for fever, an anti-infective in dressing wounds, a remedy for snakebite, and a vermifuge. Psychologically, it was used as a stimulant and sometimes a tranquilizer, and this use continues today without medical sanction.

The effects of nicotine are variable. It can act as a tranquilizer, a stimulant, or a depressant. For all regular users, its effect can vary with the time of day, the social circumstances, and the need of the moment. Effect does not seem to relate directly to the form in which nicotine is used: smoked, chewed, or snuffed; cigar, pipe, cigarette, or cud.

Many double-blind studies of the effects of nicotine have been conducted, and all kinds of devices used, to determine if its demand is physiologic, rather than psychologic. Volunteers smoked cigarettes of different strengths, and their needs were measured in terms of the number and frequency of cigarettes smoked. Tests have been made with ingested nicotine to see if the need to smoke was lessened by this manner of use. It apparently was. Once the user had become dependent on nicotine, he accommodated to any form in which it was administered. All of the tests were double-blind, and when placebos were used, there was not the usual and expected placebo effect. The body was only comfortable when it got nicotine; nothing else worked.

Personality seems to determine the form of tobacco used. Psychologically, a pipe is often a security blanket or a stalling device for the ill-at-ease individual. The elaborate routine of cleaning, filling, tamping, and lighting allows a lot of time for wit gathering. On the other hand, the tense and uptight can quickly grab a cigarette and, in one or two deep pulls into the lungs, regain composure. Today, chewing tobacco is a macho thing for many males who, unsure of their masculinity, need support. Snuff is no longer *la mode*, as it was in the eighteenth century, but its use continues, and it is often the crutch of the so-called closet smoker.

We spoke earlier of the price nicotine demands in suffering and of the pocketbook, but it demands another price which smokers often fail to recognize. It is demeaning; it demands a price in terms of human dignity. The affluent socialite, who would be appalled at seeing a starving Biafran or Indian eating garbage, would still sort through the ashtrays the next morning if she were out of cigarettes. And if it were liquor-stained, coffee-stained, lipstick-stained, or just plain dirty, she would still smoke it. During World War II, this author commanded the Trobriands. Once in a while our cigarette ration would fail. Have you ever seen soldiers scratching through the grass like so many rooting pigs, trying to find a butt thrown away a few days earlier? It lacks all dignity and self-respect.

Tobacco was at one time the economic mainstay of the New World. It became the prerogative of government to control its sale, and to this day in many countries, its distribution and sale is a function of government rather than of business. Tobacco became so important to the economy of the islands of the southern and western Pacific that it substituted for coin. The common currency of the islands was stick (or trade) tobacco, and goods were measured in value as related to stick tobacco. The stick was a constant: 8" long, ¼" thick, and ½" wide. The most popular was Emu Twist from Petersburg, Virginia.

We are so familiar with tobacco that to say more in this chapter might belabor its importance. Like all of the mind-influencing drugs, it was in and out of fashion and legality, but no government has successfully banned its use. In every country where its prohibition was attempted, it failed, in spite of the most severe penalties. Our last hope lies in education and enlightenment.

Medically this is very important. Not only does nicotine engender disease, but it also hinders many therapies. Every physician should know his patient's tobacco habits completely (and don't forget snuff) before he makes any therapeutic decision. He must remember that nicotine reacts with most psychotropics. Above all, he must understand that smokers are not very likely to stop smoking without a lot of help that goes beyond scare tactics. Perhaps every physician should remember the positive effectiveness of being able to say, "Do as I do, or at least as I have done—stop smoking!"

CAFFEINE

A good secretary makes a good cuppa coffee,
and doesn't bother me till I've had it.
    An American executive

Coffee, cola, tea, South American maté, cocoa, hot chocolate—no matter what name we give it, it is caffeine. It's the great waker-upper and, for many, a bedtime drink. The inconsistencies of its use are numerous. Children are usually forbidden coffee and tea, which encourages a curiosity to try them. At the same time, they are encouraged to drink cocoa and hot chocolate. These latter two, in the conviction of most North Americans, are children's beverages. Of course, in other cultures, hot chocolate or cocoa are wake-up drinks, often brought to your bedside in the morning if you are a house guest.

In Britain, Ireland, and Australia, the great waker-upper is tea, and in Australia, the coffee break becomes tea stop, or, as called by the workers on the waterfront, "tea oh." One remembers taking the overnight from Sydney to Melbourne and being wakened in his berth by the conductor, who automatically had brought a sizable mug of hot tea. Perhaps it was to compensate for having to awaken early at Albury, where you had to change to another train because the rail gauge changed. This was a nuisance, but the tea was hot and strong—so strong to this American palate that the tanning of one's gullet to leather seemed a likelihood.

The use of caffeine in one form or another is common in all cultures. Even among the members of the Church of the Latter Day Saints (Mormons), for whom coffee, tea, and alcoholic beverages are forbidden, caffeine is accepted in cola-type beverages. The Eskimo, who had never had any of the mind-influencing drugs (for none could grow where they lived), became confirmed tea drinkers soon after European explorers introduced them to it. Early Russian explorers of the Arctic carried their samovars with them and taught the Alaskan Eskimo, the Aleuts, and the Indians the pleasures of tea. Later, Scandinavian explorers introduced these peoples to coffee, but tea remains more popular.

Caffeine belongs to the group of chemicals called the xanthines. It occurs naturally in both hemispheres as coffee and originated in the Ethiopian area of Africa. It grows as tea in eastern Asia; as yerba maté, a shrub of South America; as cocoa, a tree native to Mexico, Central America, and the islands of the Caribbean (not to be confused with the coco palm); as the kola nut in Africa; and as the yaupon in North America. The Cassena yaupon (*Ilex vomitoria*) was used as a source of caffeine by all the Indian tribes of what is today our South.

The xanthines, which include theobromine and theophylline as well as caffeine, are all mind-influencing drugs. In addition to their action on the central nervous system, they are diuretic and they provide some cardiac stimulation. Of the xanthines, caffeine is the most commonly used. It occurs in varying strengths in the forms already mentioned. Cocoa also contains theobromine.

Who can say when some native first discovered the pleasant effect of drinking a beverage made of the tea leaf, the coffee bean, or the cocoa bean? We know that when Columbus discovered the Americas, the Caribs, Mayans, and Aztecs had been using cocoa for many years. Cortez reported it and called it the favorite drink of Montezuma. DeSoto found the Indians of the areas of Florida, the Carolinas, Alabama, and Mississippi all using a drink made from the yaupon tree. Tribes as far north as Virginia and west as Texas also used the drink.

This drink of the Indians was later often the drink of choice of our early colonists, even when coffee and tea were available. Some of the early settlers also adopted an Indian drink called the Noble Black Drink. Among the Indians, this drink, made of fermented yaupon leaves, was reserved for the chiefs and important warriors. The leaves of the yaupon were fermented, dried, and then steeped into a kind of tea. The settlers, mistaking the yaupon for the Dahoon holly, often called the drink Dahoon.

The drinking of coffee had spread from Ethiopia to the Arab world and from there to Europe. The Arabs were the first to welcome it as a way of staying awake. The early Moslems would use it as a stimulant so they could stay awake during long religious ceremonies.

Coffee also became the target of many who found it morally offensive. For a while Moslem leaders considered it to be intoxicating and therefore forbidden by the holy writings of the Prophet. It was considered sinful to use any artificial means of staying awake through the lengthy religious services, and the use of caffeine was outlawed. But as with all things that men find pleasurable, the prohibitions could not be made to stick, and today we associate coffee drinking with all Arabic societies. We also speak of mocha, and in American slang we use it as a substitute term for coffee, or java, another slang term.

Not long after the Crusades, coffee came to Europe and became a popular drink. Until tea and coffee became known in Europe, the many societies there had known only alcohol as a mind-influencing agent. In Alt Wien, coffee bibbing was so sophisticated that one had a choice of at least sixteen varieties in every Kaffee Haus. Coffee is as popular today as ever. One need only consider the coffee houses of Vienna, each with its display of a Moor serving a steaming cup.

In the United States we have the American version of the German Kaffee Klatsch, an informal social gathering with coffee and conversation. Coffee breaks are a regular ritual of American workers, and our popular cafés take their name from the French word for coffee.

The English and their tea drinking brought many things: a tea tax that became a cause célèbre and pushed us toward revolution; a good reason for expanding the Empire into Asia, where the tea plantations became a great factor in England's economy; and, of course, the delights of tea and crumpets. Anyone who experiences "having tea" in one of the tea salons of the older, more gracious London hotels cannot help but become a teaphile.

Cocoa and its derivative, chocolate, have been as important to world economy as coffee and tea. They, too, have helped us develop some happy customs: hot chocolate before a roaring fire after sleigh riding or skiing; hot chocolate with marshmallows after the football game; and, every teenager's delight, the chocolate shake after school. In Mexico and Central America, there is nothing nicer than having your room maid tap at your door to wake you and bring in your mug of chocolate.

All of the caffeine-containing herbs have found their way into our lives, and of all the mind-influencing drugs, they seem to be used with the greatest benefit and propriety. Perhaps this is because they have suffered least from legislation, prohibition, and, maybe, politicians.

Of all mind-influencing drugs, there is probably no other that is used as graciously as is caffeine. It is the drug of civilization. In one form or another, it is caught up in the very weft of our life-styles. It is legal, pleasant, usually not too expensive, and, unless used in unbelievably large excesses, apparently safe.

This last does not mean it is completely safe, and historically there were learned men in medicine who preached that coffee and tea were evil. Of course, some of these same teachers taught that opium in some form was safer, and that its use should be encouraged to help people stop the coffee or tea habit.

Let's examine this. As in all dogmatic teaching, there is value and dross. Caffeine is a stimulant. Reliable, current pharmacologic opinion holds that caffeine stimulates all portions of the cerebral cortex. It allays drowsiness and tends to produce a more clear and more rapid flow of thoughts. Tests indicate that, with caffeine, one can associate ideas better, one has an increased capacity for intellectual exercise, and that the effort can be expended for longer periods. One can also respond better and quicker to sensory stimuli. If we translate this to the office coffee break, secretaries who drink one or two cups of coffee in the morning work better. Their motor activity is improved; they type faster and with greater accuracy. However, the beneficial effects of one or two cups of coffee are negated if too much coffee is consumed. It is the old story: a little is good, but too much is bad.

Coffee, or rather caffeine, has been implicated as a cause of gastric distress. It increases the flow of gastric acids and in this way is related to peptic ulcers. It is a diuretic and in relatively small amounts can affect heart rate and rhythm. Large doses in test animals (or even smaller, regular doses) appear to produce pathologic changes, among which is the development of peptic ulcers. In excessive doses, caffeine is a potent poison. It can kill test animals in a relatively short time. They first convulse and then suffer respiratory failure.

The excess of caffeine consumed by the heavy coffee drinker can produce nervous states, chronic fever, anorexia, insomnia, and irritability. These symptoms also go hand in hand with the diet in which coffee is substituted for food, and they are also often noted in cola drinkers who develop a habit of substituting a soft drink for food and water. It is not unusual to find some cola drinkers who consume more than 10 (serving size) bottles daily. Since coffee and tea usually accompany meals or are drunk after meals, the effect is usually less untoward than, for example, the effect of alcohol, ordinarily taken before meals. The cola drinks are also often taken into an empty stomach and can, in excess, be of greater potential harm than are coffee or tea.

A definite caffeine dependency develops, producing many familiar jokes: "She's a witch until after her coffee," or, "He's a bear," or, "I can't get started till I've had my coffee." We sometimes forget about this aspect of habituation, or dependence, as we meet and work with people. It is sometimes difficult to understand why everything has to wait for coffee or a coke, but it does happen, and it happens often.

Caffeine is readily available as an over-the-counter drug in pill form. Physicians sometimes prescribe it as a stimulant, but more is sold without prescription as a waker-upper. As such, it is used by truckers, students cramming for exams, and others who, for one reason or another, want to stay awake. The usual dose of caffeine in a stay-awake pill is 100 mg. Carelessly used, a toxic dose could be easily ingested. Sometimes, in "pepping up" for a party or other event, there is temptation to take more than the dose recommended on the label. This can lead to tragedy.

Every physician is aware of the nature of caffeine; there is no need to elaborate on its pharmacology. It cannot be disregarded as a mind-influencing drug. It is one. It interacts and interferes with the action of other psychotropic drugs in many ways. The greatest danger with caffeine probably lies in the fact that it is so commonplace we tend to forget about its effects and its potential for harm. We shouldn't. Every medical history taken should include inquiry about the patient's use of caffeine.

RETROSPECTION

So reihte sie die Mutter,
die mächt'gen Zaubertränke.
Für Weh und Wunden
Balsam hier;
für böse Gifte,
Gegengift.

Richard Wagner, *Tristan und Isolde*

As Brangaene sings this, she mentions the chest of magic potions, poisons, and antidotes left by Isolde's mother. Keeping such a chest of balms and medicines was the custom of the Dark and Middle Ages. Handed down with all the incantations necessary to make the contents useful, it was part of a dowry. The secrets of curing and of the healing draughts were also part of the lore handed from witch to warlock son or from a Merlin to his apprentice. The correct incantation was often more important than the agent if the therapy were to work, for believing that it would work was most often the secret. In another chapter, Dr. Goldberg writes of the art of prescribing and the positive use of the placebo. In an older time, it was the incantation which was the art of prescribing and which often made some medicinally inactive weed a cure-all.

One remembers that Isolde became confused as to how many scratches on the vial identified the one she wanted, and so instead of a poison, it was a magical elixir of lust and love that compelled her and Tristan into their tragic elopement.

Such legends give us insight into the rationale of the use of mind-influencing agents before there was a medical science. Today we try to achieve all manner of influences on the psyche scientifically, by way of the many synthetics available, and some physicians forget that there is both art and science in healing. This is particularly true of therapy for the emotionally disturbed patient, and we hope this book will bring this clearly to mind. Our modern medicines are the real magic of therapy today, but only when used with good counsel.

Perhaps the best example of a naturally occurring drug that

links today's psychopharmacotherapy with the past is rauwolfia, or botanically, *Rauwolfia serpentina*. The snake-like appearance of its root suggested the second part of this name. Rauwolfia grows commonly in many areas of the hill country of India, and its medicinal properties have been recognized for thousands of years by the several groups of people who have occupied the huge subcontinent. In spite of its recognition and use by the healers of India, Western medicine ignored it. The physicians who went to India with the British colonization were either not sufficiently curious or, suffering the raj mentality, took the attitude that there could be nothing of real scientific value in the concoctions and mumbo-jumbo of the herb doctors, fakirs, and witch doctors. This attitude denied the Western world the knowledge and benefits of this remarkable herb until well into the twentieth century. In the United States, it was in the second half of this century that we finally discovered its benefits.

For countless centuries, rauwolfia was used as it occurred in nature: the root was chewed, or cut into pieces and eaten, or compounded into the concoctions of the herb doctors. As with all natural drugs, its use is surrounded, and perhaps confounded, by legend, superstition, and stories of magic. Its uses are chronicled in ancient Sanskrit manuscripts, and it is mentioned in the earliest Hindu literature. The popular folklore of India had the mongoose eating rauwolfia, thus making him impervious to the fatal venom of the cobra. Actually, the mongoose is faster and a better in-fighter than the cobra, but the legend was popular and gave support to the use of rauwolfia for snakebite.

The author remembers social evenings spent in the company of, and almost under the spell of, the eminent Dr. Yellapragada Subba Row, who had pioneered the concept and use of the folic acid antagonists. Dr. Subba Row, at one time a professor at Harvard and later the distinguished director of research for a major United States pharmaceutical company, was from Madras and had had much of his scientific education in India. He was familiar with the herbal medicines of India and would delight us with all manner of stories about the native herb doctors. He would recount all of the folklore and often spoke of rauwolfia, but he had so completely adopted the Western attitude toward folk medicine that he neglected to investigate this potential source of a useful agent. He was interested in rauwolfia, but he was caught up in the time of the work with anti-infectives and could not apply or expand his basic knowledge of the Indian herbs. Had he not met an untimely death, the benefits of rauwolfia might have been available in the United States years earlier.

Serious investigation into rauwolfia in the United States was delayed until the early 1950s. Then it was investigated principally as an extract of the root, called reserpine. Dr. Nathan S. Kline has written a fascinating history of the early investigation of reserpine in his book *From Sad to Glad*. It is well worth the reading for any person interested in the progress made in the care of the mentally disturbed by way of the advances made in the field of psychopharmacotherapy. The history of the use of rauwolfia in its natural form is probably less important than the more recent history of the use of its extract, reserpine. Here lies its true importance; it was the breakthrough to the whole concept of tranquilizers. It commenced a revolution in the care of the mentally ill, particularly in the institutional setting, where they had traditionally been kept under restraint.

Better tranquilizing agents have come to the fore, but rauwolfia (reserpine) was the first. In the hands of such pioneers of its use as Dr. Kline, it became a drug of major importance and provided us with another good example of the therapeutic resources available from the wonderful chemical compounder we call Nature.

We have not discussed alcohol in this chapter. It does occur naturally, as is evident by the observance of yellow jackets attracted to fallen, fermenting fruit. Ordinarily, the yellow jacket is a very aggressive insect, but after dining on the fermenting fruit, he is stupefied. One can step on him easily, for he is so intoxicated he makes no effort to fly away.

Alcohol as used by men is really the result of human ingenuity in observing nature and imitating her. It would have been fun to write about the many forms of alcohol man has devised. The history of wine would take up several volumes, and just as much could be written of spirits. What we are concerned with here is that alcohol is a major mind-influencing drug. It can be very dangerous, and because it is legal and socially acceptable, it is insidious in its potential harm. Dr. Charles Becker, Head of the Division of Clinical Pharmacology at San Francisco General Hospital, said in a recent lecture for the San Joaquin County Medical Society that of all drugs, alcohol has the greatest potential for interaction with other mind-influencing drugs.

Another thing to consider with regard to alcohol is that its legality makes many laws prohibiting other mind-influencing drugs farcical. For example, people today who want to use marijuana see that alcohol is acceptable and legal and that marijuana is not. Can one wonder if they flaunt legislations that are exercises in ambiguity and inconsistency?

There are other naturally occurring mind-influencing drugs which are not of sufficient importance to be dealt with at length but whose use, nonetheless, should be considered by a physician whose patient may be a drug experimenter. The nutmeg is native to subtropical America and is a relative of the Asiatic *Myristica fragrans*. Both are hallucinogenic. There is yurema, prepared by certain of the Indian tribes of Brazil from *Mimosa hostilis*, and though uncommon, it cannot be disregarded. Some drug cultists suggested that bananas had a certain hallucinogenic factor, but the hallucination may well be in the suggestion. And, there is ololiuqui, a kind of wild morning glory that grows in Mexico and is called *badoh negro* by the Zapotec Indians. This too may have found its way into the hands of a youngster seeking a new thrill.

In this chapter, we have already mentioned the loco weed, *Datura inoxia*. There are other members of the *Datura* family, and all have toxic properties and cause hallucinations. The jimson weed (*Datura stramonium*), a pest plant of our southeastern states, and Angel Trumpet (*Datura metel*), a favorite of old-fashioned flower gardens in the South, are both dangerous. Ingestion of either can be fatal, and both can cause hallucination. Even as this was written, there were news reports of a fad that had spread among children in the Chicago area. They were using Angel Trumpet for its hallucinatory effect, and while no deaths were reported, a number of children required hospitalization.

Nature has been generous in her supply of plants that influence our minds. Few are used today in medicine, but more and more are used in our drug subcultures, and they present a problem for all physicians. In spite of her many useful gifts, Nature seems to have failed to provide us with the gift of good sense in making use of her bounties. Certainly a method of rational evaluation makes more sense than ignorant condemnation of people who are as ill in their own way as is the alcoholic. And surely adopting such an approach would be more ethical than supporting by default of knowledge a system which makes crime so profitable that it invades every aspect of our daily life, and which feeds itself by adding to the numbers of drug users, who can benefit only their illegal suppliers. There has to be a better way.

SUGGESTED READING

Castaneda, C.: *The Teachings of Don Juan: A Yaqui Way of Knowledge.* Berkeley, Calif.: University of California Press, 1968.

Castaneda, C.: *A Separate Reality.* New York: Simon & Schuster, 1971.

Castaneda, C.: *Journey to Ixtlan.* New York: Simon & Schuster, 1972.

Goldberg, M.: *Psychiatric Diagnosis and Understanding for the Helping Professions.* Chicago: Nelson-Hall Publishers, 1973.

Kline, N. S.: *From Sad to Glad.* New York: G.P. Putnam's Sons, 1974.

Michigan Department of Social Services. *Overdose Aid* (Manual No. 11). Ann Arbor: Michigan Department of Social Services, 1973.

Rowe, C.J.: *An Outline of Psychiatry.* Dubuque, Iowa: William C. Brown Company, Publishers, 1970.

Schoenfeld, E.: *Natural Food and Unnatural Acts.* New York: Dell Publishing Co., Inc., 1967.

Smith, D.E.: *The New Social Drug.* Englewood Cliffs, NJ:Prentice-Hall, Inc., 1970.

2 Psychopharmacologic Treatment Decisions and the Assessment of Patient Behavior

Edward Stainbrook, M.D., Ph.D.

DIAGNOSIS

To diagnose is to "see through" the patient's symptoms and complaints. The diagnostic achievement is a more or less successful translation of the patient's complaints into problems that may be defined in medical terms and solved by medical methods. Effective problem-solving may require biomedical resources and technology, psychologic methods, or social and cultural intervention. With our rather deeply entrenched either-or predilection in medicine for a biologic or psychologic interpretation of disease and distress, we too frequently decide that the definition of the problem of disease and its adequate resolution require only biomedical formulation and treatment or only psychosocial techniques and considerations.

Indeed, a typology of physicians which matches the heavily reinforced historical dichotomy of body and self has been created

38

in the designations biomedical and psychosocial. But it has long been obvious that human biology is always psychobiology and that every medically interesting disorder is psychosomatic. Hence, contemporary comprehensive medicine makes increasing use of those particular patterns and combinations of biomedical and psychosocial intervention needed to deal most rationally and effectively with medical problems as collaboratively defined by the physician and the complaining patient.

Put into the language of general scientific investigation, the diagnostic task is to describe the dependent variables which are to be controlled or altered and to search out and define the independent variables which can be demonstrated to have a high probability of influencing the dependent variables. In clinical practice, dependent variables are usually regarded as the symptoms, signs, complaints, and the troubled or troublesome behavior of the patient. Rational intervention, ordinarily directed at changing or controlling independent variables, may then be decided.

However, with particular reference to behavioral control and change, the crucial influencing variables are frequently outside of the body, in the social and cultural surrounds of the person. The disturbance of gastrointestinal function or of the cardiovascular system may be due to the look on the face of another, or to conflicting values and attitudes, or to the psychosocial behavior conditioned by the life-style of the person. Frequently, the independent variables influencing psychobiologic disorder reside in the past experience of the patient. Behavior learned long ago at another time and in another place may constitute maladaptive stressing and distressing responses in the present. The past cannot really be relived, but it can be remembered, reconceptualized, and reorganized. To remember the past, either spontaneously or by invitation, is to reconstruct it. Psychotherapy may be indicated to ensure that the reconstruction will be adaptive to the present and will liberate the patient for continuing and new interpersonal and intrapersonal learning.

The patient's forecast of his future should also be considered as an independent variable: whether distorted or relatively realistic, it may influence the behavior and the biology of the present. The troublesome adolescent, for example, may be troubled not only by his past learning and his present developmental tasks and problems but also by a conception of his future as uncertain, uninviting, or meaningless. Hence, future, past, and present independent variables, within and outside the person, may all evoke, influence, or maintain the present dependent variables of symptom, complaint, biologic process, and behavior.

PSYCHOPHARMACOLOGIC TREATMENT OR PSYCHOTHERAPY?

The exhibition of psychopharmacologic agents is based usually on the assumption that the independent variables influencing or evoking the patient's symptoms derive from the physiology of the central nervous system. As already indicated, if the situation were no more complex than this, the therapeutic decisions of whom to treat and for and with what might be relatively simple. If the biologic responses of the patient which are detected as clinically interesting and as seeming to be the sources of the patient's complaints or symptoms are considered to be primary, then psychopharmacologic intervention is the treatment of choice. On the other hand, if these biologic reactions have been created and are being maintained by psychosocial situations, then attempts to alter the patient's behavior within a psychosocial context should become the therapeutic focus.

It is apparent, however, that even if the disturbed biologic processes are dependent on the psychosocial behavior, these processes may in themselves serve as stressors to the integrative functioning of the body. They may also, in turn, frequently evoke and maintain impairment of psychosocial behavior and evince withdrawal, avoidance, or other behaviors designed to protect the person from added stress or to achieve relief from stress. In such a circumstance, both psychopharmacologic and psychosocial treatments are indicated.

The immediate influence of drugs on psychophysiologic symptoms and on tension, anxiety, distress, and depression, or on cognitive information-processing defects, not only gives psychophysiologic relief, but may also alter the symptomatic behavior which is interfering with more effective psychosocial problem solving. The depressed patient, who is reacting to actual or anticipated psychosocial loss or separation, may be benefitted by pharmacologic restoration of the neurobiology which underlies emotional interests. Such a patient may then be able to experience a sense of pleasurable interest or a subjectively experienced reinforcement which will reward and sustain reparative interpersonal and socially interactive re-engagements and recommit-

ments. With concomitant psychotherapy, the situation which precipitated the depression may be reorganized more effectively and,
perhaps, preventively.

Psychopharmacologic treatment may reduce cognitive impairment in the acute schizophrenic person by normalizing the
neurophysiology of perceptual and conceptual thinking. Concurrent interpersonal psychotherapy given in a supportive environment may help alter the behavioral conditions which precipitated
the psychosocial breakdown and may provide for the learning of
more adaptive social and personal behaviors.

There is an additional consideration in the use of the "both-
and" rather than the "either-or" biomedical and psychosocial position in respect to both the diagnosing and the treating of patients which is becoming increasingly important. Experimental
evidence is accumulating which suggests that the on-off controls of
neurometabolic processes, mediated (among other influences) by
hormonal responses to psychosocial stimuli, may have intrinsic
regulatory characteristics which escape a directly correlative response to the psychosocial stress. A psychobiologic depressive
process initiated by demonstrable psychosocial stimuli may not
"switch-off" when the psychosocial stress has altered but, instead,
may continue and may maintain some of the behavior of depression after the disappearance of the evoking events. Proponents of
the endogenous depressive reaction believe that an intrinsic initiation of the neurophysiology of depression, which then becomes the
independent variable evoking and maintaining the behavior of
depression, may occur. In these last two instances, psychopharmacologic intervention would be indicated.

With respect to the possibility of the endogenous production
of behavior symptomatic of illness, physicians should also be
aware that behavioral scientists' contemporary interest in oper-
ant conditioning emphasizes the need to analyze behavior labelled as symptomatic from at least two points of view: what
evokes the behavior and what is maintaining it. Whether the
primary cause of symptomatic behavior is considered to be organic
or to be reactively psychophysiologic, the independent variables
which brought the symptomatic behavior into being may not be the
same variables that are now maintaining it. During the course of
an illness, a shift may occur from an internal-organic to an
external-environmental causation without necessarily producing
any change in some of the symptomatic behavior originally
thought to be associated with the illness. Symptoms evoked by an

organic condition now remedied by biomedical methods may continue because of their psychologic payoff in the social environment of the hospital, the clinic, the doctor's office, or in the broader life setting. In this phase of the course of illness, frequently described as convalescence or rehabilitation, psychosocial considerations of behavioral change must be applied.

PSYCHOBIOLOGY OF EMOTION

Much behavior which doctors identify as symptomatic of illness and which they choose to treat with psychoactive drugs is commonly called emotional behavior. Indeed, psychiatric illnesses are generally considered emotional disorders. Unfortunately, both the psychiatrist and the nonpsychiatric clinician may operate with a rather ambiguous concept of emotion. Extensive, interdisciplinary information about the psychobiology of emotion has accumulated in recent years. For our purposes in assessing the emotional behavior of patients and in making treatment decisions on the basis of our evaluations, we must put this knowledge together in some clinically helpful ways.

An analysis and definition of the psychobiologic components of what we experience as emotion is, perhaps, the first task. We can now feel reasonably sure that the neural structures and processes of emotion belong to specific, genetically determined anatomic and physiologic systems in the central nervous system. These systems are "prewired" regionally and integratively into the total neural organization. Their intrinsic processes are genetically programmed to produce specific expressive and behavioral outcomes in facial expression and body posture, or in vocal or other overt movements. Specific subjective feelings, describable generally as fearful, distressing, or pleasurable, are evoked by the activation, or arousal, of the various systems.

A specific neurophysiologic organization, a specific postural, expressive behavior, and a specific subjective feeling can be associated with at least the emotions of fear, distress, anger, and joy and, with less certainty, of shame, contempt, and interest. With the advent of social learning, the information from assimilated and accommodated-to life experiences will be superimposed upon the innate control of the emotional systems. Learned patterns of action, response, and expression will be imposed upon the original, inherited action outflow, or behavior.

The emotion subjectively experienced as depression, for

example, seems to be genetically organized to produce a subjective sense of distress and crying in response to the loss or lack of being mothered. This "deep structure" of the anguished feeling of distress and the psychophysiology of crying form the basis of all subsequent depressive behavior of the person. The response of fear of being harmed or injured because one is unprotected or helpless soon becomes closely associated with the experience of distress. Clinically encountered depressive behavior is thus almost always some combination of anxiety, the learned transformation of the fearful response to physical threat into an anxious response to symbolic threat, and distress. Distress is the emotional feeling evoked by actual or anticipated loss, and anxiety is induced to varying degrees by the person's appraisal of his own helplessness, or the lack of help from others, in restoring or preventing his loss.

Other emotions, such as anger at oneself or at others, and shame and guilt, also usually form some part of the pattern of depressive behavior, and the emotional elements of this pattern are constantly changing in response to the psychosocial conditions of the patient. Indeed, probably no other emotional problem points up a greater need for continued, knowledgeable evaluation of behavior than does the rational and effective management of depression. In what is too often clinically simply called depression, much other emotional behavior is also present. We look to both pharmacologic treatment and pharmacologic research to further specify the individual components of the general pattern.

The specificity of the various emotional responses is, then, genetically determined. These reactions have been "selected-in" because of their past adaptive value. Whether some of these emotional responses may be, in some ways, maladaptive in our contemporary environment is an interesting question. The deep-structured anguish evoked by loss or separation, for example, may be doing more harm than good in contemporary society, where frequently changing personal relationships, geographic mobility, and the need to be an independent individual are cultural characteristics.

INTERRELATIONSHIP OF EMOTION
AND BEHAVIOR

Apart from the genetic aspect, there have long been two basic positions from which to consider the relationships of emotion to general behavior. From one standpoint, emotion has been considered to be the cause or motivation of behavior; the other position posits emotion as the result or effect of behavior. In an open-system concept of psychobiology, both of these viewpoints are relevant, and they are not mutually exclusive. For clinical applications, they can be put together in an interesting and helpful conceptual model for the understanding of emotional behavior.

First, let us suggest a categorization of the functions of the central nervous system. These may be described broadly as: 1) arousal and amplification; 2) information processing, cognition, and memory retention and organization; 3) emotional appraisal and evaluation of information and experience; and 4) motor-behavioral execution of decisions.

Emotional behavior is initiated by the evocation of psychophysiologic arousal to any internal or external stimulus or happening that changes the ongoing orientation and attentional processes of the person. The initial response may be a sudden, startled amplification of attention with an emotional appraisal of fright or fear. This may lead either to an overt or to a movement-inhibited execution of a behavioral reaction which may have been genetically programmed as well as strongly reinforced and transformed by early learning for specific adaptability to the social environment. Such primitive overt behavioral responses to acute fear may be called hysterical and be expressed in actual movement, or they may occur as dissociative cognitive attempts to "gait out" and to deny the frightening information. Frequently, the physiologic aspect of the psychophysiology of acute anxiety constitutes the major part of the response.

In contrast, attention may be activated and be sustained at a moderate level of arousal by the emotion of pleasurable anticipation. The emotional quality of what is called interest may be so subtle or so infused with other emotional components as to be excluded from general recognition as emotional behavior. Nevertheless, interest is the emotional reinforcement which maintains intellectual and personal exploration and interaction.

The subjective feeling of emotional behavior is, in any event, brought into being and maintained by the ongoing integration of cognitive interpretations and decisions about the situation the person is in. Adaptive or maladaptive behavior performed on the basis of those interpretations and decisions, in turn, feeds back information about its psychosocial consequences; which information may abolish, change the intensity of, or alter the components of the emotional behavior. The important concept here is that the intensity, frequency, duration, and character of emotional behavior depend largely on cognitive evaluations of self and situation and on one's ability to transform emotional behavior into effective problem-solving and conflict-resolving behavioral action. If one is "hung-up," then distressing or disturbing emotional behavior has not been resolved by effective thinking alone or by thought and action together.

Since the emotional testing and appraisal of psychosocial information is constantly going on, and since both subjective feeling and physiologic responses are components of the emotional process, emotional behavior may be monitored both by subjective self-report and by the measurement of physiologic variables. As previously indicated, motor-expressive behavior and conduct may also be components of the emotional process. The current popularity of the phrases "listening to your feelings" and "getting in touch with your feelings" indicates the value of emotions as psychobiologic intelligence in modulating adaptive and effective behavior. The idea that the subjective perception of emotional responses constitutes crucial information, not only about how the patient's body "feels" about the life-situation but also about the psychosocial characteristics of the life-situation itself, forms the basis for informed decisions about psychopharmacologic treatment.

A patient complains of disturbing emotional behavior. The emotional feeling is a result of the way the patient is behaving in the life-situation, and such a complaint is an indication that the patient has not been successful in transforming his hung-up emotional behavior into effective and gratifying adaptation. The patient attempts to use behavior, usually learned in the past and strongly reinforced by past success in avoiding stress or in reducing tension, to evade or reduce more current stress. This behavior expresses itself as the clinically described symptoms of anxiety or depression. These symptoms usurp the attention and energy the patient should be devoting to interpreting and solving the problems in his life-situation which are the primary source of his distress. Designed for defense against these problems, the symptomatic behavior may actually further impair and interfere with their resolution.

What, then, is suggested in clinical diagnosis and treatment? First, the clinician should be convinced of the fact that feeling is basic information. The self-report on feeling will better inform the physician about how the patient is in his life than will any directly demanded history. Sensitive and facilitating interview behavior is obviously necessary to enable the patient to allow emotionally associated imagery, memories, and thought to be communicated. Initially, the patient may not even be aware of psychophysiologic tension, or he may only be able to express the feeling, "I'm tense, that's all." But tension is unlabelled, uninformed feeling. The skill one needs in diagnosing is to make it possible for the patient to translate tension into its psychosocial meaning in the here and now.

When the emotional behavior has been allowed to add its intelligence to the diagnosis of the patient's problems, psychoactive drugs may then be used, if necessary, to alter the biology of the emotional behavior and to control the symptoms produced by the patient's efforts at containing and reducing stress. The physician may then direct therapeutic efforts at increasing the patient's capabilities for effective behavior, at engaging significant others in collaborative problem solving, and at drawing upon supportive social and cultural resources in the patient's environment. Obviously, in clinical situations of acute, greatly incapacitating distress—whether normal, neurotic, or psychotic—drug-induced control of emotional or cognitive behavior may be necessary before the subjective psychologic content of emotional behavior may be used resourcefully in diagnosis and management.

A rather general consideration follows from this view of emotional behavior. We tend in our society to have a rather pejorative attitude toward emotions, particularly the dysphoric ones of anxiety and depression. These emotions are to be tolerated as little as possible. Perhaps we may increase our tolerance for being anxious or depressed if we understand depression and anxiety as necessary and inevitable psychophysiologic responses to the experiences of life. No person can be fully informed about what he is doing and about what he is being and becoming without listening to his frequently dysphoric and distressing feelings. Before putting them too quickly out of mind or seeking a drug-induced counterhigh, all of us, particularly the physician and his patient, should listen to their message.

3 Recognizing the Depressed Patient

Martin Goldberg, M.D.

DISTINGUISHING BETWEEN NONPATHOLOGIC DEPRESSION AND DEPRESSIVE DISORDERS

Depression is said to be the most common of all psychiatric disorders (Ayd, 1961). Certainly any physician in virtually any type of clinical practice encounters depressed patients every day. Some of these patients are undergoing mild, transient reactions of depression; others are involved in substantial, moderate-sized depressions; a few are sunk in deep depressions. The last group is seldom a diagnostic problem. The deeply depressed person presents himself with an overwhelming feeling of hopelessness and despair; with slowed speech, thinking, and gait; with tremendous feelings of guilt; and often with delusions and suicidal ideas. Encountering such a group of symptoms, virtually anyone can quickly make a diagnosis of depression. But there are many other patients in whom the symptoms of depression only peek through, so to speak.

47

There is some evidence that depression is underdiagnosed in clinical practice (Raft et al, 1975). If this is so, it undoubtedly results from the fact that many physicians conceive of depression only in its most classical sense and in the severe form described above. Medical school courses in psychiatry are apt to emphasize only this concept of depression and to fail to stress the relative ubiquity of this disorder. The problems of nomenclature also add to the confusion. Diagnostic distinctions include: psychotic depression vs neurotic depression; agitated depression vs retarded depression; reactive depression vs autonomous depression; exogenous depression vs endogenous depression; and unipolar depression vs bipolar depression. In addition, there are such classifications as involutional depressions (once called involutional melancholia), manic-depressive diseases, depressive equivalents, schizo-affective disorders, psychotic depressive reactions, and neurotic depressive reactions. For the most part, all this terminology is of little or no help to the busy clinician, and he is only hindered by attempting to understand these various diagnostic entities. It is sufficient, in practice, to classify depressions as mild, moderate, or severe. Severe depressions very often require hospitalization and should always be treated by a psychiatrist if one is available. Mild depression can very often be treated on an outpatient basis by the primary care physician. Moderate depressions fall between these two situations and the best therapeutic approach has to be gauged by the particular circumstances of each case.

Unfortunately, we use the term *depression* in two different senses: to refer to an emotional disorder and also to refer to a normal emotion that we all experience with considerable frequency. In the latter sense, depression is an emotion of sadness which may vary in intensity, but which does not persist for very long. We may feel depressed, in this normal sense, for minutes or hours, or conceivably even for a day or two. But a feeling of depression persisting for more than a day or two suggests that we are dealing not with a normal emotional reaction but with depression as an emotional disorder or disease. Whether the feelings in depressive disorder differ only quantitatively from the feelings of normal depression is uncertain; there may be real, qualitative differences also. Patients in depressions of any severity emphasize statements such as, "I never felt anything like this before"; "You can't imagine how awful this feels unless you've been through it"; and even, "This must be something more than a depression, because it feels so horrible." (It is worth noting also that patients in deep depression often complain, "I don't feel *anything*." Evidently, this is the most distressing sensation of all.) These descriptions would support the view that the person suffering from a depressive disorder is undergoing unpleasant sensations which are not only excessive in amount, but probably different in nature from any of the feelings of a normal individual. Still, we have to use terms such as "blue," "blah," "down," "depressed," "sad," and "lonely," because these are the only words available to us in attempting a description.

There is a condition that may represent a sort of half-way point between feelings of depression in the normal individual and those of depressive disorder. That is the state of mourning that ensues when we have lost someone close or dear to us. In mourning, we may feel blue and sad for a relatively prolonged period. Moreover, we may experience more than just disturbance of mood per se. Our activities and appetites may be slowed, so that we lack energy, verve, and vigor and have difficulty in eating and sleeping. We generally expect that mourning will abate considerably with time, however. A few weeks after the loss, the feelings of sadness and loneliness may persist, but our bodily processes are usually returning to normal.

In depressive disorders this is not the case. In fact, as Beck (1973) has pointed out, depressive disorder must be defined not just in terms of an alteration in mood, but in terms of five different attributes:

1. Specific alteration in mood This may be characterized by sadness, loneliness, or even apathy. (In severe depressions this mood alteration will often be described as *hopelessness*. This is a particularly sinister term for a patient to use and may bode ill for prognosis.)

2. Negative self-concept This is associated with self-reproaches and self-blame. In other words, the depressed patient is apt to dislike himself, to feel extremely and excessively guilty, and to feel at fault in many different ways. This may be reflected in statements such as, "I don't see how my wife can stand living with me"; "I'm ruining everything for my family"; and "If people ever find out what I'm really like, they will see what a fake and phony I am."

3. Regressive and self-punitive wishes The depressed patient may desire to escape, hide, or die. These wishes are quite prominent in most depressions of any severity. Far more common than overt suicidal desires are the drives to hide and escape from contact with other human beings and the outer world. Thus, the depressed patient often insists on staying at home, avoids social or work obligations, and even minimizes contacts with other members of the family. Self-punitive wishes may find expression, short of suicidal attempts, in actions or omissions which are calculated to harm the patient. For example, the author recalls several depressed patients who refused to file their income tax returns. They protested, in each case, that they did not have the energy to do so. That may have been so, but it was also true that they refused to allow anyone to help them with their returns or even to ask the government to give a legal extension on the deadline date for filing. Clearly they were using this means to hurt and punish themselves.

4. Vegetative changes Depression may bring about anorexia, insomnia, loss of libido. These are changes of particular importance to the physician concerned with recognizing the depressed patient, and a good deal more will be said about them subsequently.

5. Change in activity level Retardation or agitation may be evident. Actually, Beck's description of the change in activity level seen in depression as retardation or agitation may be slightly in error. The change might be better described as retardation with or without concomitant agitation, as virtually every depression involves a retardation: a slowing of thinking, of speech, and of gait and associated movements. In some patients one sees an agitation superimposed on this, but this agitation is not a speeding up of speech and thinking, such as is seen in manic states. Rather, it consists of repetitive and purposeless movements designed to reduce the tremendously high tension level of the depressive. Thus, the agitated depressed patient may repeatedly wring his hands or pace the floor back and forth, but at the same time, his thinking and speech will show the slowing and retardation characteristic of any depression.

These five different attributes are probably present to some degree in every depressive disorder. Their visibility varies greatly from case to case, however. In some patients with depression, the alterations in mood will be quite apparent, but the other factors will be hidden. Other patients, although suffering from some slight mood alteration, will display only the vegetative symptoms. The varieties of symptomatology possible will become more evident later in this chapter with the description of some typical cases.

PREDISPOSING FACTORS

In my clinical experience I have found three predisposing factors to depressive disorder which occur with sufficient frequency to aid in making a diagnosis. These are: age of onset, a family history of depression or of manic disorder, and an underlying personality which is of the obsessive-compulsive type. Other factors, such as body build or habitus, endocrine and somatic factors, gender, race or ethnic origin, and season of the year for time of onset, may have some relevance to the incidence of depression but are too inconsistent to be of help to the clinician.

Age of Onset

Depressions tend to occur most often after the age of 30 and are particularly common in the years between 40 and 60. This age distribution accounts for the popularity of diagnostic terms such as involutional depression, menopausal depression, and post-menopausal depression.

Depression can occur at any age. Childhood depression, while rare, does happen on occasion and may be precipitated by separation from the mother. Adolescent depressions, unfortunately, have become increasingly common in recent years. Not unusually, they are masked by delinquent or addictive behavior. Manic-depressive disease often has its onset with an episode in the late teens or twenties. Depressions in older individuals (past the age of 65) are not extremely common, and when they do occur, one should consider the possibility that some other disorder (eg, an organic brain deficit from cerebral arteriosclerosis or other brain damage) is hiding beneath the depression.

The psychosocial reasons for the age distribution of depressive disorders seem relatively clear. In the forties and fifties, all of us are confronted with awareness of our diminishing vigor, prospects, and life-expectancy, and we have a tendency to take stock of our personal accomplishments and failures. Such a time obviously furnishes fertile soil for the development of depressive symptoms.

Family History

It is quite common to find that patients suffering from depression have a family history of one or more other members of the family having suffered from this disorder or from manic episodes.

The actual genetic background of depression is not so clear. It seems to be fairly certain that the particular type of depressive disorder called manic-depressive disease is a hereditary disorder. Other forms of depression may not be transmitted on a genetic basis at all. Studies indicating that most depressives have family histories showing relatives with "psychiatric illness" (Ayd, 1961, p. 3) are misleading. "Psychiatric illness" is an extremely broad and vague label and it would be reasonable to expect that any person has at least one relative to whom such a dubious diagnostic epithet may be applied.

Nonetheless, a history of depressive disorder in the family may be obtained from a significant number of depressed patients.

Premorbid Personality

The premorbid personality which seems to predispose to the development of depressive episodes is that type which we loosely call the *obsessive-compulsive* personality. Actually, the diagnostic label is a serious misnomer: the obsessive-compulsive personality displays neither obsessions nor compulsions in the true sense of these terms. In fact, the obsessive-compulsive personality type is the personality type par excellence in our society; it is the type very often found in successful individuals, be they physicians, politicians, bankers, lawyers, skilled or unskilled workers, or homemakers. This type of person is generally conforming in his behavior and tends to be quite responsible or even perfectionistic. If he is obsessed at all, it is with the idea of doing things right and well; and if he is compulsive, it is about being somewhat neat, orderly, and organized. And this is the type of person who, somehow or other, seems a bit more apt to suffer from depressions.

What this means is that the patient who presents himself in a physician's office because he is suffering from a depression will generally not have a disturbed or chaotic personal history or a past record indicative of emotional instability. Quite the contrary, he or she may appear as someone who has always been seen as a steady, well-organized, responsible individual, often well-liked by family and friends.

Case Example 1

Mr. A is a 55-year-old man who has been employed by a large public utility company for some 30 years and has worked his way up to a vice-presidency. He presents himself in the psychiatrist's office reluctantly and only at the insistence of his company physician.

When he walks into the office, he does so very slowly and seems to collapse in a chair. His manner is pleasant on the surface, but he speaks very slowly and only in response to direct questions.

When asked what is troubling him, Mr. A states that he has some pretty severe difficulties, but that they are nothing that would concern the physician and nothing that the physician could possibly help him with. Prodded to explain this, he mutters, "I'm finished—done. I'm wiped out completely and I have nobody but myself to blame for it. I don't want to involve you in it. You seem like a nice enough person. If you get involved with me, it will be the end of you, too. That's what is happening to my wife. She'll be ruined by me and she certainly doesn't deserve it." More than a full five minutes is consumed by Mr. A's articulating these few sentences in an extremely slow, broken, painful manner. After this, it becomes impossible to get any more information from him. To any and all questions or comments, he either says nothing or simply replies, "I'm finished. Done. It's over with."

Fortunately, Mr. A has been accompanied to the office by his wife. She is quite able to fill in the details of her husband's situation. It all seemed to start about two months ago; up until then, Mr. A had been fine. He was always a healthy man, "strong as a bull—never missed a day's work. Aside from a cold once a year, he was never sick." But two months ago he began to act strangely. He was very quiet around the house, "just sat around a lot." He ignored things he had previously been very interested in: hobbies like gardening, his woodworking, and his stamp collection. His condition worsened slowly but steadily, and he started to have difficulty in sleeping and in eating. Then he began to become very hesitant and indecisive. He seemed reluctant to go to work and it was a struggle to get him out of the house in the morning. Finally, he refused to go to work at all. After missing several weeks of work, he finally made it in to his office one morning. Later that day the company physician called Mrs. A to tell her that her husband was ill and was being sent home from work, and he recommended the consultation with the psychiatrist. Mrs. A volunteered one additional bit of information. Recently she had learned that just prior to the development of his symptoms, Mr. A had been informed that a promotion to the presidency of his company, the position he had always coveted, was being given to a younger man instead of to him.

Mr. A is a typical example of the patient suffering with a severe depression. Even after only a brief examination and even with the paucity of his comments, the history obtained from his wife indicates that he has symptoms in all five areas described by Beck: alteration in mood; self-reproach and self-blame; regressive wishes; vegetative changes; and a change in activity level. Because of the severity of Mr. A's condition, because of his inability to recognize that he is suffering from an illness, and because of the strength of the regressive and self-punitive drives in this man, recommendation is made that Mr. A come into the hospital for inpatient psychiatric care. Mr. A takes this recommendation in sanguine fashion. He smiles slightly and he shakes his head negatively. He has no objection to coming into the hospital, he says, but it is useless; it won't help his problems. More important, says Mr. A, is the fact that he can't afford hospitalization. "I'm broke—I don't have a cent, and I don't have any insurance. If I come into the hospital, I'd only stick them and you for the money and ruin you, just as I've ruined my wife." That good woman explains that all this protestation of poverty is totally untrue. They are very comfortably fixed financially, and Mr. A has all sorts of insurance coverage through his company to pay all hospital and medical bills. "She's only saying that to try to cheer me up," Mr. A protests. "It isn't true. We're finished. We don't have anything."

Subsequently, it becomes necessary to commit Mr. A to the hospital legally in order to obtain his admission. In a brief hospital stay, he proves to be insufficiently responsive to antidepressant medication (at least, his response is not pronounced and rapid enough to indicate the likelihood of recovery with this treatment). A course of six electric shock treatments is given, and with these Mr. A shows rapid and dramatic recovery. His depressive, delusional system of being ruined and impoverished fades away, and he is able to leave the hospital and return to work in the matter of a few weeks' time.

In passing, it is worth commenting on the nature of Mr. A's delusional system. Patients in severe depressions do develop delusions which are of a depressive nature. Some patients will develop *somatic delusions*. These may include ideas such as, "My body is rotting away, and I am all empty inside," or, "I have a cancer obstructing my intestines so that nothing can pass in or out." In other cases, *nihilistic delusions* occur. An example of a nihilistic delusion is an idea such as, "The world is coming to an end—everything is burning up." Thus, in somatic delusions the depressive ideation is *internalized*, and the body is seen as eroding or being destroyed; and in nihilistic delusions the ideation is *externalized*, and the outer world is perceived as rotting away.

Mr. A's delusional system presented a slight variation on these themes. He had worked in the world of money and finance all his life, and his ascendancy to a vice-presidency had been accomplished by starting in accounting and eventually becoming controller of the company. Hence, his delusions were expressed in terms of the world he knew best and felt most: the world of money. He pictured this world at an end for him and that he was "finished, done," and he imagined that all his financial resources and security had evaporated.

Case Example 2

Mrs. B is a 38-year-old housewife and the mother of four children. She comes to her family physician asking for help "because I don't know where else to turn." She is quite articulate in the office and reasonably composed, but she dissolves into tears on a few occasions. As her chief complaint she states, "I'm bored stiff. I really can't stand the way my life is going." She proceeds to say, "My husband is a very nice person, but we really never did have anything in common. I'm afraid the truth is that he's dull. We've been married for 17 years and it seemed good enough at times, but maybe I was just kidding myself and putting up with it." How is her sexual relationship with her husband, the physician asks? "It's like everything else—dull, dull, dull," is the quick reply.

Mrs. B goes on to say that she probably ought to be seeing a lawyer rather than a doctor. Or maybe the doctor might suggest a good marriage counselor for her. She just doesn't know. It seems sort of hopeless, and maybe she and her husband should just recognize that and call it quits. Her physician is not quick to jump to any conclusions, however. He begins to take a little personal and family history on Mrs. B. How did her parents get along in their marriage? "Well, they got along fine," Mrs. B says. Were there any problems at all? "The only problem had nothing to do with marriage," Mrs. B opines. "It was just that mother did have to go away a lot." Further questioning clarifies that her mother's "going away" was occasioned by "nervous breakdowns" which necessitated her going into a mental hospital for treatment, including electric shock therapy. At this point, the physician begins to pick up a diagnostic scent. "What did they diagnose your mother's illness as?" he asks. "Something like manic-depressions," Mrs. B replies. A bit more probing serves to indicate that Mrs. B had "sort of a depression" herself when she was 18 years old. She became very moody and unhappy for a number of months, lost her appetite, and lost a good deal of weight. Eventually the condition passed off without any medical attention or specific treatment. And how is Mrs. B's appetite now? Well, as a matter of fact, not very good. She has lost 15 pounds in the past month or two.

Mrs. B then returns to complaining about her husband's drab personality, but by now she is in tears. Her physician suggests to her that maybe her problems aren't all marital. Maybe, just maybe, she is suffering from a bit of a depression. He suggests a trial of a tricyclic antidepressant (in this case, amitriptyline). Mrs. B is a bit reluctant at first, but finally agrees to try it. Over the course of several weeks, the physician gets Mrs. B up to a daily dosage of 150 mg of amitriptyline. He sees Mrs. B in his office after she has been on this dosage for a week, and he has a pleasant surprise. She is no longer tearful, and her appetite has returned with a vengeance. Her problems and discontents with her husband? "I really don't know what I was talking about. He is a quiet sort of person, but we find plenty of things to do and say together. I guess I was just bored and depressed with myself and was blaming it on him." Mrs. B's physician recommends that she stay on the amitriptyline at 150 mg per day for a number of months and then remain on a small daily dosage as prophylaxis against further depressive episodes.

Mrs. B had a depression of moderate intensity, characterized by some mood alteration and some vegetative change (loss of appetite), but not much else. As happens not uncommonly, she tended to cover up her alteration in mood by projecting it on her husband and her marriage ("My husband is dull and my marriage is boring," rather than, "I feel dull, bored, and depressed"). With the help of some hints from her family history and past personal history, her physician was astute enough to recognize the possibility of depression as the correct diagnosis. His therapeutic trial of the tricyclic antidepressant served to confirm the diagnosis; no antidepressant drug is going to transform a poor marriage into a satisfactory one. In clinical practice it is often appropriate to attempt such a therapeutic trial of antidepressant medication when the diagnosis is in some doubt but depression is strongly suspected. Scientific purists may well argue that in such cases, even if the patient improves markedly on the antidepressant medication, there is no proof that he was suffering from a depression. This is unquestionably true, since improvement may be due to the placebo effect (see Chapter 16), spontaneous remission, or other fortuitous factors. However, both the physician and, more importantly, his patient will be satisfied to find that recovery has indeed occurred, even if precise diagnosis remains uncertain.

SIGNS AND SYMPTOMS OF DEPRESSION

Having considered two examples of cases of depression, let us now review systematically the signs and symptoms of the disorder. Since these are apt to vary considerably with the severity of the illness, it will be most useful to break the symptomatology down into subdivisions for the various categories of severity.

Severe Depression

Chief complaints The following are the chief complaints commonly elicited from severely depressed patients:

"I feel terribly sad."
"I feel hopeless."
"Everything is awful."
"Everything is ruined."
"I feel completely empty."
"I can't feel anything."
"I'm totally exhausted."
"I can't stop crying."
"There is no point to living."
"I don't care about anything."

We must also note that in some cases of severe depression the patient comes to the physician only at the urging or insistence of family and friends, and in these cases the patient may insist that he has no chief complaints. Usually such a patient will clearly indicate that he does not mean that there is nothing wrong, but rather that the physician could not possibly be of any help to him.
Additional symptoms The severely depressed person may describe his mood as depressed, despondent, dejected, blue, or

melancholic. He may also indicate that nothing gives him pleasure anymore, and that his main desire is to avoid other people
and all activities—to escape or to hide. He is apt to express very
negative views about himself: "I'm no good"; "I don't deserve to
live"; "I'm ruining my family." He may complain of frequent
crying spells, or he may indicate that things are so bad that he
"can't even cry anymore." Very often he will describe many or all
aspects of his life in negative terms that are obviously grossly
exaggerated: "Everybody is sick of me"; "Everybody has given up
on me"; "I'm finished at my job. I've ruined it"; "My kids hate me."

Energy and interest are described as minimal or totally lacking: "I don't have the strength to do anything"; "Nothing appeals
to me"; "There is nothing that I want to do or can do, except get
away from everything and everybody, including myself."

Intellectual functioning is described by the patient as grossly
impaired, although this may again represent a distorted, negative self-view. "My mind is slipping"; "I can't remember anything
anymore"; "I can't concentrate." True memory loss is indicative of
organic brain damage and does not occur in depression. However,
the severely depressed patient is so concerned that his memory
and mental functions are impaired that he may do very poorly on
any kind of formal intellectual testing, simply because of this
performance anxiety. If the physician observes closely, he will
catch indications that such a patient really is impaired only by
the depressive's extreme preoccupation with self. Bear in mind,
also, that some severely depressed patients may have received
electric shock treatments during previous episodes of depression.
In these patients, some memory deficit may be an aftereffect of
shock therapy.

Physical symptoms generally abound and are of particular
importance since they are so often the reason for the depressive
presenting himself to the physician. Marked loss of appetite,
pronounced weight loss, severe insomnia, and localized pains of
all sorts are extremely common. The pain or pains are apt to be
quite persistent, resistant to any and all analgesics, and, of
course, not caused by any underlying physical pathology. Sexual
functioning is likely to be nil during severe depressions, but this
is seldom complained of by the patient because his sexual interest
has evaporated.

A total self-absorption in the severely depressed patient leads
to an obvious lack of genuine concern or interest for other people.
The patient usually realizes this, even though he is unable to do

anything about it. It only serves to make him feel more guilt and self-hatred, and he may complain, "I don't seem to really give a damn about anything or anybody but myself. I know I should control myself for my wife's sake and for the kids', but it doesn't seem to matter."

An extremely important symptom of severe depression is suicidal ideation or intent. This is sometimes volunteered by the patient, who protests, "I have nothing to live for. I'm going to kill myself"; "There's nothing left for me but death"; or "I won't be around to make everybody miserable much longer." More often, the physician must draw out suicidal ideas or feelings where they are present (this will be discussed later in the chapter).

In general, it is important to keep in mind that most of the symptoms of severe depression must be elicited by the physician. The patient characteristically will volunteer but little, so it is up to the alert clinician to ask the appropriate questions and to persist in the questioning until the diagnosis is established.

Signs The severely depressed person often presents an appearance so distinctive as to be virtually pathognomonic. The face is relatively immobile and tends to have either a woebegone expression or no expression at all. Gait is slow and often shuffling, and associated movements of the arms and trunk are limited. A marked slouch or stoop is frequently characteristic of the posture on standing, and upon sitting the patient tends to slump or almost collapse in his chair. In agitated depression, as mentioned before, there is a restlessness superimposed on the signs already described. This may be evidenced by pacing back and forth, wringing of the hands, purposeless movements of the legs while sitting, or other similar activities.

Signs of the depressive's underlying sadness may include constant weeping, spells of crying, or a more subtle manifestation of tears in the eyes. The eyes are generally reddened as a result of this. The effects of marked weight loss may be seen in the face, neck, and limbs.

Speech is definitely slowed down from a normal rate and is generally infrequent. Thinking is slowed also, as are all the patient's responses. An underlying lack of spontaneity is evident in a number of the signs of severe depression. It is this lack that results in a paucity of movements associated with gait and in a lack of gestures, body movements, and facial expression. All the nonverbal and bodily aspects of communication are lacking or are as though delivering one stereotyped message: "I am paralyzed; I am inert." Conversation is rarely initiated by the depressed person.

As mentioned before, delusions may be elicited and are often of a nihilistic or somatic type and reflect depressive ideation.

Moderate Depression

Chief complaints The typical chief complaints of the moderately depressed patient include:

"I'm sad a lot of the time."
"I've lost my pep and my zest for life."
"I'm worried about almost everything."
"I've had quite a few crying spells."
"My energy seems to be gone."
"I just feel blue all the time."
"I've lost my sense of humor."

Additional symptoms In moderate depressions these parallel the symptoms described for severe depression, but they are less pronounced. The mood is described as blah, blue, down, depressed. Although low self-esteem is more subtly manifested in moderate depressions, feelings of guilt, shame, and remorse for past transgressions, real or imagined, are likely to plague the patient.

Energy is impaired and deficient, but to a lesser degree than in severe depression. Consequently, the patient may say that he just doesn't seem to have the zip or the steam he once had. Concern may be voiced that this is part of growing old. Even more frequently, the patient will attribute this lack of energy to some underlying physical ailment and will seek some explanation in terms of a hidden physical disease.

His interests will be similarly diminished. In moderate depression the patient is often attempting to somehow keep up with his work or social activities but is finding this increasingly difficult to do.

Intellectual functioning may be somewhat disturbed in moderate depressions due to the underlying slowing and retardation of thought processes. The patient is particularly apt to notice and complain of this if he is involved in a job or profession which requires considerable intellectual sharpness. Quite often the patient will have great difficulty in making decisions and will vacillate a great deal.

Physical symptoms are quite common. Appetite and sleep will both be affected, reflecting varying degrees of anorexia and insomnia. Other complaints may concern persistent pains and headaches, as well as vague symptomatology which the patient may attribute to the cardiovascular, gastrointestinal, or pulmonary systems. Sexual functioning is also disturbed, and in moderate depressions the patient is quite likely to complain of this, particularly if the physician is alert enough to inquire about the sexual realm. In men, impotence secondary to depression is the common complaint, while in women there occurs a corresponding lack of sexual energy which results in a disinterest or lack of pleasure in the sex act and which may well produce secondary orgasmic dysfunction (ie, a woman who has previously been able to have orgasms may well lose that capacity while in a depressed state).

Signs These are considerably less pronounced than they are in severe depressions. However, the physician should be alert to crying spells and moist or reddened eyes. (A valuable clue may be picked up by observing the expression in a patient's eyes, which in depression tends to be a look of deep and ineffable sadness.) Because of the patient's sadness, he has generally lost his sense of humor. If any humor is manifested by the patient, it is apt to be of a self-deprecating kind.

Gait, thinking, and speech may be slowed, but this is not necessarily marked, so the physician has to look hard for these indications. The same is true of physical signs of weight loss. Again, the spontaneity of speech, gestures, and actions is apt to be definitely reduced from normal.

Suicidal ideas or intentions are not uncommon. Despite the fact that we term these conditions "moderate" depressions, suicides can and do occur. A physician should bear this in mind and should never hesitate to probe the extent of such thoughts and feelings.

Mild Depression

Mild depressions may occur in two different forms. (1) They may be characterized by all or most of the symptoms and signs already described for severe and moderate depressions; however, these symptoms and signs will be quite mild or incipient in nature, and hence will be all the more difficult for the physician to detect. (2) In many other cases, mild depressions will occur in a form that has been described as *masked depression*, or *hidden depression*. (The terms "depressio sine depressione" and "depressive equivalent" have also been used to describe this same syndrome [López-Íbor, 1972]).

Case example Dr. C is a 42-year-old dentist who is highly successful, both professionally and financially, in his work. He was born and raised in a small Pennsylvania Dutch town outside of Philadelphia. His childhood was basically happy and ordinary, although people in the town did remark that Dr. C's mother "went a little queer" when she was in her early forties. However, the townsfolk attributed that to the "change of life," Dr. C's mother got over it after a year or so, and nobody thought much more about it. Dr. C went through the local school and was a brilliant student and a model boy. He had no trouble in getting a scholarship to college, where he again did extremely well. Four successful years at dental school followed and then a three-year hitch with the military service as a medical officer. After this, Dr. C came back and opened his dental office in his hometown. Along the way, he had married his childhood sweetheart, a woman of similar background and temperament. As years went by, Dr. C was successful in his work, where he built up a huge dental practice, and prolific at home, where his wife and he managed to have seven children in the course of 12 years.

At the age of 42, Dr. C seemed to be sitting on top of the world. His practice was booming, his wife and children were thriving, and he had a rewarding life in his community and with his friends. Dr. C indeed seemed to be happy, although he noted a few small problems. One involved his sleep pattern, which seemed to be just a bit off. Because of this, he consulted his local physician and was given a prescription for some barbiturates. In addition, Dr. C began to feel a bit bored with his practice, but he attributed this to simple overwork and fatigue and thought he should get away more on vacations. Finally, there was a small problem known only to Dr. C and his wife. Dr. C was approaching his wife for sexual intercourse less and less often, and when they did have sex, they both could not help but notice that his erections were somehow not quite as strong as they always had been. On this matter Dr. C kept his own counsel, discussing it neither with his wife nor with his physician.

As luck would have it, Dr. C happened to hire a new employee for his office at about that time. She was a beautiful young woman of a very tender and sympathetic nature who took a job as one of his dental assistants. To make a long story short, within just a few months Dr. C and his new assistant were involved in a flaming love affair, complete with a sexual relationship. Truth to tell, Dr. C did not find that his potency was up to normal, even with this attractive young woman, but the thrill and novelty of the romance stimulated him enough to compensate for that.

The affair continued for about six months, and Dr. C's difficulties in sleeping and his boredom with his work continued also. Now, however, Dr. C had a new problem: a tremendous feeling of guilt. Raised in a strict, religious atmosphere, he could not really accept the infidelity in which he was involved. After six months, he felt that he could live with his guilt no longer and decided to break off the affair. This he promptly did. Moreover, he decided to make a clean breast of the matter to his wife, and he told her all about it. She accepted the revelation of his indiscretions with great empathy and the deepest understanding and promptly told him to pack his bags, get out of the house, and never contact her or the children again.

He then sought help from his clergyman, who told Dr. C, in effect, that Mrs. C was basically quite right in her position, that Dr. C was a miserable sinner, and that he should repent and seek forgiveness for his sins. Since Dr. C had already done that (with no success), he finally turned to his physician for help. But, characteristically, Dr. C did not arrive at his doctor's office down and depressed and obviously despondent. Rather, Dr. C was his usual, smiling, affable self. He admitted he was "having a little trouble at home with the wife" and thought it might be getting on his nerves a bit. Could the physician help any? Yes, the physician thought so, and he gave Dr. C a prescription for meprobamate: 400-mg tablets, two tablets four times per day.

Several hours later, Dr. C did indeed take the meprobamate tablets, but unfortunately he ingested fifty of them at once, along with all of the barbiturates that remained at his disposal. He was hospitalized in a coma and was fortunate to emerge from it some 36 hours later.

Dr. C had a *masked depression*, and the striking characteristic of these disorders is that the patient presents virtually no evidence at all of any pathologic alteration in mood. He does not seem sad, melancholic, blue, or unhappy; he has a *smiling depression*. Dr. C's smiling depression eluded diagnosis by anyone. His physician missed it originally and just attempted to treat his insomnia with barbiturates. Then he missed the diagnosis a second time when he gave Dr. C the meprobamate for symptomatic relief. Rather than being critical of these errors, however, we must realize that masked depressions are most difficult to diagnose unless one is alert to the fact that they occur with considerable frequency.

Symptoms and signs In masked depressions, careful questioning and examination by the physician will elicit some or all of the following symptoms and signs, which are present even in the absence of any visible mood disturbance.

Insomnia The patient will complain of a difficulty in sleeping, and questioning by the physician will reveal that the pattern of this insomnia is one typical of depression. That is, the main difficulty will not be falling asleep, but early morning awakening. Thus, the patient is likely to say, "I wake up at 5 AM (or 3, or 4 AM) and I can't get back to sleep, no matter what I do, and I'm miserable."

Along with this early morning awakening, there is a characteristic pattern to the patient's day. Thus, if the physician asks him, "What is your worst time of day?" or "When do you feel your worst?", the patient will generally answer, "First thing in the morning." This is because he awakens early, can't get back to sleep, has to face a day he is not eager for, and is apt to have worries and fears running through his mind. Similarly, if the doctor asks, "What is the best time of day for you?", the answer will very likely be, "In the evening." By then the worries of the day have abated somewhat, and the patient with a depression can at least look forward to some temporary relief in a brief period of sleep. (In a small minority of depressions, the patient may show hypersomnia rather than insomnia and tend to escape into sleep, so that he sleeps an excessive amount of time.)

Loss of appetite This may be denied by the patient or may be attributed to purely physical causes by the patient. Resultant weight loss will be evident in poorly fitting clothes and in hanging skin folds on the neck and limbs. In a minority of cases, depression, rather than causing a loss of appetite, causes just the reverse. Here, the patient seems to overeat to cover up or relieve the inner, hidden depression.

Lack of energy Again, the patient is apt to ascribe this to some physical cause or is apt to feel that it is an indication of the aging process.

Lack of interest This involves work, social activities, family relationships, and personal interests. In our case example, Dr. C manifested just such a lack of interest in terms of the vague boredom he was feeling with his work, work that he had previously always relished.

Sexual dysfunction due to depression includes impotence and/or loss of sexual interest in the male, and orgasmic dysfunction and/or loss of interest in the female. In not a few cases, sexual dysfunction will be denied by the patient, who will attempt to disprove its existence in some way. For example, Dr. C reacted to his underlying sexual impotence by seeking to deny it: a new woman and the excitement of an illicit affair served temporarily to bolster his failing libido.

Because of the frequency with which such cases occur, they should be better understood. Sudden development of "promiscuous" sexual behavior may well occur in the person suffering from a masked depression. Since the depressive is guilt-ridden and possessed of considerable self-hatred, his situation becomes quite precarious when others heap criticism and condemnation on him. This was precisely Dr. C's position. Scorned and blamed by his wife and by his clergyman, Dr. C's guilt and self-hatred overflowed to result in his attempt at self-destruction.

Constipation of a chronic and troublesome nature is another tell-tale symptom of masked depression. The slowing and retardation of all bodily processes extends to the gastrointestinal tract to produce this disturbance. Here again, a small minority of depressives will show the opposite gastrointestinal symptom: chronic diarrhea or colitis.

Chronic or recurrent aches and pains These may occur in the extremities or in the neck and are very common in the lower back. Persistent, recurrent headaches are equally common.

If the physician can keep these seven sets of symptoms in mind, he may be able to diagnose many cases of masked depression. When there is a family history of depressive illness, and/or when the patient is of the obsessive-compulsive personality type, the likelihood of making this diagnosis increases. (Note that both these factors were present in Dr. C's case.)

Those forms of masked depression in which the patient may complain of only one symptom (such as severe anorexia, recurrent headaches, or chronic neck or back pain) are sometimes referred to as *depressive equivalents*. No doubt this diagnosis may be overused or misused at times and applied casually to any case of unexplained insomnia, anorexia, or chronic pain. However, it is generally worth prescribing a therapeutic trial of antidepressant medication in these cases. Not a few of them will respond dramatically after all other therapy has failed.

Although the term masked depression is generally used to describe the sort of cases we have been discussing thus far, it can also be accurately applied to another syndrome. In this latter instance, an underlying depression is masked by the presence of another disorder. Drug addiction is, far and away, the most common disorder that masks depression in this fashion, and the most common type of drug addiction is, of course, alcoholism. For this reason, the physician should take a long, hard look at any alcoholic patient. The question to ask is: does a depression lurk beneath the exterior symptoms of alcoholism? Is the patient hiding an alteration in mood by resorting to drink, or is he attempting to cure the ravages of depressive insomnia and lack of energy by artificially stoking his fires with alcohol? A depressive disorder may be recognized in a seemingly alcoholic patient if the physician considers all the various, telltale signs and symptoms we have already described, plus any family history of depression and the patient's premorbid personality.

If it is established or strongly suspected that the patient's alcoholism does indeed cover up a depression, treatment should proceed as follows: first, as for any alcoholic problem, the patient must completely stop the intake of any alcohol. Then, and only then, the patient may be treated with antidepressive medication to reach the underlying pathology. Attempting to treat the depression of an alcoholic who is still drinking simply does not work. Worse, the combination of antidepressant medication plus alcohol can be a deadly one, as is pointed out elsewhere in this book. Carrying out the program of stopping alcoholic intake and then treating the depression generally requires a period of psychiatric hospitalization.

HOW TO RECOGNIZE THE SUICIDAL PATIENT

The case example of Dr. C brings out the fact that there is danger of suicide with the depressed patient. As a matter of fact, virtually any patient who is suffering from a depression represents a suicidal risk, regardless of whether his depression is severe, moderate, mild, masked, or hidden in nature. Recognizing and estimating the severity of suicidal risk is, therefore, a task in which every physician needs definite skill. Fortunately, the task is neither impossible nor extremely difficult if it is pursued systematically, as in the following steps (Goldberg, 1973).

(1) Always *ask* the depressed patient about suicide! There are some old myths to the effect that asking a person about suicide may put the idea into that person's head or may aggravate any suicidal intent that is present. That is pure nonsense. Asking directly about suicide cannot produce any harmful effects. It can only bring out the facts and feelings that are already present and perhaps even help to defuse the latter somewhat.

Many of us hesitate to ask about suicide because we really are afraid to know. It is the old ostrich psychology: what we don't see or don't know will not bother us. And indeed, if the physician asks a patient about suicidal intent and determines that such intent is present, he should be ready, willing, and able to take appropriate action.

(2) When you do ask about suicide, use plain and direct language. Don't be evasive and don't beat around the bush or use euphemisms. "Have you thought about killing yourself?" or "Have you thought of committing suicide?" are the appropriate questions.

(3) In most instances, patients will answer honestly and directly if they are questioned in such a manner. In other words, the physician can believe his patient; and if the latter clearly states that he has not been thinking of self-destruction, the issue may be put aside. On the other hand, if the patient says something like, "Yes, I must admit I have been thinking about killing myself," then the physician's questioning must continue.

(4) If the patient admits to suicidal thoughts, the next question is, "How *much* have you been thinking about suicide?" If the patient then says, "Oh, the thought has occurred to me once or twice, but I would never do anything like that," then it would appear that the suicidal threat is not very great. But if the patient says, "I've been thinking about it a good deal" or "I think about it all the time," then the indications are ominous and the physician proceeds to the next question.

(5) "Have you thought about *how* you would kill yourself?" Again, if the patient replies with something like, "Things aren't that bad—I haven't really made any plans," that is somewhat reassuring. On the other hand, indications of definite suicidal plans are very alarming. Such plans may be revealed by an

answer like, "I've got some pills put away for just that purpose," or "I think I would lock myself in the car in the garage with the motor running and the garage door closed."

(6) The last question the physician needs to ask is, "Is there anything or any reason to keep you from killing yourself?" If the patient offers any strong reason whatsoever, such as, "I'd never do it because of my religion," or "I couldn't do something like that to my wife and kids," then the suicidal threat may not be overly grave. If, however, the patient says, "There's no reason in the world why I shouldn't kill myself," or "I can't think of anything; my family will be better off without me," then it must be recognized that the danger of self-destruction is extremely strong.

(7) While asking these various questions, the physician should bear in mind that *hopelessness* is the most consistent and ominous warning sign of possible suicide. The more hopeless the person seems, the more likely it is that he will make some attempt at self-destruction.

(8) Once it is recognized that a patient has suicidal intentions, two steps should be carried out immediately. First of all, the physician should contact the closest relative or friend of the suicidal person and share with him or her the knowledge of the patient's condition and danger. Secondly, a referral for psychiatric consultation should be arranged as quickly as possible. Not every suicidal patient requires psychiatric hospitalization, but every such patient should be seen by a psychiatrist to determine if hospitalization is needed.

(9) Do not give medications or prescriptions for medications in any substantial amounts to the suicidal patient. Be especially aware that tricyclic antidepressants (amitriptyline, imipramine, desipramine, etc) and MAO inhibitors (see Glossary) are especially effective in producing death by overdosage. If it is necessary to give the suicidal patient medication, he should be given small supplies that will last only for a few days.

MANIC BEHAVIOR AND EPISODES

Patients with recurrent depressions are sometimes also susceptible to developing episodes of manic behavior. In some ways, the manic state is just the opposite of the depressed state. There is a mood alteration, but instead of being down or despondent, the person experiencing a manic episode is excessively cheerful, elated, or even euphoric. Instead of being slowed in his speech, gait, and thinking, as the depressed person is, the manic patient is speeded up. He talks very rapidly and is apt to walk quite rapidly and move around a good deal. He will move around a good deal in his thinking, also, jumping from one idea to another with such rapidity that his speech reveals a flight of ideas. The manic person's judgment is often very poor; he is *too* decisive (ie, impulsive). He may suddenly engage in behavior quite foreign to his previous personality: reckless spending of money, promiscuous sexual behavior, complex business deals. Like the depressed patient, the manic patient is apt to eat little and get insufficient sleep.

On the surface, at least, the manic seems to have an exaggerated self-concept. He is apt to describe himself as ultra-superior in all respects, and if he has delusions, they may be delusions of grandeur (eg, seeing himself as a famous leader, a messiah, or even a God figure). Again, this seems diametrically opposed to the low self-concept held by the depressed patient.

Despite these polar differences, the manic and depressed states are really closely related. Psychologically, the manic condition seems to represent a supreme effort on the patient's part to deny an underlying depression. Thus, manic states have a tendency to deteriorate into frank depressions. Some manic patients, in the full bloom of their excitement and elation, can be brought to tears or to the verge of tears by sharply worded questions aimed at their underlying insecurities. The inflated self-opinion of the manic is really only a thin veneer: it covers up the same low self-concept and morass of guilt found in the depressed patient.

Moreover, manic patients also can be self-destructive. Their impulsive behavior in financial, sexual, and family matters may produce many partially self-destructive effects. Then too, sleep and appetite are interfered with in the manic state, as the patient's excitement preempts his attention to his bodily needs. A severely manic patient may ignore food, drink, and rest to the extent that a dangerous, or even fatal, condition of malnutrition, dehydration, and/or exhaustion results.

Diagnosing the manic patient may be difficult, particularly if the condition is mild and the patient is not previously known by the physician. In such instances, diagnosis is often made by obtaining a history from a close relative of the patient which describes the development of his mood alteration and behavioral changes. Severely manic patients, with their clinical picture of excitement, restlessness, and constant talk and physical activity, are less difficult to diagnose. However, the physician will have to differentiate between the severely manic patient and the patient in a state of schizophrenic catatonic excitement. Generally this distinction can be made on the basis of the doctor's interpersonal reaction to the patient. In interacting with a manic patient, one generally feels somewhat amused by and definitely sympathetic to him. In contrast, interaction with someone in a catatonic excitement will call forth a very threatened feeling. The doctor will not feel at all amused; he will feel frightened for his own safety—and rightly so, since the state of catatonic excitement is an extremely dangerous one that is apt to produce violent behavior.

When a patient recounts that someone in his family has had a manic episode or episodes, this can be taken as an indication that manic-depressive disease may run in that family, and it is perhaps more significant than a family history of simple depression per se.

RECOGNIZING DEPRESSION IN THE ADOLESCENT

Adolescents do suffer from depressive illness, but they are apt to show symptomatology different from adult patterns. In perhaps the majority of cases, alteration of mood is not apparent or is only slightly apparent in the adolescent patient who is depressed. The following symptoms and signs quite commonly mask an underlying depression:

1. Poor school performance or a sudden, unexplained drop in performance level
2. Rebellious behavior at school
3. Rebellious behavior at home
4. Disturbed sleep, lack of appetite, and persistent, recurrent headaches
5. Use of "hard" drugs, psychedelic agents, or alcohol

We cannot say, of course, that every teenager who shows some or all of these signs is suffering from a depression. There are thousands of adolescents showing poor school performance, rebellious behavior, and drug usage who are not really depressed. Nonetheless, when these symptoms do occur, the possibility of an underlying depression in the adolescent should be considered.

DIFFERENTIAL DIAGNOSIS

For the practicing physician the most important differentiation to make is that between depressive illness and the anxiety states. On the face of it, such a differentiation would seem to be relatively easy. The depressed patient is down, blue, despondent, and slowed; whereas the anxious patient is jumpy, jittery, tense, and hyperalert. Unfortunately, these conditions cannot be compartmentalized quite so neatly, since very often there is considerable anxiety mixed in with depression. Consequently, most depressed patients will show some symptoms of anxiety along with their depressive features. From a practical standpoint, the physician can follow this rule: where a patient shows features of both anxiety and depression, presume that the depression is the basic problem and treat the depression first and foremost. (Quite possibly, the anxiety will clear up as the depression lifts.)

In older patients, depressive illness must be differentiated from organic brain syndromes, in which there is actual brain damage from cerebral arteriosclerosis, cerebral atrophy, brain tumors, and the like. Organic brain syndromes are much more likely to cause real memory deficits; often, recent memory will be impaired while remote memory is intact. Patients with organic brain syndromes will also show confusion, impairment of concentration, disorientation, and poor judgment at times, and may confabulate in an attempt to cover their defects. Neurologic examination, skull x-rays, electroencephalograms (EEGs), and EMI-scan (cerebral tomography) techniques may be needed to establish the diagnosis.

In younger patients, depressive illness may sometimes be confused with certain physical disorders, such as infectious mononucleosis or hepatitis. This confusion occurs because these physical disorders produce lethargy and a plethora of vegetative symptoms that are similar to those seen in depression. Appropriate physical and laboratory examinations will serve to make the differentiation.

SUMMARY

The essence of all we have said in this chapter could probably best be summarized by, "Depression is a very common, everyday, garden-variety disease." Be alert to that fact and be on the lookout for depressions in your patients.

As with any disease, early recognition is highly desirable. Most depressions are self-limiting; that is, even if left untreated, they will probably run their courses and disappear after three to nine months. But early diagnosis and treatment of depression serves several important purposes. (1) It helps to reduce the intensity and the duration of the patient's suffering. (2) By shortening the depressive episode, we can minimize the social, occupational, and family disruption that the depressed patient may produce. (3) Most important, the sooner the depression is ended, the sooner any danger of suicide is removed. Patients do recover from depressive illnesses—if they don't kill themselves first. Consequently, the early recognition and treatment of depression not only alleviates suffering but it may in some instances be a life-saving accomplishment.

REFERENCES

Ayd, F. J.: *Recognizing the Depressed Patient.* New York: Grune & Stratton, Inc., 1961.

Beck, A. T.: *The Diagnosis and Management of Depression.* Philadelphia: University of Pennsylvania Press, 1973.

Goldberg, M.: *Psychiatric Diagnosis and Understanding for the Helping Professions.* Chicago: Nelson-Hall Publishers, 1973.

López-Ibor, J. J.: Masked depression and depressive equivalents. In *Depressive Illness*, edited by P. Kielholz. Baltimore: The Williams & Wilkins Co., 1972.

Raft, D., Davidson, J., Toomey, T. C. et al: Inpatient and outpatient patterns of psychotropic drug prescribing by nonpsychiatrist physicians. *Am J Psychiatr.* 132:1309, 1975.

4 Diagnosing the Psychotic Patient

Doris Berlin, M.D., M.P.H.

When a patient walks into your office and sits down next to your desk, your first question usually is, "What seems to be the trouble?"

If the patient replies, "I just can't sleep at night," you might pursue a line of questioning leading to a physical diagnosis such as hyperthyroidism, or, failing to find a history or suggestive evidence of physical disease, you might discover that your patient is worried about losing his job. In such a case, further inquiries and examination could well lead to a diagnosis of acute anxiety or a neurotic personality.

On the other hand, your patient may be vague; he may be evasive and talk about other things. He may talk about how his neighbors keep him awake because they want to get his money, despite the fact that you know he is unemployed and quite penniless. Or he may even tell you that an old friend has reported him to the FBI and that the "feds" are trying to force him to confess to something that he did not do. Under such circumstances, it

73

wouldn't be long before you would say to yourself, "This man is crazy!"

And you would probably be right. The extremely disturbed person who is so mentally ill that he suffers from delusions and/or hallucinations is relatively easy for the professional, and even for the layman, to identify. It is the "walking-around" psychotic—the one who is not so obviously mentally ill—who is not as easy to spot. This chapter, therefore, is aimed at helping you diagnose such a patient. He may be one of the 300,000 people who have been discharged from mental hospitals in the last 10 years (Ozarin, 1976). Or he may be a person who has had multiple admissions to psychiatric inpatient services and is currently in "controlled remission" (ie, he is able to function marginally, or even better, as long as he is kept on sufficient psychotropic medication).

Recent evidence indicates that mental patients rarely need to be hospitalized for long periods. In fact, they do better when discharged (and usually, maintained on psychotropic medication) as soon as the disturbance in thinking is sufficiently corrected to make this possible. Thus, the desocializing effects of being "away" (loss of friends, loss of jobs, alienation from family) are lessened. Moreover, there is less of a tendency for patients to become apathetic, withdrawn, and lacking in initiative. The average length of stay in a mental hospital is about 18 to 30 days at present, and it is getting shorter all the time.

As a result of the advent of psychotropic drug treatment and of new concepts concerning patient care, the mental patient now most frequently resides in his own home or in a nursing care home, family care home, halfway house, or similar residence. He is no longer banished indefinitely and left to his fate in a mental hospital. The basis of care for the psychotic is mostly outpatient rather than inpatient. We cannot yet "cure" the majority of cases of mental illness, but we can enable most patients to function. Some will do so surprisingly well, while others will show residual disabilities such as social isolation, difficulty in holding a job, or inability to adjust to family life.

Many psychotic conditions are chronic in nature, but in today's world most patients with chronic psychoses will spend the greatest part of their lives in the community, with one or more periods of hospitalization when necessary. Twenty years ago, the situation was often the reverse: patients with chronic psychoses spent most of their lives in hospitals, with only occasional periods of living in the community.

Because of the situation we have just described, more psychotic patients are presenting themselves to any and every practicing physician. Mental illness confers no immunity to physical illness, of course, so the ambulatory psychotic patient may come into your office because of his cardiovascular, gastrointestinal, pulmonary, or genitourinary dysfunction. Or, such patients may present themselves with physical complaints that turn out, on careful examination, to actually be mental in origin. Finally, many patients prefer to be followed by a private practitioner rather than an outpatient clinic after they leave a mental hospital. Such patients may come in with requests for renewals of prescriptions for psychotropic drugs, with symptoms indicative of adverse drug reactions, with requests for reassurance, and for help when having difficulty coping—not only with some of the situations they face as "ex-mental patients" but also with those problems all of us have as ordinary human beings in the course of living, loving, and working.

The walking-around psychotic may also be someone who has never been hospitalized for mental illness. It is probable that there are more people with various forms of psychoses outside of hospitals than in them. According to one researcher, the ratio of untreated to treated "cases" in the general population is staggering (Dohrenwend, 1970). It has been estimated that as many as two million people may be walking around in our country suffering from some degree of a psychotic condition.

It is also true that more people with hypertension, heart disease, and diabetes are outside of, rather than in, hospitals, yet we have failed to realize that the same situation pertains to mental illness. It has never been true that all psychotic people were hospitalized, nor that all those "outside" were free of psychosis. Since psychoses are chronic disorders, they may require varying degrees of inpatient care: none, infrequent, periodic, or only intermittent, just as is the case with hypertension, heart disease, diabetes, and all other chronic diseases.

Latent psychosis is another form of walking-around psychosis. People with this type of disorder ordinarily function adequately, but they may temporarily "break down" under unusual stress. Prompt treatment with counseling, reassurance, and the appropriate neuroleptic medication may well enable them to readjust in a short time without any need for hospitalization. Overt psychosis, thus, can quickly become latent again through prompt, concerned, and adequate care.

DEFINING A PSYCHOSIS

With the trend toward emphasis on outpatient treatment of the mentally ill, you will be seeing more and more psychotic patients in your office. Since the average physician sees a total of 156 patients a week (Wechsler, 1976), recognizing the psychotic patient as easily and rapidly as possible becomes important in handling them correctly. But what is a psychosis?

Psychosis is defined by some as "serious" mental illness. This is in contrast to neurosis, defined as less serious and less incapacitating. Unfortunately, there are no blood tests, no laboratory methods, no measurements available to diagnose a psychosis (discounting psychologic testing, which is a complicated and expensive procedure). In the absence of objective tests, the clinical examination is our main tool for making a psychiatric diagnosis. We will be discussing this examination in more detail shortly. It is quite useful in uncovering the less blatant forms of psychosis. A consultant may be needed to help in determining the more specific diagnostic subcategories.

A psychosis is characterized by disturbances in feeling, thinking, communicating, and behaving. Recent studies point to a hereditary tendency toward manic-depressive psychosis, and possibly toward schizophrenia, with the hereditary features involving biochemical changes in the transmission of brain impulses. No such tendency has yet been demonstrated in neuroses, which are generally believed to be due more to psychologic than to biologic causes.

In general, when patients are aware of difficulties in functioning, when they complain of something foreign to their personality which is making them tense or making them do things they otherwise would not do, they are more likely to be neurotic than psychotic. The person with a psychosis is less apt to complain of "something inside" causing difficulty and is more likely to place the source of his trouble outside himself. He is not likely to say that he is upset or feeling tense or highly nervous, but rather that there is some plot against him; someone is trying to harm him; he is being subjected to "rays," etc.

Perhaps the concept of *distortion* may best convey our use of the term psychosis. There are distortions of thought, as when a person thinks he is some historical or great figure; distortions of behavior, such as sitting for days looking out a window, not eating or drinking; distortions of communication, as in abnormally rapid speech with increasing irritability and intolerance of interruption; distortions of perception, such as interpreting standard symbols in personal terms.

Along with distortion, psychosis may also involve impairment, particularly in regard to memory, concentration, and orientation. These types of impairment of thought are indicative of the presence of an organic psychosis. Later in this chapter, when we discuss the identifying characteristics of psychosis which are disclosed in the mental examination, our concept of psychosis will become clearer and more complete.

HOW PSYCHOSES DIFFER FROM OTHER PSYCHIATRIC CONDITIONS

There are ten main diagnostic classifications listed in the *Diagnostic and Statistical Manual of Mental Disorders* (American Psychiatric Association, 1968). To distinguish psychosis from other mental conditions, however, we usually need to consider just two other categories: neuroses and personality disorders.

Patients with neuroses feel uncomfortable with and within themselves. They are tense or nervous and experience a sort of mental discomfort, as opposed to physical pain. The cardinal feature of all neuroses is *anxiety*, which may be experienced directly, may be converted into physical symptoms, or may be linked with depression. Despite the disturbances in emotion, however, there is no disturbance or distortion of thinking with the neuroses. Consequently, the neurotic person knows that something is wrong with him and knows that the difficulty lies inside himself, although he may very well misidentify this trouble as being physical rather than mental in origin. The neurotic person worries about being crazy, but he is far from it; he fears "losing his mind," but virtually never does.

In personality disorders, patients do not complain of discomfort with themselves. In fact, the individual with a personality disorder rarely, if ever, recognizes that he has a problem. Rather, he causes difficulties for other people, especially those close to him, through his behavior. He *acts out* his inner conflicts in addictive, destructive, antisocial behavior. Such people are brought into your office, at the insistence of a family member or friend, because of alcoholism, sexual disorders, or a broken nose after a fight. They are often irritable, demanding, and impulsive. They include the antisocial personalities who spend time in jails, seemingly without remorse. They do not show anxiety, as the neurotic does, unless they are thwarted in their behavior. (Only when they cannot act out their conflicts in aberrant behavior do they become anxious or upset within themselves.) On the other hand, people with personality disorders do not distort reality or substitute their own inner worlds for outer reality, as the psychotic patient does. Thus, the individual with a personality disorder may do wrong, but he knows very well what is wrong and what is right.

If anxiety is the cardinal feature of neurosis and acting-out behavior the cardinal feature in personality disorders, then the cardinal feature of psychosis is *distortion of reality*. The psychotic finds the real world too painful to bear, so he retreats from it by withdrawing into himself and into his own reality. Tony J., whose wound you sutured yesterday, robbed a grocery store to have money to fly to the Orange Bowl game. He showed no remorse at his crime, just anger that he missed the game. Clearly, he is an antisocial personality who seeks enjoyment regardless of cost. Helen O., on the other hand, seems unable to enjoy anything and is preoccupied with other matters. She thinks about robbing a bank as a way of "getting even" with the bank manager for slighting her when she was a teller. Instead of accepting social invitations from her friends, Helen has spent the past two months sitting in her room brooding about the fancied rejection. Although she is contemplating an antisocial action, she is not suffering from a personality disorder; she is immersed in a psychosis in which her world has become one of hurt, pain, and a desire for revenge.

To sum this all up in another fashion, we may say that the neurotic knows where he wants to go, but he's very anxious and tense about it. The antisocial person also knows, and he just goes, without fear of consequences. The psychotic patient, on the other hand, often does not know where he wants to go. In fact, sometimes the poor person is not even sure of where he is!

IMPORTANCE OF DIAGNOSING PSYCHOSIS

On a typical day in your office, you probably see at least 30 patients, 2 to 5 of whom may be severely mentally disturbed.

Because of your heavy workload, your goal is to treat all of your patients as expeditiously as you possibly can. The neurotic and the psychotic patient are included in this goal, of course. Diagnosing their conditions enables you to handle them to both your and their satisfaction with greater ease.

There are many treatments available for neurosis and psychosis, and new ones are appearing regularly. Many of the new medications have highly specific applications; hence, diagnosing the condition accurately will enable you to give the most precise medication available for its alleviation. Once you have stabilized your patient on the correct medication—and this may require a period of trial and error as to the exact drug and the correct dosage—then you must consider the fact that medication alone cannot effect complete rehabilitation.

Medication alone does not give the patient support, motivation, esteem, or trust; nor does it give him a job. Medication alone will not enable the patient to avoid getting upset when there is conflict within the family. It does provide a baseline stability which enables the patient to respond more normally and more effectively to various opportunities. These opportunities may include job retraining programs, socialization programs, psychotherapy, group psychotherapy, and family therapy. Where the physician does not have time to do psychotherapy or provide the rehabilitative social and ongoing care needed by such a patient, it is recommended that he become informed of available community resources so that he may refer the patient to those that are appropriate. Medication, generally on a continuing and long-range basis, remains essential, as without it the patient will not be able to successfully avail himself of all the other, varied treatment modalities.

Ideally, the patient who is referred to community programs will come back to your office for periodic checkups. During such visits, one might look for intercurrent illnesses which require treatment; side effects might require readjustment of medication. Most important of all, these visits should build a relationship of trust that will enable the patient to feel he can come to you when he cannot deal with his problems anywhere else.

Furthermore, you may sometimes find that a patient who has been doing well on a particular medication suddenly becomes worse. This may or may not be related to some stressful incident that has occurred. If you are familiar with such a patient's history and diagnosis, you may be able to prevent rehospitalization and assist the patient in dealing with his crisis by making a modest change or increase in the medication. Whether you increase the dosage of psychotropic medication fairly rapidly to prevent rehospitalization or decide to refer the patient for consultation will depend on many factors. In assessing these factors and handling such a case you would be performing *triage*. Triage implies that you not only have a tentative diagnosis in mind, but that you are also estimating the future course of the illness—that is, making a prognosis. As a part of doing this, you send the patient to the most appropriate place at the most appropriate time. Hospitalization may or may not be indicated. Even where it cannot be avoided, it is likely, with today's methods of treatment, that your patient will be in the hospital for only a month or less and will soon be seeing you as an outpatient again for continued care.

Some recent studies indicate that there may be a higher than normal prevalence of certain emotional disorders among the families of mentally ill patients. For example, there are more alcoholics in the families of manic-depressives than in other families. In light of this, you may want to be especially alert to the possibility of discovering mental illnesses in other members of the patient's family when and if they come to you for checkups. You may also take advantage of the opportunity to practice primary preventive medicine by counseling family members on handling unnecessary guilt feelings, problems in child rearing, marital problems, and, of course, the difficulties of living with a former mental hospital patient.

Knowing the history and the diagnosis of a patient's condition enables you to formulate a prognosis. In cases of very severe, or "core," mental illness with a history of multiple hospitalizations, the prognosis might be that the patient will be disabled for life, no matter what drugs or additional therapeutic methods are applied. Under such circumstances, your expectations concerning the patient's progress may be lower. You may encourage periodic visits to your office to maintain him at his highest possible level, and you may find it desirable to counsel his family, so that they do not have unrealistic expectations of him. With all this, you will expect that from time to time he will be likely to require brief periods of rehospitalization.

In other cases, where a patient with a diagnosis of mild psychosis has had no hospitalizations and has been able to function adequately despite his disorder, you may prescribe appropriate medication and proceed with relatively high expectations of renewed performance on his part.

The primary care physician is today the main treatment source for all forms of mental distress, as indeed he has been for many years. Rewards in the treatment of psychotic patients may be great. As one patient recently told her family doctor, "Maybe you should be worried for me—because I'm not, and you are the only link I have with reality." This is a tribute to the ability of one physician to bridge the gap between the real and fantasied worlds of his patient. Such an accomplishment can be a source of satisfaction for any doctor and points up the importance of diagnosing and treating the psychotic.

CONDUCTING A MENTAL STATUS EXAMINATION IN DIAGNOSING PSYCHOSIS

The primary care physician knows very well how to do a physical examination of his patients; he has not been nearly as thoroughly trained in conducting a mental status examination. Nonetheless, making a diagnosis of mild or severe psychosis is not such a different process from making a diagnosis of anemia or diabetes by clinical examination alone. In some cases it may actually be easier.

Similarities between physical and mental examinations include the following:

1. Negative findings are just as important as positive findings.
2. In most cases, no single finding makes a diagnosis, and a combination of certain specific findings is necessary to establish the diagnosis.

A brief mental status evaluation suggests that the examiner *look, listen,* and *think.* This sort of evaluation can provide sufficient information for a tentative diagnosis, if not a specific and final one. Where more detailed examination is required to clarify or substantiate a diagnosis of psychosis, consultation with a psychiatrist is helpful. Generally, one accomplishes the looking part of the examination by closely observing the patient from the minute he walks into the office until he leaves. The listening part takes place primarily during the history taking and the discussion period after the physical examination. Thinking goes on all the time as one puts together the various items seen and heard, and forms a tentative diagnosis.

We will now go into some of the things to be covered in the mental status evaluation. Keep in mind that this is being discussed from the viewpoint of diagnosing psychosis, and not other mental states. As a result, the discussion will concentrate on what to look for and what to rule out in diagnosing psychosis.

When we *look* at the patient, we study his attitude and manner, gait, dress, and appearance. Bizarre or inappropriate dress may be observed in the psychotic; a generally unkempt or disheveled appearance in a patient of reasonable economic means may kindle our suspicions. We observe the attitudes the patient communicates nonverbally: is he hesitant, friendly, depressed, excited, angry, aware, confused? Both distant, withdrawn behavior and inexplicably hostile and aggressive behavior may indicate the possibility of underlying psychosis in the patient.

It is most important to *listen* and to let the patient tell his story. How he tells his story—what aspects he stresses and what aspects he minimizes—is a key in judging the content and flow of his thought processes. If the flow seems to be rather strange, with one idea following another with no apparent logical connection and for no apparent reason, we detect another of the symptoms of psychosis. In order to best evaluate this flow of ideas, we try to avoid interrupting the patient. Interruptions make it difficult or impossible to estimate the quality of the flow and may also keep the patient from revealing some significant parts of his history. When we encourage the patient to communicate in his own way, it is easy to pick out those patients who are quite unable to do this. If we try to cut corners by just asking questions, we may remain unaware that a patient cannot communicate in a coherent and relevant manner. Also, by posing questions we divert information into channels which we consider important, rather than into those which the patient considers important.

We must, of course, ask some questions in order to be able to rule out certain diagnoses. For instance, it is important to know if the patient is oriented; that is, does he know who he is and where he is, and does he know the date? If the patient's general conversation clearly indicates that he is oriented in these three spheres of person, place, and time, we don't insult him by asking any questions relative to orientation. But if his orientation seems unclear, we investigate with appropriate inquiries. It is surprising to have a seemingly composed patient of about 85 years tell you that she is 33, and that she is in the city of Milwaukee rather than Scranton! Such signs of disorientation are an important indication that an organic psychosis may be present.

Memory is also often adversely affected in the organic psychoses, particularly memory for recent events. Therefore, questions are appropriate: does the patient remember what he had for breakfast, what the weather was like yesterday, what holiday recently occurred? If we are unsure about recent memory, we can ask the patient to remember any three words (eg: red, table, Broadway), and then ask him to recall them five or ten minutes later. A person with unimpaired memory should remember all three with no difficulty.

Questions about the sensory perceptions of the patient are important for eliciting reports of hallucinations and illusions. (Hallucinations are false perceptions in which a patient perceives something that does not exist; illusions are misperceptions in which a patient misidentifies what he sees, hears, smells, or feels.) The patient should be asked directly if he has heard or seen anything unusual, or if he has experienced any unusual smells or tactile sensations. Many physicians hesitate to ask such questions because they fear the patient will be offended. Usually, though, the patient is glad of the opportunity to confide these experiences to someone who is interested. Auditory hallucinations—hearing voices uttering threatening, derogatory, or persecutory remarks—are quite common in schizophrenic psychoses. Visual hallucinations also occur fairly frequently in these *functional psychoses*. Olfactory and tactile hallucinations, on the other hand, are rare in schizophrenia and should alert you to the possibility of either an *organic* or a *toxic psychosis*. Bear in mind that toxic psychoses caused by drug usage may produce a plethora of hallucinatory experiences encompassing the auditory, visual, olfactory, and tactile modes.

As already mentioned, while direct questions may be necessary in assessing orientation, memory, and sensory perceptions, evaluation of the patient's stream of thought can only be made by listening as the patient speaks spontaneously. Note whether his speech appears to be under pressure and seems to pour out in a veritable gush—a telltale symptom of *manic psychoses*—or if it is slow and blocked, with the patient stopping repeatedly in the middle of a thought—a symptom often seen in *depressive psychoses*.

In evaluating the patient's thinking, we are also concerned with the content of his thought. Does he have any *delusions*—false beliefs not based on reality? Does he feel that he is being persecuted and that people are after him? Is he grandiose; does he have delusions in which he believes he is great, or perhaps that he is some noted person, such as the President of the United States, or even God? We also look for *ideas of reference*, which are thinking disturbances in which the patient feels that public commentary or actions are aimed specifically at him. For example, the patient may say that he saw the news on television and was certain the news announcer was addressing his comments solely to him; or he may read an article in the newspaper which says, "FBI is looking for 10 most-wanted criminals" and decide that the FBI is really after him. Delusions and ideas of reference are both indications of an underlying psychotic process.

By careful listening we may also evaluate the patient's mood. Does he complain of being depressed? Does he describe himself as blue, melancholy, despondent, down, or blah? Or does he portray his mood as one of excitement, exaltation, or even euphoria? Perhaps even more important than the patient's words may be his nonverbal communication of mood, which is roughly equivalent to what we call affect. The affect that generally accompanies severe depression is expressed by a look of sadness in the eyes, a downturned mouth, frequent tears in the eyes, furrowed brow, etc. The affect of happiness or euphoria may be seen in a sparkle in the eyes, a broad smile, or laughter.

Psychotic patients of the schizophrenic type may show two disturbances of affect. Some severe and chronic schizophrenic patients exhibit *inappropriate affect*. Thus, they may be talking about something very sad, such as the death of a close relative, and at the same time be wreathed in smiles and giggling. The second, and more subtle, disturbance seen in many schizophrenic patients is a *flatness, or shallowness, of affect*. This manifests itself in the patient's always seeming bland and unemotional, with little range of physical display for his feeling. Such flatness of affect is one important clue to watch and listen for in detecting the schizophrenic patient. One should not confuse flatness of affect with the inbred restraint of display of emotion that some people have.

There are two additional areas of concern in listening to and questioning the patient: *insight* and *judgment*. Is the patient aware that something is wrong with him? If he is, this shows a degree of insight, and it is typical of the neurotic. The psychotic, on the other hand, tends to insist that he is fine and that the difficulties come from other people or from some outside source.

The relative nature of judgment makes this process difficult to assess except by comparison with the norm. If we ask a patient what he would do if he found an addressed, stamped, and sealed letter in the street, we judge the normalcy of his response by whether he would do what most people would do: put the letter in a mailbox. The slightly sociopathic individual might say that he would open the letter. The psychotic might give a bizarre response, such as indicating that he would tear the letter to shreds or set it on fire. This sort of disturbed judgment is another clue to the presence of psychosis.

We have designated the last part of the brief mental status evaluation for diagnosing psychosis as the *thinking* part, and it involves the mental process of sifting and sorting out the data we have gathered by looking and listening. We do it continuously without being much aware of it. After having grouped the data into appropriate categories, we arrive at the most likely diagnosis and, perhaps, some alternative ones.

Summary of the Evaluative, Diagnostic Process

Again, in the mental, diagnostic process we go through, we first decide whether or not the patient is psychotic. If the patient is psychotic, we then decide whether he or she has an organic psychosis. If memory, orientation, and concentration are disturbed, we will come up with the organic diagnosis; but if they are all intact, we suspect we are dealing with a functional psychosis—either schizophrenia or manic-depressive disease. If the patient shows greatly disordered thinking with delusions and/or ideas of reference; if his affect is flat, blunted, shallow, or inappropriate; if he has auditory and/or visual hallucinations, the diagnosis would be schizophrenia. In manic-depressive disease, on the other hand, disturbance of mood is predominant. The patient will show and complain of either melancholia or euphoria. Speech, thinking, and body movements will be significantly slowed in the depressive phase and abnormally sped up in the manic phase. Delusions, when present, will be either depressive or grandiose in content. Depressive delusions include somatic delusions ("My body is rotting away") and nihilistic delusions ("The world is coming to an end"). Grandiose delusions may range all the way up to the misidentification of oneself as God or the Messiah.

Once we have made a diagnosis of functional psychosis and have decided whether we are dealing with a schizophrenic patient or with someone suffering from manic-depressive disease, we have the opportunity to institute prompt and effective treatment. (The psychotropic drugs used in that treatment are discussed elsewhere in this book.)

SOME CHARACTERISTICS OF PSYCHOSES

Now let us discuss in greater depth the criteria that guide the diagnosis of psychosis and the differentiation of the organic and the functional psychoses.

Impairment of Reality Testing

This disturbance of functioning is characteristic of all forms of psychosis. The real world is interpreted differently by the psychotic patient than by most people. The neurotic will say that the sun is shining brightly because there are no clouds to block it from view. A severely ill psychotic may believe this shining sun is a sign to "proceed full steam ahead in my mission to save the world." A walking-around psychotic will say he thinks it may be a sign from heaven, but he's not sure.

The following is another example of differences in ability to check out or cope with what is happening in the real world: a neurotic, on hearing his fellow workers talking and laughing, goes over and asks, "What is so funny?" He may fear they are laughing at his tie, but he usually checks that fear out against reality by trying to get the facts. The latent psychotic in the same circumstance also fears that others are talking about him, but he reacts by withdrawing and by isolating himself. He stays by himself during a work break, refuses to mix with his fellow workers, and buries himself in a book. The overtly psychotic person goes one step further. He is convinced that people really are talking about him in a malignant way and are plotting against him or defaming him. Usually, he, too, does nothing about this but withdraw further into himself. Very rarely, he may become sufficiently agitated to lash out at or attack his supposed persecutors. In any case, it never occurs to him that his belief is false, or even that it may be false!

We have all seen people like Jean, a childish, giggly, 85-year-old woman who comes in for her annual checkup. She tells you that the telephone calls she occasionally gets that consist of silent, heavy breathing are from an old beau of hers who is too shy to come calling directly. Of course, she could be right! But you find out from her spinster sister that neither of them have ever had any male friends and that Jean's interpretation of the calls is a bad case of wishful thinking. On further physical examination you find signs of poor oxygen supply to the brain due to arteriosclerosis, heart failure, and some anemia. You correct the latter two conditions; your patient then admits the calls are probably from some telephone crank.

Your patient Jean, then, is an example of a person with impaired reality testing due to a mild organic psychosis. Impaired reality testing will also be quite evident in any form of schizophrenia and in manic-depressive disease. In the latter, the impairment is most likely to manifest itself in two areas:

1. *Self-estimate*: The depressed patient will estimate himself as worthless, useless, nothing; the manic patient will judge himself to be virtually flawless, infinitely talented, and exquisitely intelligent.
2. *Estimate of the outer world*: The depressed patient will see the world as a horrible, meaningless torture; the manic will view it as a totally exhilarating, wonderful place to be.

Disturbances in Orientation, Memory, and Concentration

These are the disturbances of functioning which are characteristic of the organic psychoses and which differentiate the latter from schizophrenia and manic-depressive disease.

An individual's orientation is circumscribed by three spheres: person, place, and time. Thus, in testing a patient's orientation we need to find out if he knows who he is, where he is, and when it is. Through careful listening we may be able to determine whether a given patient can answer these questions. If listening alone will not give us this information, then we must ask. We can preface our questions by saying, "I know some of these things may seem silly to you, but I need to ask them as part of your examination." We then ask directly, "Where are you?"

The patient need not know the exact address of your office in the hospital where you are examining him, but he should know that he is in a doctor's office in a hospital and not at his Uncle Ben's house or the post office. Next we ask, "What is your name?" and "Who am I?" We expect the patient to know his name, of course. If he does not know the doctor's name, that is not necessarily significant; but again, he should recognize that you are a physician and should not describe you as a relative, old friend, or the greengrocer.

Memory can be tested by a series of questions that follow naturally after those on orientation. "How old are you? When were you born? Who is the President of the United States? Who was the President before him? And who was the President before him?" Also, before these questions are asked, you can inform the patient that you are going to give him three words that you want him to remember, and that you will ask him to recall those words for you in about ten minutes. Use three unrelated, easy words, such as *red, table,* and *Broadway.* The patient with an intact memory should have no trouble recalling them.

In the patient with organic brain damage, recent memory is typically impaired, whereas memory for remote events is intact. Thus, the patient may be able to tell you that Herbert Hoover was elected President in 1928, and he may even be able to name the vice-president of that time, although he may have no idea who the current President is. He may be able to tell you the prices of potatoes and beef in 1909 but be quite unable to describe what he had for breakfast that morning. If he does describe what he had for breakfast, you might check this for accuracy with a relative or with someone in attendance, as patients with organic memory defects often confabulate.

The patient's ability to concentrate can also be evaluated indirectly during your interview. Does he stick to a subject reasonably well, or is he distractable and prone to wander in his thoughts? A rough test of concentration is the "serial sevens" test. In this, you ask the patient to start with one hundred, subtract seven mentally, and tell you the remainder. Ask him to keep subtracting seven from the remainder, telling you the new remainder each time (thus: 100, 93, 86, etc). It is within normal limits to make several errors, but a patient with impaired concentration will generally have all kinds of difficulty with this test and will struggle badly and make many more errors than is normal.

Organic brain damage is seen in diverse types of physical illnesses. It may result from infection of the meninges, from trauma to the brain, or from the effects of an expanding intracranial mass such as a brain tumor. It occurs in people with arteriosclerotic cerebrovascular disease who may or may not have had strokes. Acute organic brain disturbance may follow a thrombus or hemorrhage in the brain, but a more chronic disturbance may develop through the gradual narrowing of the blood vessels to the brain, as Alvarez (1966) describes in his book *Little Strokes*.

In an organic brain disorder the pathologic process may interfere only minimally with the patient's ability to deal with the ordinary demands of life. It becomes a psychosis only when the patient develops a serious deficit in his or her ability to cope with reality. Thus, James H., 76, has a stroke; he recovers enough to return home to be cared for by his son. Mr. H. may manage for several years as a semi-invalid with moderate impairment of brain function, slow in movement and in thought. He may have difficulty in remembering recent events—something considered by most of us to be part of the normal aging process. Gradually, however, his memory impairment becomes such that he cannot remember that he turned on the gas stove; he cannot recognize his son; he regresses to the point where he hardly talks at all. At this point, we might describe him as suffering from an organic psychosis of the arteriosclerotic or senile type.

As mentioned before, organic brain impairment, whether psychotic or not, may be seen in many other physical disorders. It is a prominent effect of infectious diseases such as encephalitis and tertiary syphilis. It is seen in toxic conditions resulting from ingestion of chemicals and medicinal products, including alcohol, LSD, amphetamines, and anticholinergic medications. Brain function is impaired to varying degrees in such unusual conditions as lead encephalopathy, beriberi, and acute porphyria. Brain tumors originating in or metastasizing to the brain and cranial cavity may also be responsible for varied defects in mental ability.

Chronic organic cases are usually seen early in the history of the disease by the primary care physician, and these patients may be in his care for a long time. Ultimately these patients may deteriorate mentally to the point where they have to spend the last few years of their lives in a nursing home or mental hospital. Institutionalization and separation from family and friends usually serves only to speed the patient's decline, often by super-imposing serious depression on the underlying organic disorder.

It is quite possible, although not very common, for some patients to suffer from a mixture of organic and functional components in psychosis. A chronic schizophrenic patient may contract syphilis sometime during his life and develop psychotic manifestations from paresis. Or he may be a heavy drinker who develops an alcoholic psychosis. Some psychiatrists are now reporting cases in which a schizophrenic patient also develops episodes of manic-depressive psychosis. These are the cases where one might inadvertently overlook one aspect of a patient's problem, restrict treatment accordingly, and thereby limit the degree to which the patient improves. It has always been a dictum of medicine that where one diagnosis suffices to explain a condition, one and only one diagnosis should be made. This dictum is now open to question, as indicated by the following case example.

Jeremiah A. was a chronic alcoholic who had been on disulfiram (Antabuse) for quite a few years and had managed to function fairly effectively as a salesman, husband, and father. In his middle forties he was in an automobile accident and sustained multiple injuries which required a long period of hospitalization. After this accident, his behavior was unpredictable and bizarre at times. He almost lost his job and required large amounts of drugs such as diazepam (Valium) and chlordiazepoxide (Librium), to which he rapidly became habituated. Mr. A. had started to drink again when he finally returned to work. In the early stages of this return to alcoholism, he had an affair with a woman whom he met at an office party. He contracted gonorrhea from this liaison and underwent penicillin therapy, which was adequate to cure his gonorrhea, but which did not touch the syphilis that he had acquired at the same time. Always a heavy smoker, he developed a chronic cough in his early sixties. Within the space of a year, his behavior became increasingly inappropriate and he showed many evidences of bad judgment and confusion. Chest x-ray revealed a lung tumor, and when Mr. A. was hospitalized for the surgery that eventually revealed a bronchogenic carcinoma, serologic findings were positive.

In diagnosing a case such as this, consideration must be given to the chronic alcoholism, old trauma to the head from the automobile accident, central nervous system damage from the syphilis, and metastatic spread of the lung cancer to the brain as possible etiologies. Careful studies on Jeremiah A. revealed that, unfortunately, all four of these phenomena were involved in the florid organic psychosis that he presented.

It should also be mentioned that organic psychoses often develop in patients who have previously been treated for long-standing neurotic conditions. The psychosis always has a totally different etiology, of course, but we must be careful that we do not miss the diagnosis because of our preoccupation with the already existing neurosis. For example, in his later years, a severe hypochondriac may start to complain of memory loss and confusion. Rather than dismissing these complaints as just two more in the scores he has presented, we must be alert to their possible psychotic significance.

Abnormal Perceptions

We have already discussed the abnormal perceptions which occur in psychoses. These include illusions and hallucinations which may be visual, auditory, olfactory, or tactile in nature. Again, olfactory and tactile hallucinations may occur in organic or toxic psychoses but generally do not occur in schizophrenia or the manic-depressive psychoses. Visual hallucinations involving very gaudy, garish, brilliant colors and perceptions should also make you suspicious of a drug-induced toxic psychosis.

Disturbances in Thinking

Abnormalities here include ideas of reference and delusions. The latter may be paranoid, grandiose, somatic, or nihilistic, but the type of delusion does not differentiate the type of psychosis. Paranoid delusions, for example, are extremely common in schizophrenia but also occur frequently in senile, or arteriosclerotic, organic psychoses; in drug-induced psychoses; and in psychoses resulting from brain tumor or brain damage. They are typical of the psychoses produced by chronic ingestion of amphetamines, and they may even occur as a feature of so-called involutional melancholia.

The deteriorated psychotic patient's delusions will probably be quite evident and quite disorganized in nature. On the other hand, the ambulatory psychotic, particularly if he is a borderline case, may be able to hide his delusional system. Or he may have it so well organized that it appears extremely logical, at least at first blush. You may have to talk with your patient quite a while before you elicit a remark such as was made by Joan K. She said that she had no friends and wanted it that way because, "People turn what you say around and use it against you." A little later in her visit, Joan commented, "If I told you what is going on, I'd be dead." You do not need to know the total content of her paranoid thinking to make a tentative diagnosis and to prescribe a regimen of antipsychotic medication.

Bear in mind also that grandiosity often accompanies feelings of persecution. Paranoid people tend to explain their persecution to themselves by reasoning that others want to hurt them out of jealousy of their powers or talents. Eldon D., a psychotic who claimed the Mafia was after him, was telling his doctor that he wanted to hitchhike to California. The doctor asked, "Wouldn't that be dangerous? What if a car should hit you on the highway?" "No problem," Eldon replied. "That wouldn't matter at all, because I would just push it away!"

Disturbances in Mood and Self-esteem

Depression will not be dealt with in any detail here since a separate chapter is devoted to this very common condition. But we can consider one question: when is a depression psychotic in nature? Clearly, a depression is psychotic if it is accompanied by delusional thinking. Moreover, any depression in which there is suicidal thought and/or intent should be regarded as psychotic. In fact, it may be wise to consider any sizable depression as being psychotic, since that designation is more likely to impel us to give prompt and adequate treatment of the condition.

We should be alert to manic, as well as depressive, psychotic disturbances of mood. Manifestations include euphoria or extreme elation such as is typical of the manic state in manic-depressive psychoses. Psychotic states of euphoria may occasionally be due to ingestion of psychoactive drugs.

Low self-esteem may be an important symptom of depressive psychosis in its own right. Of course, millions of people who are not psychotic in any way suffer from low self-esteem, but if the condition is characterized by deep feelings of unworthiness and horrible guilt, it may well be a symptom of depressive psychosis.

Sergeant G. was recommended for officer candidate school but refused to go through with his application because he was sure he "wouldn't make it." Something about his refusal prompted his commanding officer to send Sgt. G. to the base psychiatrist for an examination. The sergeant had an excellent leadership record, high intelligence, and good results on all his aptitude tests, but he kept insisting to the psychiatrist that he was "unworthy" of further advancement. Some gentle probing revealed that he felt deeply guilty about having been unkind to his younger brother many years ago. At that point the psychiatrist attempted to reassure Sgt. G., telling him that none of the things in his past would keep him from getting through officer candidate school and explaining that his guilt made him feel unworthy, but that he was simply human like all of us and thus susceptible to meanness and to error in his ways. None of this moved the sergeant; he persisted that he was totally unworthy not only for officer candidate school but even to be alive! At that point, the psychiatrist rightly concluded that Sgt. G. was suffering from a latent psychotic depression.

Impairment of Social Functioning

In addition to disturbances of perception, thought, and mood, there are two other features which characterize psychosis: *withdrawal* and *passivity*. While these may be less prominent, they are quite pervasive. They are particularly striking in schizophrenic patients, although they are also observed in depressed psychotics and in many organic psychotics.

In the ambulatory psychotic patient, the processes of withdrawal and passivity may cause either minor or major impairments in functioning. The patient is apt to have few friends and to rarely go to places of public entertainment. Characteristically, he has little or no social life and spends most of his leisure time in seclusion. More disruptive impairment of social functioning may be manifested by phenomena such as frequent job changes, with the psychotic being fired or quitting for trivial reasons.

These patterns of behavior are all reflections of the difficulties psychotic withdrawal creates in the sphere of interpersonal relationships. The family of the psychotic patient does not, and cannot, have intense communication and contact with him. The psychotic's tolerance for interpersonal contact is low, and he can only handle relatively brief periods of interchange with other people.

Poor Insight and Judgment

Bad judgment seems to be part and parcel of the human condition. We witness it in all that goes on. When it occurs in high places, it provides grist for the media mills and lurid headlines. Bad judgment is hardly confined to our offices as an exclusive trait of the mentally ill. The psychotic patient characteristically evidences an exaggerated degree of bad judgment. The very fact that he has come to our office, though, is a sign of good judgment! At least someone, if not the patient, has recognized that there might be something medically wrong and has sought appropriate help.

The exaggerated degree of bad judgment characteristic of the psychotic patient may be a sign to look for in establishing a diagnosis. Again, disturbances of judgment of a severe sort can alert us to the possibility of psychosis, but they cannot serve to differentiate one type of psychosis from another. Schizophrenic psychoses, depressive psychoses, organic psychoses, and drug-induced psychoses all may cause impairments of judgment, and all are characterized by a relative lack of insight. People suffering from manic psychoses, especially, often show extremely poor judgment. They engage in promiscuous behavior that is quite out of character for them; or they may become involved in financial deals and expenditures that bankrupt them and their families.

Particularly worthy of note is the poor judgment that often constitutes one of the early symptoms of organic psychosis caused by cerebral arteriosclerosis. This may betray itself in the flagrant display of sexually seductive behavior by an elderly person; grandpa, for example, may shock and stun the family by talking about intimate sexual matters with his eight-year-old granddaughter.

ATTITUDES TOWARD PSYCHOTIC PATIENTS

At the beginning of this chapter we discussed the obviously psychotic patient whom the average person—and the average physician—think of as "crazy." There is a derogatory connotation to this label, and it may imply a number of false ideas about people who are mentally ill.

One such idea is that mental patients are inferior and inadequate. In truth, of course, they possess the entire range of human attributes. Some are subnormal in intelligence; this does not make them any less human. Other patients are normal in intelligence and endowment; still others are highly intelligent, brilliant, or markedly talented, and may be creative in the arts or in science. Not a few manic-depressive patients are actually so energetic, keen, and capable between episodes of illness that they have created huge fortunes from business endeavors.

A second commonly held concept is that persons who are mentally ill are to be feared because they are assaultive. This is true only of an exceedingly small group of patients. Most aggressive patients can be treated effectively with antipsychotic medications. Personal experience as an institutional psychiatrist suggests it is probably safer to be in mental institutions than in the communities in which they are located! Nonetheless, the newspapers and other media give considerable publicity to crimes committed by mental patients or ex-patients, and they rarely have anything to report about the thousands and thousands of such people who are totally law-abiding. This serves to reinforce our misconceptions.

Another reason people give for fearing the mental patient is that his thinking seems so different from a "normal" person's that we cannot easily anticipate how he will react. This may be true in part, especially when you do not know the patient. But when you do come to know him, his illogical thinking may make sense to you as it never did before. The film "One Flew Over the Cuckoo's Nest" gives a vivid example of this phenomenon. People watching the film identified with the patients and cheered them in their escapades because they recognized and identified with their basic humanity. Patients hospitalized for mental illness are really much more like the rest of us than they are different from us. It may even be that it is their basic similarity to us which frightens us so ("That could be me!") and makes us pretend they are strange and different.

Yet another concept about persons with psychopathology is that they have such serious afflictions that they cannot be helped. Today, this is patently untrue. New medications and modes of therapy have revolutionized the practice of psychiatry in the last 20 years. Most patients can be helped to live and function in the community, and only a very few show no favorable response to appropriate therapy. This does not mean, of course, that all patients are cured or that they may not require readmission at some later time. There is every hope and likelihood, however, that even better methods of treatment will be developed to provide more effective and longer-lasting help for the psychotic. Research in this area is active, and its progress in the past 20 years gives us hope for tremendous strides forward in the years to come.

The last point to be made is that people who fear dealing with persons who are mentally ill are often fearful of mental illness in themselves. It is as though they feel that mental disturbance is in some way contagious and that seeing others who have lost contact with reality might make them lose their own grasp. Such fears are ill-founded, of course. Contact with the psychotic makes for increased self-awareness, which may be painful at times, but which can also lead to greater depth and maturity of the personality.

The misconceptions detailed above are prevalent in all of us. It behooves every physician—family practitioner, internist, or psychiatrist—to think through his attitudes on mental illness and the mentally ill. These patients deserve no less from us than the same objectivity that we routinely give to the physically ill.

REFERENCES

Alvarez, W. C.: *Little Strokes*. Philadelphia: J. B. Lippincott Co., 1966.

American Psychiatric Association: *Diagnostic and Statistical Manual of Mental Disorders*, 2d ed. Washington, DC: American Psychiatric Association, 1968.

Dohrenwend, B. P.: Epidemiological data for mental health center planning. II. Psychiatric disorder in general populations: problem of the untreated 'case.' *Am J Pub Health* 60:1052, 1970.

Ozarin, L. D.: Community alternatives to institutional care. *Am J Psychiatr*. 133:69-72, 1976.

Wechsler, H.: What to expect in private practice. *Resident and Staff Physician* June, 1976.

5 The Anxious Patient

Martin Goldberg, M.D.

WHAT IS ANXIETY?

Although we all talk about anxiety and "being anxious," we rarely stop to define just what is meant by these terms. Anxiety is an emotional state that is closely related to fear. It is a nameless dread; it is the terrible feeling that something awful is going to happen. As such, it bears an intimate relationship to depression, which is the feeling that something awful has indeed happened.

While anxiety is closely related to fear, it differs from the latter in some significant ways. If any of us had to suddenly confront a dangerous animal—let us say, a huge lion that had escaped from a zoo—we could well predict our feelings and actions. Our hearts would start to pound wildly; we would begin to sweat and tremble; our knees would knock. Surging adrenalin would make us ready for "flight or fight," and just about all of us would promptly choose the former alternative. We would feel fear. But there are some people who might develop these same reactions—pounding heart, sweating and trembling, knocking knees—if they were suddenly confronted by a tiny toy poodle dog. This is *anxiety* rather than fear. It is a situation in which the danger that we feel is *internal*, rather than being external as it is in fear. The danger is not really a threat to life or limb (the tiny dog is harmless, after all) but is some threat to our inner security or self-esteem (we will look foolish and people will laugh at us if they see our apprehensiveness).

Anxiety is no rare phenomenon in our lives. Our forefathers may have lived with fear: fear of wild beasts, fear of ravaging diseases, fear of starvation and of death-dealing poverty. We live with anxiety: anxiety about appearing foolish, anxiety about failing in our endeavors, anxiety about being unloved, unlovable, or unloving. We all experience anxiety virtually every day of our lives, so we know its signs and symptoms well. In its most blatant form, anxiety has the following manifestations: trembling of the hands; "knocking" of the knees; quavering or "tightness" in the voice; excessive perspiration; "lump" in the throat; strong, and at times irregular, pounding of the heart; elevated blood pressure; facial flushing; stomach doing "flip-flops"; cramping or pain in the gastrointestinal tract; excessive urination; diarrhea; stuttering or stammering speech.

To check out these various symptoms in our own memories, all we need do is think back to the last time we took an important final exam. We will recall most of these phenomena quite well. The tremors, the sweating, the lump in the throat, the excessive urination and diarrhea—they were all there. So familiar are these manifestations that our folk language refers to them in numerous ways. We talk of being "all shook up" and of "clutching"; the athlete speaks of "choking up" or "taking the lump." We all live with anxiety.

Yet we must ask, where does it all get its start? What early experiences in our lives condition us for this? What is the prototype of this feeling state that plays such an important part in our lives? Philosophers and theologians, as well as psychiatrists and psychologists, have debated long and loud over this question. Freudian thinking in this matter is not totally clear. Freud's early view was that anxiety is an affect experienced whenever libidinal gratification is dammed back or denied expression. He reevaluated this view later (1926) and formulated the theory that the ego looses anxiety in the organism as a warning signal when it becomes aware of instinctual processes arising within the id which threaten the organism with destruction. The concept of anxiety as a warning signal has much value, as we shall see, but otherwise this theory is somewhat vague, and eminently debatable.

Otto Rank, one of the many followers and pupils of Sigmund Freud who broke with the master and established his own school of thought, has a different view (1952). He regards the first experience of anxiety in life as occuring very early indeed. He sees the prototype of anxiety in the experience of birth. The human infant, previously protected and nourished in its mother's womb, is expelled into the world, where its needs for nourishment, warmth, and protection will no longer be automatically taken care of by the physiologic processes of pregnancy but will be dependent on the attention and whim of another person. (More recently, others have postulated, and in some cases produced evidence, that even intrauterine life is not always serene and that the fetus may be quite definitely affected by emotional storms and anxiety in the mother.)

Neither the Freudian nor the Rankian explanation of prototypical anxiety is without merit, but neither seems totally satisfactory. A far better and simpler concept emerges from the writings of psychiatrist Karen Horney (1937). Horney defines anxiety as the result of our earliest perception that we are alone and helpless in a potentially hostile world. "Alone and helpless in a potentially hostile world"—these words seem to cover both Freudian and Rankian thinking, and the description seems all too familiar when we think back to our own very earliest experiences. (Can you recall your very first day in school? Does this sound like a fairly good description of your feeling state at that time?)

Anxiety is not a purely pathologic condition, however. It has its uses and purposes, and in proper amounts it serves all of us in a most important way. Anxiety has a signalling function: it alerts us that there is danger so that we may mobilize our inner resources and do our best to cope. A classic example of this is the stage fright that any entertainer experiences before his act goes on. Any veteran performer (actor, artist, musician, lecturer, athlete, politician) comes to realize that this stage fright—that is, anxiety—is a very favorable sign, and that its absence may be ominous. I can attest to this from my own experience in teaching and lecturing. These activities have become fairly commonplace to me, and yet I seldom face a lecture or speech without feeling a fair amount of anxiety beforehand. I know there is no real external danger; the audience is unlikely to hoot me from the podium or rush me out of the auditorium and out of town. But there is the internal danger: will they like my lecture? Will I make myself seem foolish or stupid? Will I be dull and boring? Will I lose self-esteem? For some little time, then, I do indeed feel alone and helpless in a potentially hostile world. Almost always, as I actually start a speech, my voice is a bit shaky and tight. The anxiety lingers until I am well launched into my subject, and as the audience seems not only to remain awake but to respond a bit, anxiety finally melts away.

I can recall one occasion in my life when that was not quite the way things happened. At that time, I was to give a speech at my own medical school on a subject I knew rather well; I had spoken on the subject dozens of times. The setting was known to me, the subject was known to me, even the audience was quite well known to me. As I rose to speak on that occasion I felt perfectly cool, calm, and collected. No jitteriness, no tremors, no tension plagued me. Inwardly, I congratulated myself that I had finally made it. I was no longer anxious about something silly like giving a little talk. I began to speak and my voice was deep and relaxed. My calm continued, and I spoke with near-perfect control. Halfway through this talk, however, with anxiety still a missing factor, a different feeling arose in me: I am boring myself to death! A quick inspection of the audience revealed that they were in a similar, semihypnotic trance. I had lost my anxiety and I had paid a price—my effort to communicate well was not really mobilized effectively. Since that time, I am happy to say, I have returned to my usual pre-lecture jitters. No longer do I hope for their disappearance, for I realize that the proper amount of anxiety helps me to function most effectively.

Excessive amounts of anxiety will not accomplish such a purpose. The speaker who is excessively anxious will not communicate well at all. He will continue to stutter and to stammer and to lose his train of thought and speech, or he will retreat behind some defense that separates him from his audience, such as mechanically reading his lecture while never looking at the audience, or projecting dozens of slides on a screen so that he does not really have to communicate at all.

We can conclude, then, that a certain amount of anxiety keeps us alert and ready to do our best, but that excessive amounts of anxiety swamp our systems with emergency signals, to the detriment of any performance. Moreover, since anxiety is a sort of signal, it is only of value if it is intermittent. A steady signal becomes meaningless. A fire alarm that rang steadily would have no value at all; it must ring only when there is actually a fire. Similarly, steady states of anxiety are of no use to the human organism; they only produce confusion and exhaustion.

Case Example 1

Mrs. D is a 33-year-old suburban housewife and mother of two children. She has always been a "worrier," and in recent years she has found more and more to worry about. She worries about her children. When they get slight colds or other viral infections, she is fearful that they are going to become quite ill and feels that she may not be giving them the proper medical treatment and care. At other times, when no physical illness mars the scene, Mrs. D is concerned about her children's psyches. Is she being too permissive with them? Why do they seem so disobedient and unruly? She loses her temper with them easily and then worries that she is being too hostile and punitive.

Meanwhile, Mrs. D has other worries. One of these is her husband, a rising and successful young corporation executive. He spends considerable time at his job, leaving his wife to handle the children by herself. On the occasions when he is home for any length of time, generally weekends, he promptly and steadily imbibes martinis until he either becomes bellicose or enters into a peaceful, but frightening, stupor. Mrs. D worries about his drinking and about what it is doing to him. She worries about their relationship, which seems to be nearly nonexistent. In addition, Mrs. D worries about her aged and ailing parents, many miles away in another city; about the routine boredom of her life, which she finds rather purposeless; about the necessity to entertain and carry out certain other social functions that don't really interest her; and about her sexual desires, which seem to have evaporated somewhere along the line, leaving her to suspect that she is "frigid." And if she has any time and energy left after all that worrying, Mrs. D can always worry about the deterioration of suburban private schools; the sad state of our nation, the world, and the ecology; and various newspaper and magazine articles which lead her to vaguely suspect that she may have cancer, diabetes, arthritis, or, at the very least, high blood pressure.

The effects of all this worry on Mrs. D's body are quite pronounced. Although she continues to function, and attractively so, in her role of suburban housewife, she is a smoldering volcano of chronic anxiety under this veneer. She has trouble getting to sleep, and after watching the late, late show, she may still toss and turn for several hours before she dozes. Her heart pounds so readily and so often that she is quite convinced she is going to suffer a heart attack one of these days. She frequently has trouble swallowing and worries about fine tremors in her hands, but no one else seems to notice this. Very often she is short of breath, and if someone comes up behind her suddenly or surprises her in any way, she "jumps" with the heightened startle reaction so characteristic of the chronic anxiety sufferer.

After a number of years of such suffering, Mrs. D knows that she needs help. Getting it, however, proves to be surprisingly difficult. Mrs. D chooses to confide first in her husband, telling him she feels something is wrong with her. "Not a damn thing is wrong," he replies, "that wouldn't be cured if you would just get interested in something and stop moping around doing nothing." Mrs. D takes this advice to heart and begins some volunteer work at the local hospital. But this doesn't seem to help any. In fact, she finds that she is worrying about the patients in the hospital and is overly concerned as to whether or not she has carried out her simple duties properly.

Next Mrs. D talks to a number of close friends about her problem. They are uniformly reassuring. They all have similar worries, they tell her, "Everyone does." And almost unanimously they emphasize to Mrs. D their high regard for her. She is such a competent person, they all feel; she "really has it together." This is immensely reassuring to Mrs. D, but somehow it proves to be not at all helpful in diminishing her anxieties.

Finally she takes the problem to her family physician. He is no stranger to her. She has had numerous visits and checkups with him when she was concerned about chest pains, insomnia, the lump in her throat, or episodes of anxious overbreathing. On all these occasions, her physician has been able to tell her that she is really in fine physical shape and that there is nothing organically wrong, "just a little tension." Often, he has used the occasions of these visits to give her a prescription for an antianxiety drug such as meprobamate or Valium (diazepam). The medications have proved slightly helpful for a short while, but on each occasion Mrs. D found that the drugs did not really change her situation, and she stopped taking them. Now she confronts her doctor with the idea that there must be something wrong with her—perhaps it is something emotional, something psychologically wrong. Perhaps she ought to see a psychiatrist. "Nonsense," her doctor replies with a good-natured chuckle, "You don't need a shrink. You're no more crazy than I am." And Mrs. D leaves his office with only another prescription for a minor tranquilizer to show for her visit.

Mrs. D's situation is a very common one, and there is much that we can learn from it. Her friends are correct. Mrs. D does "have it together," in that she is functioning (albeit at a considerable price to herself), and they do all have worries similar to hers, since anxiety is common to us all. Her physician is also quite correct. Mrs. D is not "crazy." She is, however, suffering from excessive anxiety almost constantly, and she would very likely benefit a great deal from seeing a psychiatrist. Chronic anxiety, as one of the mildest of all emotional disorders, is apt to respond reasonably quickly and quite well to competent psychotherapy. Yet because the patient with anxiety seems normal and resembles the rest of us so much, we often overlook the problem and fail to encourage this sort of patient to get definitive help.

Mrs. D's anxiety state was almost constant and was *free-floating*; her apprehensions seemed endless and attached themselves to all aspects of her life. In other people, excessive anxiety occurs only in periodic or sporadic outbursts as *anxiety attacks*. Such attacks, characterized by shortness of breath, hyperventilation, chest pain, gastrointestinal symptoms, weakness, and dizziness, are almost always misidentified by the patient as representing some sort of serious physical disorder, such as a heart attack or a stroke. Many such patients are misdiagnosed and subsequently treated for hypoglycemia; labyrinthitis, or Meniere's syndrome; or low blood pressure. However, careful history taking and interviewing will generally establish that such anxiety attacks occur in a particular set of circumstances in which the patient feels overly concerned about loss of self-esteem or is otherwise in severe emotional conflict, as our next example illustrates.

Case Example 2

Mr. E was a schoolteacher in his late twenties when he was referred to me some years ago. He had been suffering from attacks of dizziness and weakness which made him feel as if he were going to faint or otherwise lose consciousness (he never did faint, of course, which is the usual case in these situations). After making the rounds of otolaryngologists and neurologists, he was sent to me by his family physician. A careful history of his illness, taken over the course of several interviews, revealed the following facts. His anxiety attacks had started 18 months earlier; prior to that he had never suffered any. (Coincidentally, he had been married about 18 months ago.) His attacks always occurred in public places, generally when he was teaching in school and sometimes when he was at a large social gathering or party. These parties were invariably affairs to which he really did not want to go but which he attended at his wife's request and urging. This fact made me suspect that Mr. E's anxiety attacks might generally occur when he was in a conflict about being somewhere he did not want to be. Consequently, I questioned him closely about his feelings concerning teaching. He revealed that he had been teaching for only two years. The first year he had a small class of very cooperative pupils and rather enjoyed teaching and receiving the admiration of his students. During the second semester (which was just after his marriage) he began to have a few, very minor anxiety attacks, which consisted mostly of feelings of dizziness and weakness. In his second year of teaching, he had a large and unruly class that was generally considered to be "impossible." Mr. E had his difficulties with them and found that he could not make these students his allies, as he had done with his first class. During this year his anxiety attacks became much more frequent and severe, although he did not identify them as such but thought that he was physically ill.

Because of the interesting chronology of his sickness, in subsequent interviews I questioned Mr. E specifically about his marriage. At first he insisted that the marriage was great and that there were no problems. Gradually, though, he admitted to an area of resentment and discontent. His wife was a schoolteacher also, and it had been their understanding that when they married they both would work for at least several years. After marriage, however, his wife had simply neglected to look for a job and never did go to work. As he talked about this, Mr. E admitted to considerable anger at the fact that he had to work and face his unpleasant class each day while his wife stayed home and did as she liked. With my encouragement, Mr. E began to share these feelings openly with his wife. Strangely enough, this was something he had never done before. She proved to be not at all unreasonable and was actually quite responsive to his feelings. In fact, she soon applied for and found work as a substitute teacher.

Meanwhile, I was explaining to Mr. E that his anxiety attacks seemed to occur when he forced himself to do something he really didn't want to do. I encouraged him to avoid such activities temporarily to see if the attacks would disappear. This involved his taking a brief leave of absence from teaching. The anxiety attacks did indeed disappear during his leave of absence, with the important result that Mr. E became convinced that there was nothing wrong with him physically and that his problems had actually been entirely emotional in nature. He returned to teaching after an absence of less than a month, and although he enjoyed his class no more than before, he was quite free of anxiety attacks thereafter.

PATTERNS OF ANXIETY

In many patients (such as Mrs. D and, to a lesser extent, Mr. E), anxiety is "free-floating" and may attach itself to almost anything. In other people, anxiety is experienced largely or entirely in one particular form or in one particular area of life experience and concern. Some of the common patterns of anxiety are discussed below.

Phobic Anxiety

Characteristically, the phobic patient experiences anxiety only in very specific circumstances. He may be fearful of high places, of open places, of crowds, of crossing bridges, of flying in airplanes, of being away from home, or of some particular animal, such as dogs, cats, or snakes. There are dozens of different phobias, and fancy, Greek-derived names for each variety.

Many of us suffer from some phobic anxiety, but it is usually slight, and we can overcome it and take that airplane ride or drive across that bridge even though it makes us uncomfortable. The true phobic patient, however, cannot overcome his anxiety that easily. Also, many phobic people have multiple phobias; that is, there is more than one set of circumstances that makes them quite anxious. Yet even these people will be quite free of anxiety and able to function as long as they can avoid the anxiety-provoking circumstances. Consequently, the phobic person is not apt to bring his complaints to the physician. More likely it will be the phobic's relatives who are distressed and who turn to the doctor for help. "My wife is fine around the house, but there's absolutely no way I can get her to go out with me socially" and "My husband just won't go into the city, no matter what, because he can't stand crowds" are the sort of statements the physician will hear. The spouse of the phobic patient is forced to accept definite, often drastic limitations on his or her life-style in order to accommodate the process of phobic avoidance.

Hypochondriacal Anxiety

The hypochondriac is somewhat similar to the phobic. Here again, anxiety is limited rather than free-floating, and in the hypochondriac it is limited and displaced onto the body. The hypochondriac has excessive concern and fears about his body and his health. This type of anxious patient is all too familiar to every physician.

The hypochondriac has a basic, underlying excess of body-consciousness. He is constantly aware of his body and its functioning and hence he may be overly concerned about his breathing, his digestion, his elimination, or the beating of his heart. All bodily processes which are under autonomic control and function are, for most of us, outside of our conscious awareness as long as they are functioning properly. We only notice our breathing, our heartbeat, or our elimination if there is something going wrong. The hypochondriac, on the other hand, is always aware of these processes and is constantly fearful or imagining that something is amiss (sometimes this over-awareness may actually disturb functioning, as in the case of premature ventricular contractions). Most often there is no organic lesion and no physical problem present in the hypochondriac. In other cases, there is a genuine physical difficulty, but the patient's concern and anxiety about that difficulty are far out of proportion to its significance.

Case example Mr. F is a 60 year-old attorney who has survived four marriages and three divorces. He has done so despite his own dire, repeated predictions over the last 30 years that he was not long for this world.

In the course of an ordinary week of his life, Mr. F averages two office visits and five telephone calls to his general practitioner; one office visit and eight telephone calls to his psychiatrist; a varying number of special visits and calls to his dentist, podiatrist, ophthalmologist, dermatologist, and other specialists; several discussions with his neighborhood pharmacist; and innumerable telephone calls and discussions with family, friends, and acquaintances. The purpose of all these calls and visits is to obtain reassurance. Mr. F knows, at least intellectually, that he is a severe, chronic hypochondriac. Nevertheless, he cannot control his behavior. Moreover, as with many people who suffer from this particular disorder, Mr. F uses his illness to gain a maximum amount of dependence upon and attention from all those around him.

Like most hypochondriacs, Mr. F uses far too many medications. He regularly takes sedatives, analgesics, antihistamines, antispasmodics and anticholinergics, muscle relaxants, and minor tranquilizers. Moreover, he has a tendency (again, common in many hypochondrical patients) to continue using a medication indefinitely once it has been prescribed for him. Thus, he will take a newly prescribed analgesic along with several previously prescribed pain-relievers, rather than replacing one with the other. Not infrequently, Mr. F develops some symptoms due to side effects and interactions of the various medications he is taking, and this is often further aggravated by his excessive consumption of alcohol.

Mr. F is a rather extreme example, but most of his features are quite typical of hypochondriasis. He would be best managed therapeutically if he were encouraged to seek remedies and palliatives other than drugs or medications for his condition (such nondrug remedies for anxiety will be discussed later in the chapter). Mr. F's disorder is a *panhypochondriasis*; that is, his excessive concern about his health is quite general and includes over-attention to his respiratory, cardiovascular, gastrointestinal, and skeletomuscular systems. Other hypochondriacs may tend to focus their anxiety on one particular bodily system, as is the case with patients suffering from cardiac neurosis. Alternatively, they may develop anxiety about some particular disease, as happens with people who have have phobic concerns about cancer, veneral disease, or some other disorder.

Anxiety about Sexual Functioning

This is a pattern of anxiety which is not generally considered in diagnostic classifications, but it is included here because it is quite common and is rather closely related to hypochondriacal anxiety. Like the latter, this particular type of anxiety is expressed in the patient's excessive awareness of his body and its functioning. Sexual arousal and sexual performance are, normally, rather spontaneous and automatic events, just as are the gastrointestinal and cardiovascular processes. When, for some reason, a person becomes too aware of or concerned about his sexual abilities, functioning is inevitably disturbed. Many cases of secondary impotence result from the fact that some men, for various reasons, become excessively concerned about their ability to have and sustain a penile erection. Masters and Johnson (1970) have pointed out that such men are suffering from "performance anxiety." (Compare this sort of performance anxiety with the beneficial pre-performance anxiety of the actor or speaker discussed previously: acting or speaking is volitional and is facilitated by a certain amount of pre-performance anxiety, while sexual arousal is basically not volitional, but automatic, and is consequently impaired by performance anxiety.) Similarly, women who become overly concerned with achieving orgasm are apt to develop enough anxiety to actually interfere with their relaxation, their sexual arousal, and their eventual orgasm. Anxiety is also a factor in cases of premature ejaculation, where it may interfere with a man's ability to delay ejaculation in intercourse, and in cases of vaginismus and dyspareunia, where it may prevent a woman from relaxing the perineal musculature to allow the easy introduction of the penis.

Anxiety with Psychosomatic Disorders

Anxiety plays a key role in psychosomatic disorders such as bronchial asthma, essential hypertension, peptic ulcer, and ulcerative colitis. It has not been demonstrated that excessive anxiety is the cause of these conditions, but it is certainly a contributing factor.

We are all familiar with the various effects of anxiety on the body. Every time I take a blood pressure reading on one of my patients, I am struck by the role of anxiety in elevating the systolic pressure. I always take an initial reading and then, leaving the sphygmomanometer cuff in place, chat with my patient for a few minutes in a relaxing manner. Then I take a second reading, which very often shows the systolic pressure to have dropped 10 to 30 mm as anxiety diminished and the patient relaxed. Similarly, but with a far more scientific approach, Wolf and Wolff (1947), Margolin (1950), and many others have studied the effects of anxiety in patients with surgical openings into the stomach, where it can be observed that anxiety causes hypersecretion, increased gastric motility, and increased vascular congestion.

Patients with psychosomatic disorders often find themselves caught in a vicious circle. Anxiety is an important contributing factor in the etiology of their disorders, but as they become aware of the disturbance in functioning, they become increasingly anxious about being diseased or abnormal. Hence, a cycle of anxiety—disease—anxiety develops, and it is often very difficult to interrupt.

Case example   Mr. G, a 19-year-old college sophomore, was referred to me by his internist. The physician had made a diagnosis of a duodenal ulcer and this was confirmed by upper gastrointestinal x-ray studies. In addition to the recommendation for psychotherapy, Mr. G had been given a regimen which included a careful diet, the elimination of smoking and of alcoholic beverages, and the use of antispasmodic and sedative medications.

Mr. G was sufficiently frightened by the diagnosis to adhere quite strictly to this regimen as he embarked on psychotherapy with me. We met regularly, twice a week, to talk about the possible sources of his anxiety and to attempt to get them into perspective and reduce them. After three months of this therapy, Mr. G again underwent radiologic examination of his upper gastrointestinal tract. The examination showed that the duodenal ulcer was considerably larger! Alarmed and confused by this news, I had a session with Mr. G in which I attempted to confront him with the facts: despite all our efforts, his condition was worsening. Was he actually violating the regimen and not telling me? Did he have any idea why he was worse? "I'm no doctor, so I don't claim to know the answer," Mr. G responded, "but, yes, I do have a theory about this. For the past three months I've been totally miserable. I'm not supposed to drink at all, so I can't go to the fraternity parties where everybody is guzzling beer. I can't eat anything like pizza or chili, so when all my buddies are going off to get a snack, I just have to sit in the dormitory and stew. I can't even smoke a damn cigarette, so I just get more and more tense. And taking the medicine just makes me feel that I'm really sick and abnormal."

Mr. G's theory made a great deal of sense to me. He was trapped by a "therapeutic" regimen which actually fed into and augmented his anxiety and was really quite anti-therapeutic. I talked the matter over with his internist and we decided to take a totally different tack. Mr. G was told to stop his medication, to smoke when he wanted to, and to eat and drink what he liked. "Just be a little sensible," I counseled him, "but go ahead and live your life the way you want to." Three months later Mr. G again had an upper gastrointestinal series, and, lo and behold, his duodenal ulcer was so completely healed that no radiologic evidence of its existence remained.

While I would not advocate this particular sort of management in every such case, Mr. G's response exemplifies the importance of interrupting the anxiety—disease—anxiety cycle in treating any psychosomatic disorder.

Neurasthenic Anxiety

This type of anxiety is closely related to the hypochondriacal sort. The neurasthenic patient, however, rather than being fearful of disease or overly concerned about various parts of his body, expresses his anxiety in the form of generalized weakness and physical fragility. He never feels strong enough to do much of anything and he overreacts to any activity that is the least bit strenuous, to even mild variations in temperature, or to any circumstances that are the least bit discommoding. Obviously, some care must be taken to differentiate patients suffering from hypothyroidism or other endocrine disorders from those who are true neurasthenics. The neurasthenic patient, complaining of lack of energy, must also be differentiated from the depressed patient. The latter will lack energy, but in addition will be much more likely to show alterations in mood (feeling blue or melancholy), true and severe anorexia, and a type of insomnia characterized by early morning awakening (see Chapter 3). The neurasthenic, on the other hand, is more likely to present an almost lifelong history of complaints that contains no real evidence of mood alteration. If there is insomnia, it will be of a type characterized by difficulty in falling asleep rather than by waking up early.

Obsessive-Compulsive Anxiety

The true obsessive-compulsive patient is a highly interesting subtype of the neurotic, anxious person. In this rather complex disorder, the patient's anxiety manifests itself in *obsessions*: persistent, unwanted thoughts which intrude on the patient's consciousness and which are generally of an antisocial or unacceptable nature (for example, "I wish my mother would die" or "I'd like to commit some sexually perverse act"). In reaction to these obsessive thoughts, the patient then has *compulsions*: ritualized actions that the patient feels he must carry out (for example, repeated washing of the hands or repeated counting of certain numbers).

The obsessive-compulsive person has been referred to as a sort of "psychic bookkeeper" (Goldberg, 1973). On the debit side of his mental ledger are the bad, nasty, obsessive thoughts, and on the credit side are the ritualized, compulsive actions, offered up as a form of mental penance and expiation. Thus the obsessive thought "I want to kill my father" can be balanced and cancelled out by the washing of the hands: an attempt to wash away the mental crime and the guilt. Because the obsessions return again and again, though, the compulsions must be carried out repeatedly also, and the net effect is a person who is always at least somewhat hampered by his mental symptoms, and in severe cases, badly crippled by them.

The case of a man I knew many years ago, a chronic patient in a mental hospital, illustrates how debilitating an obsessive-compulsive anxiety can be. This man suffered from a compulsion in which for every four steps taken forward, he had to take three steps backward. To see him attempting to walk a few hundred yards from one hospital building to another was to realize the extent to which his symptoms rendered him an invalid, for it could take him several hours to accomplish that short trip.

Hysterical Anxiety

There are two subclassifications of hysterical anxiety, and these are generally referred to as *dissociative anxiety* and *conversion anxiety*.

Dissociative anxiety The patient suffering from dissociative anxiety will show one or more of the following symptoms: freezing, fugue states, amnesias, or multiple personality. All of these symptoms involve altered states of mental consciousness.

Freezing is the simplest and by far the most common dissociative symptom. It is a phenomenon in which the person reacts to a particularly intense anxiety-provoking situation by literally "freezing." He becomes motionless and speechless and is out of contact with the environment, although he does not lose consciousness. The entire reaction lasts only a matter of minutes, after which the person returns to a normal state of consciousness with no recollection of the episode.

An example of this phenomenon may be seen in Mrs. H, a 20-year-old woman who has been married for only five or six months. These months have been unhappy ones for her because they have been marked by repeated, severe quarrels with her new husband. Mrs. H comes to her physician for help at her husband's urging—not because of the marital conflict, but because of a curious circumstance that he has noted during their many fights. At the height of the battle, when he is locked in furious argument with his wife, her eyes cloud over, she does not speak or move, and she does not appear to hear what her husband says to her. After five minutes or less, this reaction disappears as suddenly as it came on, and Mrs. H returns to her normal self but has no memory of the brief interlude.

Mrs. H is, of course, manifesting a typical hysterical freezing reaction. Such reactions always occur, as hers do, at times of severe emotional stress. They are easily differentiated from the catatonic reactions of schizophrenia, as these last for days, weeks, or months and the freezing reactions persist for only a few minutes. Differentiation must also be made from petit mal seizures. This distinction can be made on the basis of an electroencephalogram, which will be quite normal in the patient with a freezing reaction, but which will show the characteristic "dart and dome," three-per-second waves and generalized high voltage in petit mal.

Fugue states are a more complex sort of altered state of consciousness and may also occur as a manifestation of hysterical anxiety. In a fugue state, a person carries out a whole series of actions that generally take him far away from where he started. These actions, usually involving geographical movement, are done in an automatic manner and are carried on outside of the individual's usual state of awareness. Thus, the patient may "wake-up" after a fugue state to find that he is in another location—even another city or another state—with no real memory of how he got there. Fugue states characteristically last longer than freezing reactions and are apt to persist for many hours or for several days. As a psychiatric symptom, fugue states are rare, and since in certain instances they may also be caused by organic brain damage, the diagnosis of fugue state as a manifestation of anxiety should be made only after careful neurologic examination, skull x-rays, and electroencephalograms have ruled out an organic basis for the disorder.

The patient in a fugue state carries out actions and movements without recalling them, but at least he does know, throughout his altered state of consciousness, who he is. In contrast, patients with *amnesias* are unable to recall their personal identities. They do not know, for a period of time, who they are, where they have been, or what they have done in life. It is as if their minds were temporarily wiped clean of all memory and recall. Again, these very rare altered states of consciousness may be a reaction to overwhelming anxiety and may sometimes persist for many weeks. Here, also, differentiation must be made from states of amnesia which stem from organic brain damage.

It should be noted that acute alcoholic intoxication, particularly in the chronic drinker, is also likely to produce "blackouts"—that is, periods of memory loss, fugue state, or amnesia. Such blackouts, which are organic or toxic rather than hysterical in nature, are a well-recognized warning sign of impending severe alcoholism.

The psychodynamic factor that is common to freezing, fugues, and amnesias seems reasonably clear: an altered state of consciousness seems to protect the individual from overwhelming anxiety. Thus, the patient removes himself temporarily from an unbearable mental conflict. The person who cannot remember who he is or how he got where he is does not want to remember, because the knowledge is tied in with excessively painful amounts of anxiety.

The condition known as *multiple personality* is an extremely rare and complex disorder in which hysterical anxiety alters consciousness in such a way that two or more separate personalities coexist within the same individual. The classic example of this is, of course, an actual case which became well known to the general public in the book and movie *The Three Faces of Eve* (Thigpen and Cleckley, 1957).

Before leaving the subject of altered states of consciousness, we might mention two examples of such altered states which occur very commonly in normal individuals. These are *somnambulism* and *somniloquism*, or sleepwalking and sleeptalking. The sleepwalker is very much like the person suffering from a fugue state, but on a smaller scale. Some sleeptalkers can carry on long, seemingly meaningful conversations with another individual while they are sound asleep, and on awakening they have no recollection whatsoever of the conversation.

Conversion anxiety In patients suffering from this syndrome, overwhelming anxiety is somehow converted into a physical paralysis or dysfunction. The paralysis always involves either the voluntary musculature of the body or the special senses. Hence, in this category we encounter patients with hysterical paralysis of the arms or legs, hysterical inability to walk, hysterical blindness, hysterical aphonia, or hysterical deafness.

We speak of the anxiety as being "converted" in these patients because once they develop their physical dysfunction, they are remarkably free of anxiety. The genesis of the symptoms always involves a conflictful situation which produces marked anxiety, but once the paralysis emerges the patient is singularly calm and unconcerned. This characteristic has been referred to as "la belle indifference," the beautiful indifference of the hysteric. He may calmly tell the physician, "both my legs are paralyzed and I can't move," while showing no sign of apprehension or dismay. Conversion paralyses are apt to develop quite suddenly and may disappear just as abruptly, often responding to treatments based on the power of suggestion (including faith healing).

The various conversion paralyses should be differentiated from true psychosomatic conditions. In the latter, anxiety is a causative and/or aggravating etiologic factor in the disorder, but it does not abate or disappear as the physical disorder develops. In fact, as was pointed out previously, the psychosomatic patient becomes increasingly anxious about his dysfunction. The hysteric with conversion symptoms becomes calm as the dysfunction appears. You will also note that psychosomatic ills affect those parts of the body under the control of the autonomic or involuntary nervous system, such as the stomach, intestines, heart, and lungs, whereas conversion reactions involve the special senses (sight, smell, hearing) and those parts of the body under the control of the voluntary nervous system.

Before leaving the subject of hysterical anxiety, some comment on the reaction of these patients to medications and drugs is in order. All of these patients, whether they suffer from the dissociative or the conversion forms of the disorder, are extremely suggestible. They are apt to show all sorts of reactions to medications, and these reactions are often based not on physiologic effects but rather on what the patient imagines the medication is going to do to him or even on his personal reaction to the physician. For this reason, and on the basis of my experience with many such patients, I would strongly advise against prescribing sedatives, tranquilizers, or any antianxiety medications for the hysterical neurotic. These patients will do far better if other means of anxiety reduction and control are prescribed by the physician, and the latter will not have to contend with such protestations as "Your medicine made me sick" or "That medicine ruined me."

THE MASKING OF ANXIETY

Anxiety can be masked or temporarily relieved by the use of sedative drugs. Unfortunately, our society (like a great many societies) accepts and propagates this method of dealing with anxiety. The drug which is used for this purpose most often is, of course, ethyl alcohol, in all its various dilutions, forms, and brews. We learn to reach for a drink at every party, at every social gathering, and in every situation where we are apt to encounter a bit of anxiety. A striking example of this phenomenon is one that I have encountered over and over on the commercial airlines. Occasionally while flying these airlines, I am on a flight that is for some reason delayed en route or unable to land as scheduled. In such a situation the passengers naturally become quite anxious: the buzz of conversation in the plane rises; people begin to ask what is wrong and to come up with speculations; one can feel the tension mounting at a rapid rate. Generally, however, the airline will quickly come to the rescue and a stewardess will announce, "We are going to be delayed for a while, but why don't you all just relax? We're going to serve free cocktails and will be around shortly to take your orders." Thus the perfect "solution" is applied to the problem. For the next half hour or more virtually everyone on the plane drowns his anxiety in free alcohol and all is well. Only a confirmed skeptic like myself sits there soberly thinking that I still don't know why the plane has been delayed. Moreover, I certainly hope I don't run into any of my inebriated co-passengers after the landing when we all take to our automobiles in the airport parking lot.

With this strong, culturally endorsed pattern in existence, it is not surprising that one encounters many patients who are habitually masking rather excessive anxiety with alcohol or some other drug, be it Valium (diazepam), meprobamate, or a barbiturate. Any person who needs a "three-martini lunch," or three martinis on the train home from work, should be considering what the sources of that need are, rather than blindly indulging it. The physician can often be helpful in pointing out very honestly to his patients the danger of drug abuse, particularly alcohol abuse, as a means of covering or masking anxiety. Going from this kind of drug abuse to genuine alcoholism is a very short step for almost anyone. We shall soon consider other methods of anxiety reduction that may be recommended to the person who is relying on drugs to ease his tensions.

DIFFERENTIAL DIAGNOSIS OF THE ANXIOUS PATIENT

The physician's first task is to differentiate the anxious person from the normal one. Since anxiety is a normal reaction in all of us, it is easy to dismiss the anxious person as perfectly normal and merely overly concerned. After all, he's only complaining of the same symptoms that we ourselves suffer with at times! To avoid falling into the trap of such reasoning, we must recognize two factors. First, many, or perhaps most, of us are overly troubled with anxiety ourselves. The fact that we also suffer with this common disorder, however, does not make it normal and does not lend validity to dismissing a patient's complaints with an "Oh, everybody feels that way" sort of remark. Second, the anxious patient is often complaining of a feeling that, in extent and amount, is far in excess of what we are accustomed to feeling and is far in excess of normal. As pointed out before, a minimum amount of anxiety is desirable for effective functioning, but an overwhelming amount of anxiety cripples performance and impairs personal relations and satisfaction.

The anxious patient must also be differentiated from the depressed patient. This is not always an easy distinction to make, because many depressed people have a good deal of anxiety mixed in with their depression. However, the following points will often help to differentiate these two very common disorders:

1. The anxious patient is apt to complain of feeling jittery, tense, nervous, and restless, whereas the depressed patient is more likely to complain about his alterations of mood and to describe himself as sad, blue, lonely, unhappy, or despairing.
2. The anxious patient generally will not show the retardation of thought, speech, and gait which is so typical of the depressive.
3. While the anxious patient may complain of insomnia, it will generally prove to be of a type in which he has

difficulty in falling asleep or in which he awakens during the night but can get back to sleep; the anxious patient then tends to sleep late in the morning. The depressed person, on the other hand, may experience a type of insomnia in which he awakens in the very early morning and cannot get back to sleep.

4. The "worst time of day" for the anxious patient may be any time, depending on the situations that provoke his anxiety. The "worst time of the day" for the depressive is almost inevitably the early morning, when he is awakened prematurely and has to face a day and a world which he dreads.

5. Suicidal thoughts or intentions virtually never occur in the anxious patient, but they are relatively common in the depressive.

6. Delusions are never present in the anxious person, whereas they are frequently an aspect of severe depressions.

Taking these factors into account may make the differentiation of these two disorders easier. In those cases where doubt remains, it is wise to prescribe an antidepressant medication on the likelihood that the person is depressed. A good therapeutic response to that medication may confirm the diagnosis.

Certain physical disorders may produce symptoms resembling those of anxiety. Hyperthyroidism is particularly likely to produce such a similar symptomatology. Hypoglycemia, although often diagnosed, is probably a much less common cause of anxiety-like symptoms.

Finally, we must differentiate the anxious patient from the person who is using and abusing stimulant drugs. Caffeine is by far the drug most commonly involved. Not a few patients will present themselves to the doctor with classical symptoms of anxiety—tremors, excessive perspiration, palpitations of the heart, and jitteriness—and will prove to be people who are consuming 8 to 10 or more cups of coffee each day. Careful history taking and questioning about consumption of tea, coffee, hot chocolate, and soft drinks containing caffeine should be carried out with any patient whose complaints resemble the symptoms and signs of anxiety. Where excessive intake of stimulants is detected, a recommendation for stopping this should precede any other therapeutic measure and may well solve the entire problem.

Needless to say, stronger stimulants such as amphetamines, methylphenidate (Ritalin), and sympathomimetic drugs can produce anxiety-like conditions even more readily than caffeine, but their use is less common.

MANAGING AND REDUCING ANXIETY

The management and reduction of anxiety with mind-influencing drugs is considered at length in another chapter in this book. It is my belief that the use of such drugs should be a last resort for the anxious patient and should be the last thing that the physician recommends. Therefore, I will briefly describe some nondrug approaches to and recommendations for the management and reduction of anxiety.

Understanding

This is an approach that seems to have lost popularity in recent years, yet I believe it is still the most valid. If we can understand what we are anxious about, if we can name the "nameless dread," then we are greatly relieved and relaxed.

As an example, consider the situation mentioned before in which the passengers in an airliner become excessively anxious because there is an unexplained delay en route. We have already noted how the drug alcohol is used to deal with this anxiety. Now consider an alternative. Suppose the captain of the airliner comes on the intercom and announces, "Folks, we are going to be delayed about 30 minutes in landing at Philadelphia. They have had a snowstorm and they are now clearing the landing areas at the airport. By the time we do land, everything will be clear and we won't have any problem. Sorry about this delay, but we'll get you all down in good shape." What the captain has furnished is understanding, and just as surely as the tension in the plane was mounting before, it will now dissolve and disappear, without the use of drugs.

It is not always, or even generally, that simple for the patient to understand the sources of his anxiety, but our first efforts should be made in this direction. Why is he anxious? What overloads of conflict or concern are operating within him? By taking a bit of time, by listening carefully, and by encouraging our patients to examine such questions, we may be of considerable help.

Encouraging Tranquility and Equanimity

People become overly anxious because they are worrying about what *might* happen: what might happen today; what might happen tomorrow; what might happen next year. They also brood about the past, fretting and grieving over that which is long done and gone. In addition, they worry about matters that are not really relevant to them and about matters that simply cannot be changed or controlled.

Borrowing a leaf from Alcoholics Anonymous, we can prescribe some wiser approaches for our anxious patients. They should be encouraged to "live their lives in day-tight compartments," to concern themselves basically with matters that have to be dealt with in the here and now and to eschew the problems of the remote past or remote future. To worry about tomorrow and the day after and the day after that is far too overwhelming for any of us. Our patients should also be advised to change that which can be changed and to accept that which cannot. I frequently give my patients some advice from the late, great New England psychiatrist Austen Fox Riggs (1922), and I tell them to put these questions to themselves about any problem that seems difficult:

1. Is it *your* problem?
2. Is it your problem *now*?
3. If it is your problem and it is your problem now, what are the possible things you can do about it? Consider them and make a choice.
4. If it is your problem and it is your problem now, but there is nothing that can be done, then tell yourself that and assert all your faith and acceptance.

Meditation and Relaxation

A number of self-administered techniques are available which tend to reduce anxiety by inducing a state of relaxation and/or meditation in the body and mind. Transcendental meditation (TM) is currently the most popular of these. It embellishes the processes of relaxation and meditation with various metaphysical or quasi-religious trappings, such as the use of the mantra. In medical practice, it is quite useful to recommend a simplified meditation-without-metaphysics technique to the anxious patient. The following steps may be suggested:

1. Meditate for 20 minutes, twice a day. Don't skip any sessions and don't add any, do 20 minutes of meditation, neither more nor less.
2. Do not meditate within two hours after eating.
3. Find a comfortable chair or couch on which to recline.
4. Close the eyes and progressively relax the muscles of the body. Do this by contracting the muscles of each part of the body, then relax them and leave them relaxed. Start with the toes and work up through the feet ankles, calves, thighs, hips and pelvis, abdomen, chest, neck, arms, forearms, wrists, fingers, and facial muscles.
5. Breathe deeply and slowly and repeat a nonsense syllable to yourself on each expiration. Use a syllable or sound like *oom, rahm,* or *oan.*
6. Concentrate on the breathing and on the nonsense syllable. Don't try to think about anything or not to think about anything. Don't try to relax. As much as is possible, don't try at all!
7. When the 20 minutes are up, keep your eyes closed for a minute or two, then open them. Remain reclining for another minute or two, then get up.

Just why a technique of meditation such as the one described (or such as TM) is helpful in reducing anxiety is unknown. But lest we think that such approaches are new and strictly modern discoveries (or, at least, new in the West), it is well to recall the methods of Coue, used in the early 1900s. Most of us know that Coue taught people to think and say, "Every day in every way, I'm getting better and better," but what we don't realize is the method that Coue advocated to propagate this way of thinking. According to one novelist of that era (Galsworthy, 1926), one was instructed to lie down on a comfortable chair or couch, minimize all outside stimuli, relax the body, and repeat the catch phrase ("Every day . . . .") over and over to oneself for a period of 15 to 30 minutes.

Change in Life-Style

Many patients with patterns of chronic and excessive anxiety are suffering because their style of living is incompatible with their personal needs. For such patients, a well-thought-out change in life-style may be far more helpful than all the drugs in the pharmacopeia.

Case example Mr. J is a 35-year-old accountant. He has been happily married for 10 years, has two small children, and enjoys his work, which he finds lucrative and stimulating. Mr. J, however, is a chronic worrier. He worries quite excessively about any minor illness, such as a cold, that he develops. He worries that his wife does not eat enough and that she will suffer from malnutrition. He worries profoundly when either of his children develops one of the many fevers or ills that beset any childhood. In addition, Mr. J has generally had a high level of nervous tension, reflected in a constant physical restlessness and "the jitters."

Mr. J consulted me for psychiatric treatment and we embarked on a course of psychotherapy in which he came to understand a good deal about himself and his inner conflicts. Despite this increase in understanding, however, his hypochondriacal worries and jitters did not diminish appreciably. Consequently, we decided to evaluate how Mr. J had adjusted his life-style according to his new understanding of himself. In our psychotherapy we had determined that Mr. J tended to be overly passive and a bit too dependent on other people. After gaining these insights, though, Mr. J had not really changed any of his living patterns.

We arranged for him to have a complete checkup with an internist. Then the internist, Mr. J, and I had a conference in which we agreed on some possible changes in life-style. As a result, Mr. J, who had been quite inactive physically, began to bicycle for a half hour each day and to visit his local "Y" three times each week to play handball and basketball and to work out on the track. These activities were chosen because they were ones that Mr. J felt he could really enjoy. He also decided to spend one evening a week away from his family to participate in sports, go to a show, or do whatever suited him. Finally, Mr. J also undertook to become more healthfully self-assertive, both in his work and in his social relationships.

After three months on this regimen, the change in this man was most striking. He was far more relaxed, and his restlessness had virtually disappeared. Even more impressive was the fact that he felt well and was not thinking about illness or breakdowns in his body, but was rather intrigued with how well his body could function when given the chance. Five years later, Mr. J continues to thrive in his new pattern of living.

This example clearly indicates how a change in life-style which emphasized physical activity and a reasonable degree of independence served to dispel a pattern of chronic anxiety.

Of course, there is a place for the use of antianxiety drugs in therapy. When other measures fail, when patients lack the motivation for nondrug therapies, and when anxiety is so overwhelming as to necessitate some very immediate and temporary surcease, then the use of medications becomes appropriate. Much more will be said about this in the chapter on antianxiety drugs.

REFERENCES

Freud, S.: *The Problem of Anxiety*. New York: W. W. Norton & Company, Inc., 1936.

Galsworthy, J.: *A Modern Comedy*. New York: Charles Scribner's Sons, 1926.

Garre, W. J.: *Basic Anxiety*. New York: Philosophical Library, Inc., 1962.

Goldberg, M.: *Psychiatric Diagnosis and Understanding for the Helping Professions*. Chicago: Nelson-Hall Publishers, 1973.

Horney, K.: *The Neurotic Personality of Our Time*. New York: W. W. Norton & Company, Inc., 1937.

Margolin, S. G., Orringer, D., Kaufman, M. R. et al: Variations of gastric functions during conscious and unconscious conflict states. In *Life Stress and Bodily Disease*. Baltimore: The Williams & Wilkins Co., 1950.

Masters, W. H. and Johnson, V. E.: *Human Sexual Inadequacy*. Boston: Little, Brown & Co., 1970.

Rank, O.: *The Trauma of Birth*. New York: Robert Brunner, 1952.

Riggs, A. F.: *Just Nerves*. Cambridge, Mass: Riverside Press, 1922.

Thigpen, C. and Cleckley, H. M.: *Three Faces of Eve*. New York: McGraw-Hill, Inc., 1957.

Wolf, S. and Wolff, H. G.: *Human Gastric Function: An Experimental Study of a Man and His Stomach*. 2d ed. New York: Oxford University Press, Inc., 1947.

6 Fitting the Medication to the Patient

A Pharmacologic Viewpoint
for the Clinician

Henry H. Swain, M.D.

INTRODUCTION

The decade of the 1950s saw the introduction into medical practice of four new families of mind-influencing drugs: (1) the phenothiazines and related antipsychotic drugs which ameliorate the thought disorders of schizophrenia; (2) the monoamine oxidase (MAO) inhibitors, which, in many cases, can elevate the mood of depressed patients; (3) the tricyclic antidepressants, likewise effective in the management of psychiatric depression; and (4) the benzodiazepines, which lack antipsychotic and antidepressant properties, but which are highly effective antianxiety and anticonvulsant drugs.

The availability of these new drugs has increased both the capabilities and the responsibilities of the physician who chooses to use them. These new substances offer the doctor a much broader range of therapeutic possibilities than was available to him when he was limited to such classical mind-influencing drugs as morphine, alcohol, and the barbiturates. However, there has proved to be a large patient-to-patient variation in the type and magnitude of effects which these new agents produce; the drugs cause side effects which are both serious and surprising, and the interactions with other drugs are subtle and complicated. In short, the new mind-influencing drugs have complex pharmacologies.

These antipsychotic, antidepressant, and antianxiety agents make it possible for the general practitioner and family physician, not just the psychiatrist, to offer effective pharmacotherapy to patients who have moderately severe emotional and psychiatric illness. However, in order to use these therapeutic tools safely and effectively, the physician must know more about the varieties of mental and emotional illness and the symptoms and diagnosis of his particular patient, as well as the pharmacology of the drugs involved.

During the first half of this century, if a patient were suffering from insomnia, anxiety, or agitation, it is quite likely that he would have been given a trial of phenobarbital. The drug has a simple pharmacology and is reasonably safe and well tolerated by most patients over long periods. Predictably, the major side effect of its use was excessive sedation, and if this became troublesome, the dosage of phenobarbital could be reduced, or the drug could be discontinued completely. The major drug interaction potential of phenobarbital (its ability to induce in the liver those enzymes which are responsible for the metabolism of other drugs) was not known at that time. In some cases, phenobarbital did offer the patient useful relief from his symptoms. Specific psychiatric diagnosis was not as essential as it is today; phenobarbital was practically the only drug available, and a trial of its use seemed to offer far more help than harm.

With the appearance of the newer mind-influencing drugs, accurate diagnosis of the patient's illness became much more important. With appropriate use, each of the new drugs offers a therapeutic effectiveness previously unavailable, but the range of patients which can be benefitted by each drug is narrower than before. The axiom of the therapeutic trial—"treat first, think later"—became less likely to be helpful and more likely to be harmful than it was in the days of phenobarbital.

Accurate psychiatric diagnosis is important for predicting the natural course of the patient's illness and for evaluating the therapeutic effectiveness of a drug. A careful history taking and physical examination are necessary before therapy is initiated if the physician is to be able to distinguish between those signs and symptoms which are a part of the patient's illness and those which are the consequence of drug administration. Potent mind-influencing drugs can produce, as well as alleviate, mental and emotional symptoms.

A patient's mental illness can alter his response to a drug. The actions of a drug may be perceived very differently by a so-called normal individual than by one who has a particular psychiatric illness. For example, a tricyclic antidepressant does not raise the spirits of a normal individual, but it has a striking effect in this regard in a patient with endogenous depression. Similarly, chlorpromazine is often perceived as dysphoric by normal individuals, but as comforting by schizophrenic patients.

The mind-influencing drugs also influence the body in important and, often, complex ways. For each of these agents, it is important for the physician to know which organs and systems are likely to be affected, which tissues will show the first signs of toxicity, and what somatic disease conditions predispose an individual to toxicity from a particular mind-influencing drug. These and related pharmacologic aspects of the drugs will be discussed in this chapter; the problems of drug interactions with other prescribed and nonprescribed agents will be discussed in a later chapter.

ANTIPSYCHOTIC AGENTS

Substituted Phenothiazines

This is a remarkable family of drugs. Its members exert a bewildering array of effects upon the body, but in spite of this they are reasonably safe drugs. Though the number of patients who regularly receive phenothiazines is large, the number of clinical conditions for which they are used is quite small. The major use of these agents is in the control of the symptoms of schizophrenia. Other psychiatric uses include their occasional employment in the control of manic reactions and, still less commonly, depressions. Formerly, they were used to treat "bad trips" caused by LSD, amphetamines, or other psychedelic agents. As antiemetics, the phenothiazines are effective in controlling nausea and vomiting from a number of causes, though not that arising from motion sickness. Intractable hiccough often responds to these drugs.

Phenothiazines have no place in the management of anxiety or other nonpsychotic forms of emotional illness. Though they are effective as antiarrhythmic agents, their use in the control of disturbances of cardiac rhythm is not recognized clinically. In the earliest days of their availability, they were used to prolong and intensify the effects of other drugs upon the central nervous system, but this use of the phenothiazines has been discarded therapeutically and remains only as an undesirable drug interaction.

Convulsions, either epileptic or drug-induced, represent a relative contraindication to the use of phenothiazines, which, despite early reports to the contrary, actually lower seizure threshold.

The pharmacology of the phenothiazines involves the central nervous system, the autonomic nervous system, the cardiovascular system, and certain endocrine functions. In the central nervous system, the most-utilized property of these drugs is their ability to ameliorate the thought disorders which characterize schizophrenia. Patients become less withdrawn or belligerent. Perceptual disturbances and paranoid projections tend to disappear. Affect appears to become more appropriate. These antischizophrenic effects are relatively slow to develop, requiring several weeks or even months to produce maximum improvement. Tolerance apparently does not develop to the antischizophrenic actions of the phenothiazines.

Sedation, on the other hand, is an immediate effect in normal individuals and schizophrenics alike, but tolerance to it develops. Thus, with continued administration of a phenothiazine to a schizophrenic patient, the initial sedative action becomes less prominent and the antipsychotic effect becomes more apparent with the passage of the first few weeks.

Extrapyramidal signs are produced by prolonged administration of high doses of any of the phenothiazines, though this effect is more prominent with some members of the drug family than with others. Parkinsonism, akathisia (the need to move about constantly), dystonia, and tardive dyskinesia are all recognized extrapyramidal manifestations of phenothiazine action. Of these, tardive dyskinesia is the most feared, because discontinuing the phenothiazine does not relieve the condition. In fact, it may appear for the first time only after the drug has been discontinued, and the condition may persist indefinitely thereafter.

Conditioned avoidance is an experimental technique which has been used repeatedly to identify drugs which are related pharmacologically to the phenothiazines and which differ from the classical sedative-hypnotic agents such as the barbiturates. In this technique, an animal is trained to respond to a tone in order to avoid an electric shock. The administration of a phenothiazine or related drug, in a dose so small that the animal's physical ability to escape from the shock is unimpaired, causes it to ignore the warning tone. A barbiturate, on the other hand, interrupts the animal's response to the tone only when given in doses so large that its physical ability to escape from the electric shock is impaired by sedation and ataxia.

Phenothiazines exert a variety of blocking effects on the autonomic nervous system. Alpha-adrenergic receptors are blocked, so the pressor effects of epinephrine and norepinephrine are reduced. In fact, after a large dose of a phenothiazine, epinephrine may actually cause a fall in blood pressure (epinephrine reversal). On the other hand, phenothiazines block the re-uptake of catecholamines by adrenergic nerve endings, so that under certain circumstances the effects of sympathetic nervous system stimulation are enhanced. The muscarinic actions of acetylcholine are blocked by the atropine-like properties of phenothiazines. These drugs also block the actions of serotonin. The histamine-blocking properties of the antipsychotic phenothiazines are minimal, even though chlorpromazine was originally investigated as a potential antihistamine.

The major cardiovascular side effect is orthostatic hypotension, which is probably a consequence of the alpha-adrenergic blockade. Another cardiovascular effect of the phenothiazines is a quinidine-like depression of the intracardiac impulse, a condition which may be responsible for the cases of sudden death which are occasionally encountered in patients receiving large doses of the phenothiazines. Within the phenothiazine family there is considerable difference between the relative incidences of cardiovascular and extrapyramidal side effects, as will be discussed below.

Endocrine effects appear to be the result of actions of the phenothiazines upon the hypothalamic regulatory hormones. Lactation can be a troublesome side effect in female patients receiving phenothiazines. Gynecomastia and amenorrhea occur occasionally. Furthermore, phenothiazine administration can lead to decreased adrenocorticotropic hormone (ACTH) release and, therefore, to decreased cortisol levels. Pituitary growth hormone is suppressed, which has led to the suggestion of using phenothiazines to control acromegaly.

Temperature regulation is impaired by phenothiazine administration in that the individual's body temperature moves toward the ambient temperature. Thus, under most circumstances the body temperature falls, but in a hot environment, heat stroke and fatal hyperthermia can occur.

Other well-recognized side effects of the administration of phenothiazines include intrahepatic cholestatic jaundice, ocular changes, blood dyscrasias, and dermatologic reactions.

Tolerance, physical dependence, and drug abuse are not problems with the phenothiazines. Tolerance develops to the sedative effects but not to the antipsychotic actions. Physical dependence is minimal if it exists at all. There is no evidence that patients abusively self-administer these drugs; in fact, the problem is quite the opposite—some patients are reluctant to take their prescribed medication. The danger of suicide from an overdose of a phenothiazine is small because of the flat dose-response curve of this family of drugs.

Not all of the substituted phenothiazines which are used in therapeutics have the antipsychotic and other properties described above. The exceptions include promethazine (Phenergan), which is employed as an antihistaminic; ethopromazine (Parsidol), which is a centrally acting anticholinergic drug used in parkinsonism; and methotrimeprazine (Levoprome), an analgesic. The parent molecule, phenothiazine, is of no particular pharmacologic interest.

The antipsychotic phenothiazines are divided into three groups based upon the nature of the chemical substitution at the 10-position (ring nitrogen) of the phenothiazine nucleus: (1) the aliphatic group, (2) the piperidine group, and (3) the piperazine group of drugs. Table 1 lists some of the important members of each of these groups.

There are significant differences among the groups in the relative incidence and severity of the various side effects. Specifically, extrapyramidal side effects are more prominent and cardiovascular side effects are less so with the piperazine derivatives (fluphenazine, prochlorperazine, perphenazine, trifluoperazine, acetophenazine). Conversely, with the aliphatic group (chlorpromazine, triflupromazine, promazine) and the piperidine group (thioridazine, mesoridazine), it is the cardiovascular actions which are more apparent, while the extrapyramidal changes are not as pronounced. The members of the piperazine group are significantly more potent than the members of the other two

Table 1
Antipsychotic Phenothiazines

Substitution Group	Member Drugs
Aliphatic	Chlorpromazine (Thorazine)
	Triflupromazine (Vesprin)
	Promazine (Sparine)
Piperidine	Thioridazine (Mellaril)
	Mesoridazine (Serentil)
Piperazine	Prochlorperazine (Compazine)
	Trifluoperazine (Stelazine)
	Perphenazine (Trilafon)
	Fluphenazine (Prolixin)
	Acetophenazine (Tindal)

groups, so smaller total dosages are administered, but the antipsychotic effectiveness is the same for all three groups.

Substituted Thioxanthenes

The substituted thioxanthenes are chemically and pharmacologically very similar to the substituted phenothiazines and differ only in that the ring nitrogen of phenothiazine is replaced with a carbon atom. Two members of this family are available clinically: chlorprothixene (Taractan), which has the same aliphatic side chain as chlorpromazine, which it resembles closely; and thiothixene (Navane), which has the same piperazine substitution as prochlorperazine, which it resembles in its relatively high incidence of extrapyramidal side effects.

Haloperidol

This butyrophenone, known commercially as Haldol, bears no obvious chemical relationship to either the phenothiazines or the thioxanthenes. Nevertheless, it shares a number of pharmacologic properties with them, including that of antipsychotic action. With its high potency and relatively high incidence of extrapyramidal side effects, haloperidol resembles the piperazine group most closely. Its antipsychotic effectiveness is essentially the same as that of the phenothiazines and the thioxanthenes.

The multiplicity of drugs available for the treatment of schizophrenia makes it possible for the physician to choose the one that best fits the needs of the particular patient. Thus, for a patient in whom a hypotensive episode might have serious consequences (such as stroke or myocardial infarction), thioridazine or chlorpromazine would seem less desirable than a piperazine derivative or haloperidol. Conversely, if the danger from extrapyramidal side effects seemed greater, the reverse choice would be appropriate.

MONOAMINE OXIDASE INHIBITORS

Monoamine oxidase (MAO), an enzyme located in the mitochondria of many cells, oxidatively deaminates the body's biogenic amines: epinephrine, norepinephrine, dopamine, and serotonin. Drugs which inhibit this enzyme produce mood elevation in depressed patients, exert a moderate antihypertensive effect, and are effective for the treatment of narcolepsy. The considerable toxicity of these agents and the numerous interactions which they display with other drugs limit the usefulness of this pharmacologically interesting family of therapeutic agents.

The immediate effects of monoamine oxidase inhibition are less obvious than might be anticipated if one considers the central role which the biogenic amines are thought to play in both the psychologic and the physiologic functions of the body. Animal studies show that a single dose of an MAO inhibitor can produce a marked inhibition of enzyme activity and significant changes in the tissue concentrations of biogenic amines with little or no alteration in the behavior of the animal.

In man, the mood-elevating effects are slow in onset, and many days or even weeks of treatment may be required before the change is apparent. Similarly, the effects of MAO inhibitors persist after drug administration is discontinued. This is not surprising, since the drugs produce irreversible inhibition of MAO, and complete restoration of activity requires the body's synthesis of new enzyme protein, a process requiring several weeks.

Mood elevation may be accompanied by other signs of central nervous system stimulation, up to and including frankly manic reactions. Hyperreflexia, tremors, insomnia, nightmares, hallucinations, and convulsions have been noted.

The antihypertensive effect of MAO inhibitors is more apparent when the patient is in the upright position than when he is recumbent. Therefore, it is not surprising that orthostatic hypotension is a common side effect of the MAO inhibitors, whether they are being used in hypertension or in psychiatric depression. The antihypertensive action is slow to develop, with several weeks of therapy needed before the maximum effect is demonstrable, and the effect persists for a number of days after the drug has been discontinued. The mechanism by which the antihypertensive effect is produced is not understood. Among drugs of this family, there is not a good correlation between the degree of inhibition of the MAO enzyme and the extent of blood pressure reduction.

In addition to excessive central nervous system stimulation and orthostatic hypotension, side effects of the MAO inhibitors include liver damage, dizziness and vertigo, skin rashes, and inhibition of ejaculation.

The interactions between MAO inhibitors and other drugs are numerous and often serious. These drug-drug interactions, which are a source of even greater concern than the direct toxicity of this group of agents, will be discussed in a later chapter.

Four MAO inhibitors are presently used in the United States for psychiatric depression. Three of these are hydrazine compounds which are very similar to one another, with actions as described above. They are phenelzine (Nardil), nialamide (Niamid), and isocarboxazid (Marplan). The fourth antidepressant MAO inhibitor differs in chemistry and in the time course of its action. Tranylcypromine (Parnate) is not a hydrazine but, rather, closely resembles amphetamine in structure. It has a prompt onset of central nervous system stimulatory action, probably an amphetamine-like effect, in addition to the long-lasting properties of all the MAO inhibitors. Also available on the market is pargyline (Eutonyl), an MAO inhibitor that is sold as an antihypertensive drug rather than as an antidepressant, even though its properties are essentially the same as those of the other hydrazine-type MAO inhibitors.

TRICYCLIC ANTIDEPRESSANTS

The structural formula of the tricyclic imipramine (Tofranil) bears a striking resemblance to that of promazine (Sparine), a phenothiazine antipsychotic drug. A sulfur atom in the latter compound is replaced by an ethylene group in the former. However, the pharmacology of imipramine and other tricyclic antidepressants is very different from that of the phenothiazines. Imipramine is ineffective in ameliorating the thought disorders in schizophrenic patients; on the other hand, it has a distinct mood-elevating effect in many patients who are suffering from endogenous depression.

Mood elevation is effected only in depressed patients; normal individuals show neither elation nor euphoria and generally find the drug unpleasant to take. The excesses of central nervous system stimulation such as tremors, convulsions, and mania which are seen in patients on MAO inhibitors are seldom seen in patients receiving tricyclic antidepressants. Instead, sedation is the prominent effect of these drugs, in depressed patients and normal persons alike.

Atropine-like, antimuscarinic side effects are prominent with the tricyclic antidepressants, and patients are often troubled with dry mouth, blurring of vision, and urinary retention. Tricyclic antidepressants have been used in the treatment of enuresis, probably because of their atropine-like properties.

The primary effect of tricyclic antidepressants on the sympathetic portion of the autonomic nervous system is to block the uptake by adrenergic nerve fibers of norepinephrine and several other drugs. Since this uptake by nerve endings is the major mechanism by which the action of endogenous norepinephrine is terminated in the body, the administration of imipramine and related drugs causes a potentiation of some of the actions of the sympathetic nervous system. Tachycardia, hypertension, and cardiac arrhythmias are all recognized side effects of these drugs. Persons with cardiovascular disease are particularly susceptible to certain serious consequences of imipramine administration. Congestive heart failure has been precipitated in individuals with inadequate cardiac reserve. Myocardial infarction has developed, serious arrhythmias have appeared, and sudden, unexplained death has occurred in patients receiving drugs of this family.

Death from acute overdosage is more common with the tricyclics than it is with the phenothiazines, benzodiazepines, or even the MAO inhibitors (though this latter group clearly has a greater overall toxic potential). Imipramine and related drugs are effective suicidal agents, and the depressed patients who receive them are potentially suicidal; therefore, a significant danger exists. The danger is maximal shortly after the initiation of therapy. Before treatment, the patient's mood and bodily activity may both be depressed to the point where he is not energetic enough to act out suicidal impulses. When imipramine therapy is started, physical activity often improves before mood does. Therefore, after a week or two on the drug, the patient may still have suicidal thoughts and be far more able now to act upon them.

Acute overdosage of imipramine causes hyperpyrexia, convulsions, cardiac arrhythmias, and coma. Physostigmine has proved to be effective in reversing this coma and saving the lives of persons poisoned with tricyclics. (Abusive self-administration is not a problem with the tricyclic antidepressants.)

In addition to imipramine, the tricyclic antidepressants include anitriptyline (Elavil), desipramine (Pertofrane), nortriptyline (Aventyl), protriptyline (Vivactyl), and doxepin (Sinequan).

BENZODIAZEPINES

The benzodiazepines form the major chemical family within the pharmacologic group that has been labelled variously as "antianxiety agents" and as "minor tranquilizers." These substances differ markedly from the phenothiazines in that they produce neither antischizophrenic therapeutic actions nor extrapyramidal side effects. They have none of the antidepressant properties of the tricyclics or of the MAO inhibitors. The benzodiazepines share some pharmacologic properties with, but differ in other respects from, the standard, classical sedative-hypnotic drugs such as the barbiturates. Diazepam (Valium), a benzodiazepine, is said to be the most widely prescribed drug in the United States today.

The several benzodiazepines which are available clinically combine sedative, hypnotic, anticonvulsant, and muscle relaxant properties. The sedative effect may be either desirable or undesirable, depending upon the circumstances. As hypnotic agents, the benzodiazepines differ from the barbiturates in that they cause less suppression of rapid eye movement (REM) sleep, but the significance of this difference is not clear. Their anticonvulsant effectiveness is limited by the development of tolerance to this action; thus, the intermittent use of diazepam in the control of status epilepticus is very popular and effective, while for continuous administration in seizure suppression, other drugs are usually preferred. Skeletal muscle relaxation is produced by all sedative agents; under certain circumstances, the benzodiazepines appear to be more specific relaxants than the barbiturates, but often it is difficult to demonstrate such a difference. A specific action against anxiety is not only difficult to prove but is also difficult to define. However, the widespread acceptance of the benzodiazepines by patients and physicians alike suggests that these drugs exert rewarding effects, whether or not these effects can be quantified.

An important difference between the benzodiazepines and the barbiturates can be seen by comparing their dose-response curves: with the benzodiazepines there is a much wider range between the sedative dose and the lethal dose. Large intravenous doses of diazepam may cause respiratory depression or cardiovascular collapse, but by the oral route this drug almost never produces life-threatening symptoms, even when a large number of tablets have been ingested. Thus, the risk of suicide with oral benzodiazepines is very small indeed.

Tolerance and physical dependence develop to the several effects of the benzodiazepines, but when these long-acting drugs are discontinued, the blood levels fall so slowly that abstinence signs do not appear for several days, and then they are usually mild. Discontinuation of very high dosages of a benzodiazepine can precipitate seizures. Habituation is much more prevalent than is physical dependence. Patients become accustomed to taking the drugs regularly, and often the physician finds it difficult to persuade the patient to discontinue the medication, even though no physical abstinence signs develop. To what extent the continued use of a benzodiazepine over long periods constitutes drug abuse is as yet undefined.

Of the many benzodiazepines which have been synthesized and studied, four are available on the American market as antianxiety agents, two are promoted as hypnotic agents to induce sleep, and one is available as an anticonvulsant. The most widely used of the antianxiety agents is diazepam. Chlordiazepoxide (Librium) is slower in its absorption from the gastrointestinal tract than is diazepam, but it shares the latter's relatively long duration of action. Oxazepam (Serax) is a metabolite of diazepam and is shorter acting than the parent compound. Clorazepate (Tranxene) is most similar to oxazepam in chemical structure and is the least well known of this group of drugs. The benzodiazepines which are used primarily as hypnotic agents are flurazepam (Dalmane), which is available in the United States, and nitrazepam (Mogadon), which is widely employed in Great Britain. Clonazepam (Clonopin) has been approved recently in the United States for use as an anticonvulsant in the treatment of absence attacks, myoclonic seizures, and akinetic seizures.

CONCLUSIONS

The availability of the new classes of effective mind-influencing drugs creates several challenges for the physician who would use them. (1) Because these newer agents have complex pharmacologies which differ significantly from those of the classical sedative-hypnotic agents, it is incumbent upon the physician to familiarize himself with the range and complexity of their actions. (2) Accurate clinical diagnosis of the patient's mental or emotional problem is important because the newer agents are much more specific therapeutically than the classical agents are. (3) A recognition of the patient's presenting signs and symptoms, an awareness of his previous medical history, and an understanding of the natural history of his illness are necessary if the physician is to be able to distinguish the symptoms which are being treated by a drug from those which are being caused by it. (4) In the final analysis, the physician must decide not only which drug to use, but whether to employ any drug at all in a particular patient. It may well be that for certain persons the therapeutic results would not be great enough to justify the cost, the toxicity, the potential for drug interactions, and the potential for drug dependence that accompany the use of a mind-influencing drug.

7 Antidepressants

Allan B. Wells, M.D.
Myer Mendelson, M.D.

The chance discovery in the 1950s of two classes of antidepressant drugs has revolutionized the medical treatment of depression. Because of the stimulating effects of amphetamines, much of the clinical research until that time was directed toward animal screening of amphetamine-related drugs.

In 1952, while investigating the usefulness of iproniazid for the treatment of tuberculosis, clinical researchers noted that some of their patients experienced an elevation of mood long before the medication affected their tuberculosis. Dr. Nathan Kline later established the specific antidepressant action of iproniazid (Klein and Gittelman-Klein, 1975), which was related to its ability to inhibit the enzyme monoamine oxidase in various biologic tissues. These findings stimulated an explosive effort to find better and less toxic antidepressants and resulted in the development of a class of antidepressants now known as monoamine oxidase (MAO) inhibitors.

Several years later, and again serendipitously, another class of antidepressants was discovered. In the search for more effective antipsychotic agents, a phenothiazine-like agent related to chlorpromazine was tested in a group of schizophrenic patients. It was found to have no effect on psychotic symptoms, but it appeared to improve depressive symptoms in those schizophrenic patients who were also depressed. Later studies confirmed the effectiveness of this agent in nonschizophrenic patients who manifested only depressive symptoms. Again a surge of investigative work developed a whole class of medications, known as tricyclic antidepressants, of which imipramine was the prototype.

In a matter of a few years, these two unanticipated findings led to the development of a new treatment modality for one of humanity's most painful disorders.

DEPRESSIVE ILLNESS

The word depression is ambiguous. The present psychiatric nomenclature contains a variety of diagnoses referring to depression. These classifications make for some confusion and are presently being revised in a way that will more accurately reflect when antidepressants would be useful. Depression refers to an emotional state or mood which can occur in nonpathologic contexts, in a schizophrenic disorder, or in an affective illness. The actual indications for the use of antidepressants are related more specifically to the presence of *depressive illness*. Although the mood of depression is generally present in depressive illness, this disorder encompasses a wider range of symptoms than the mood disorder alone. Even though the patient may not show such physical signs as a fever, swelling, or a rash, or be diagnosed by laboratory tests or x-rays, depressive illness is a genuine illness, with its own morbidity and mortality.

Depressive illness sometimes falls under the rubric of clinical depression, endogenous depression, primary depression, or bipolar or unipolar depression. It stands in contrast to neurotic disorders, character styles, or grief reactions. Encompassed by the concept of depressive illness are the associated signs and symptoms accompanying the central mood state of depression. The extent to which these other elements are present is crucial in determining the usefulness of antidepressants.

People may describe their depressed mood in numerous ways. They may simply state that they are depressed or "feel blue." Dejection, despondency, sadness, melancholy, "down" are some of the descriptions one hears. Others may say, "I just feel awful," and not be able to attach a specific label to their mood. They may also be experiencing other affects concurrently: feelings of anxiety, guilt, and open hostility are commonly expressed. In some instances these may be the dominant feelings, obscuring or overpowering the depressive mood.

Characteristically, the depressed patient suffers a profound and painful feeling of being unable to cope, sometimes with the most trivial aspects of life. He may feel that brushing his teeth, shaving, or washing his hair is an overwhelming task. If one inquires, the patient may say that he has lost his ability to enjoy life, even in those pursuits that invariably brought pleasure before. The patient feels deadened and is often alarmed because he has lost the ability to love those persons close to him. Further inquiry reveals that there is often a change in mood during the course of the day. The patient indicates that some part of the day is more painful, that his feelings then are more intense. This nadir is commonly experienced in the morning, with improvement occurring as the day goes on. Rationalizations to explain this diurnal variation of mood are common. "The day is coming to an end," or, "I can finally go to sleep," or, "I don't have to face anyone in the evening" are some ways the patient perceives this mood change. More rarely, the situation may be reversed, with mood deteriorating as the day goes on. This diurnal variation of mood is a biologic phenomenon and is unrelated to the particular events of the day each patient may face.

Vegetative Signs

Somatic changes are important clinical signs in depressive illness. Classically, the patient complains of sleep disturbance; he awakens in the middle of the night or early in the morning and cannot fall asleep again. Some patients may complain that they have great difficulty falling asleep at all. Others experience excessive sleep; some so extreme that they sleep up to 12 to 20 hours a day and can barely be roused. Physical signs and symptoms of depressive illness are often related to a general slowing down of the bodily processes: loss of appetite, with subsequent weight loss that may be severe; loss of sexual drive; constipation; weakness; and chronic fatigue are the most common.

Less frequently, patients may experience physical pain: headache, chest pain, or gastrointestinal pain. In some cases this may be so prominent that the other symptoms, even the mood of depression, may be dwarfed by comparison, and the underlying disorder obscured.

Psychomotor Changes

The slowing down of bodily processes has its effect on motor behavior. The patient walks slowly and talks slowly (psychomotor retardation). He may sit for long periods of time in one spot, appearing preoccupied and brooding. The facial muscles are dragged downward giving the appearance of profound melancholia; even a smile on such a face appears incongruous. When the depression is severe, a stuporous state which may mimic catatonic schizophrenia may be present. Paradoxically, some patients may manifest psychomotor agitation, with restlessness, pacing, palpitations, hand wringing, and irritability.

Withdrawal from social contact with family and friends is commonly noted in depressive illness. The patient can no longer bear to cope with other people, and he retreats into isolation. Uncontrollable spells of crying and sobbing may occur and may sometimes last for hours. Occasionally a patient reports that he is so depressed that he feels unable to cry.

Perceptual and Cognitive Changes

Loss of self-esteem is a strikingly consistent finding in depressive illness and is accompanied by self-accusatory, self-critical thoughts. These may be so intense that the patient becomes delusional. Pessimism is rampant, and the world is perceived through a screen of helplessness, hopelessness, and despondency. One feels unable to obtain gratification no matter what effort he makes. If the patient is asked about his concentration, the response will usually be that this is impaired, sometimes to the point where he can't read a newspaper or follow a television program. Hypochondriacal thoughts often arise and may range from preoccupations with heart disease or cancer to the delusion that something inside is rotting away. Occasionally hallucinations may develop, and these are usually self-accusatory and self-condemning.

In view of this experience of lowered self-esteem, self-blame, hopelessness, and pessimism, it is not surprising that most patients with depressive illness think that life is not worth living. This may lead to suicidal ruminations and plans, and finally to action.

Antidepressants are not useful for the treatment of the transient unhappy or unpleasant experiences of life, nor for that of the normal grief reactions to loss. However, when signs and symptoms form the constellation described here, then definitive treatment with antidepressants becomes appropriate.

USING ANTIDEPRESSANTS

At the present time, the tricyclics and the MAO inhibitors are the most frequently utilized antidepressants. Lithium carbonate is also being used in some patients with depressive disorders and will be discussed in another chapter. Amphetamines are stimulants and have limited effectiveness in treating depressive illness when used alone.

General Principles

The following principles are those observed by the authors in their own clinical practice. The first is related to the pharmacology of these medications. Unlike the amphetamines, the minor tranquilizers, or the barbiturates, the antidepressants are slow-acting, and it takes from one to three weeks before clinical improvement is noted after a therapeutic dosage has been reached. This must be stressed to the patient to avoid the misconception that in one or two days he will have symptomatic relief. The clinician must be keenly aware that a trial of a few days is no trial at all.

The second principle is that antidepressants must be used in high enough dosages to be effective. As a class, they are often prescribed in subtherapeutic dosages. While small dosages may be effective in some cases (the elderly, for example), an adequate trial commonly necessitates much higher dosages. For example, a patient who has not responded to 75 to 100 mg of imipramine daily may show dramatic improvement if the dosage is raised to 250 to 300 mg daily. Not uncommonly, however, patients are maintained on subtherapeutic dosages and never attain an effective drug level. In our practice, an adequate trial often constitutes the highest dose that the patient can tolerate. Table 1 lists effective

Table 1
Therapeutic Dosage Ranges of the Antidepressants

Type of Antidepressant	Usual Therapeutic Daily Dosage Range
Tricyclic	
Amitriptyline (Elavil, Endep)	100–450 mg
Desipramine (Norpramin, Pertofrane)	100–450 mg
Doxepin (Adapin, Sinequan)	100–450 mg
Imipramine (SK-Pramine, Tofranil)	100–450 mg
Nortriptyline (Aventyl)	75–250 mg
Protriptyline (Vivactyl)	20–60 mg
MAO Inhibitor	
Isocarboxazid (Marplan)	20–80 mg
Phenelzine (Nardil)	45–150 mg
Tranylcypromine (Parnate)	20–80 mg

therapeutic ranges we and others have determined for both tricyclic and MAO inhibitor antidepressants. It should be noted that maximum dosages are usually higher than those listed in drug package inserts or in the *Physicians' Desk Reference*; in our clinical opinion, the dosages given by these sources are not sufficiently high for a great number of patients.

Some patients may respond to extremely low dosages. These include not only the elderly but other patients as well who probably represent a subclass of "hyperresponders." Conversely, some patients will respond only to extremely large amounts of medication: for example, 500 to 800 mg of amitriptyline daily.

The third principle holds that a systematic trial of all the antidepressants should be attempted until a good clinical response is obtained. At the present time there are six tricyclics and three MAO inhibitors available in the United States. More are on the market in other countries. There is no method as yet to reliably determine which antidepressant will be effective for a particular patient. Someone with depressive illness may respond to any antidepressant, to several, or to only one. This has an obvious corollary. If we can't predict which antidepressant will work, each of them must be tried until an effective one is found for the patient. Occasionally one reads that a clinician should be familiar with one or two tricyclics and one MAO inhibitor. Our clinical experience has been that this is not adequate. We have been impressed with the numbers of patients who do not respond until the fifth, sixth, or last antidepressant has been tried.

These three principles constitute the basis of an adequate therapeutic treatment plan: the patient must be on a medication at a high enough dosage; the duration of the therapeutic trial must be sufficiently long; and if the patient does not respond to one antidepressant, the others must be tried systematically until symptomatic relief is obtained.

It is important that these principles be shared with the patient at the beginning of the first therapeutic trial. If further courses of medication are needed, the patient will have understood from the start that this is part of the treatment plan. Otherwise, some patients will feel that there is in fact no hope for them, or that their treatment consists of repeatedly futile attempts. As part of the therapeutic alliance with the patient, the clinician should also emphasize that the medication will not work immediately and that certain side effects may be anticipated.

Administration

The maximally effective dosage should be ascertained by placing the patient on escalating daily dosages: for example, an initial 25 to 50 mg of imipramine, increased by 25 to 50 mg daily. There is a good deal of evidence that tricyclic antidepressants given as a single dose at bedtime minimize side effects. This is especially true for doxepin and amitriptyline, which have sedating side effects and which therefore often hasten the disappearance of the insomnia so distressing to depressive patients.

Which Antidepressant to Use First?

While it is true that the clinician has little guidance about which medication to use first, the sedating qualities mentioned above often make doxepin and amitriptyline useful first choices. Antidepressants cannot be considered tranquilizers, and they are not useful as antianxiety agents during the day. Patients often complain of grogginess after using them, and this must be taken into consideration.

Generally, our own clinical practice is to use each of the tricyclics before moving on to the MAO inhibitors. In depressions which have phobic features, imipramine may be the first choice.

However, the MAO inhibitors may be the drugs of choice in certain kinds of depressive illness (eg, in patients with an hysterically anxious personality). Some patients with rapid-cycling depression and hypomania also respond better to MAO inhibitors.

The fact remains that most of the time the clinician has no way of predicting which antidepressant the patient will respond to. It is important, therefore, to discover in the initial evaluation whether the patient has been previously depressed, and if so, what treatment has been received. This information is sometimes difficult to obtain, but the results are often very rewarding, for one may find that the patient has in fact been successfully treated previously with an antidepressant. Another trial on the same medication would, of course, be the initial therapeutic choice. It is surprising how often this historical information is not sought.

Similarly, inquiry should be made as to any family history of depressive illness. There is some evidence that effective clinical responses to particular antidepressants run in families. The biological basis for this is speculative, but the clinical observation would seem to lend support to the theory of a genetic component in depressive illness.

Evaluating Clinical Improvement

After the patient has been on an effective dosage for 10 to 21 days, the clinician must evaluate his progress. Some patients may assess their disorder more accurately than others. They may report that they are sleeping better; that they have a greater sense of well-being; that their feelings of helplessness, hopelessness, and social withdrawal are less acute; that they are now able to enjoy different experiences. The clinician is looking only for any sign of improvement, not for complete recovery, which may take weeks or months. He has to decide whether to continue the present medication or to prescribe another, so reports of even minor improvement are important. Some patients may improve but may not experience a sense of being less depressed. The patient may still feel depressed, but perhaps he can now concentrate better, or he may have fewer vegetative signs. Family members may provide valuable information: that the patient is more active, is eating more, or seems to be coping more effectively. It is important at this point to reevaluate this patient in terms of suicidal feelings. Although some aspects of the depression are improved, the continuing feelings of despondency may still be

144

intense. Paradoxically, the patient can now cope better with the complexities of a suicide attempt, and this must be assessed. As time goes on and improvement continues, the patient will in fact begin to experience a sense of improved well-being.

If the therapist notes no improvement after three to four weeks of medication at a sufficiently high dosage, then a change should be implemented. When one tricyclic follows another, it is probably best to raise the dosage of the new antidepressant while lowering that of the previous one. This is not usually difficult for the patient if the clinician writes out the dosage changes for the following week or so. This avoids abrupt withdrawal from medication, which in some cases can lead to nausea, vomiting, and diarrhea for a brief period. Such reactions are a rebound effect of the withdrawal of the anticholinergic effects of the tricyclics. Changing from a tricyclic to an MAO inhibitor generally involves a washout period of four to seven days before the latter is instituted.

How Long on Antidepressants?

The patient has improved; the disabling, painful depressive illness has passed. What is the appropriate therapeutic strategy at this point? The patient is only too eager to stop taking this medication with all its uncomfortable side effects. The apparent alternatives are: to discontinue the medication after the optimal therapeutic effect has been achieved; to maintain the patient at a lower dosage; or to continue treatment at the optimal dosage for four to six months before gradually decreasing the dosage over a period of several months. Patients sometimes take the first course of action without consulting the therapist. In some cases they are able to do this without experiencing a relapse. More commonly, however, they will experience a return of depressive symptomatology over a period of weeks or even months.

Some clinicians recommend continued treatment at a lower, maintenance dosage. Our own clinical experience favors keeping the patient at the high, optimal level of medication for a period of four to six months before gradually lowering the dosage. Lower maintenance dosages do not seem to support the patient when he is under stress, and often the maintenance dosage has to be raised again. Decreasing the dosage slowly over a period of months allows observation of any return of depressive symptoms and may disclose a critical dosage level. The decision to decrease the dosage is also dependent upon the patient's previous history of depression. A patient who has had several depressions in the recent past would naturally be kept on medication for a longer period. (The issue of prophylaxis against depression with lithium carbonate is discussed in another chapter.)

Managing Side Effects

To work with antidepressants is, in part, to work with side effects. The clinician should attempt to have a clear idea of which signs represent side effects, which are depressive symptoms, and which represent adverse effects. Side effects are almost invariable, they usually diminish in intensity with time, and they generally can be handled by reassuring the patient. Adverse effects, while uncommon, usually require discontinuation of the drug and/or other medical intervention. The following are those side effects associated with the tricyclics.

Anticholinergic side effects These are the most common side effects of the tricyclics; it is a rare patient who does not experience at least a dry mouth with therapeutic dosages. Urinary hesitation, frequency, or urgency may occasionally be present. Rarely, urinary retention may occur and may require catheterization or use of bethanecol (Urecholine). Constipation is a common problem and liberal use of laxatives and/or stool softeners is often necessary. This effect is completely reversible, and the patient need not worry about the "laxative habit" after discontinuing the medication. Blurred vision for fine print due to impaired accommodation is also common. This usually recedes with time. Palpitations are also associated with the anticholinergic effect of tricyclics and are usually transient. Small doses of the beta-adrenergic blocker propranolol are effective in stopping this if it is frequent.

Vascular side effects The major vascular side effect is postural hypotension, characterized by dizziness, light-headedness or feeling faint. This usually occurs when the patient is rising from a chair or bed, or going up stairs. It is usually brief, and it diminishes with time. Occasionally the effect will be so severe as to require that the dosage be decreased or the drug discontinued.

Neurologic side effects Trembling is the most common neurologic side effect and usually appears in the higher dosage ranges. Again, this usually diminishes with time, but if it should continue to be bothersome, phenytoin (Dilantin) (up to 200 to 300 mg daily) will usually reduce or eliminate it within a few days. Occasionally, incoordination, loss of balance, and slurred speech are noted with higher dosages. Paresthesias may also occur.

A slight impairment of immediate memory sometimes manifests itself. This is only vaguely annoying to some patients but may be quite distressing to others. It involves only immediate recall and is completely reversible when the medication is stopped. Patients say that they forget what they are saying in midsentence, or forget where they placed things. Reassurance is necessary, especially for older patients, who may fear that they are becoming senile.

Transient visual hallucinations, which usually involve the perception of small animals or insects, also may occur with tricyclics. Remarkably, most patients state that they are unconcerned about these hallucinations and ascribe them spontaneously to the medication.

Weight gain Patients on antidepressants (both tricyclics and MAO inhibitors) often gain weight. The gain is usually modest but may occasionally be large. This may be ascribed to one of the following: 1) patients moving out of a depressive state will experience less anorexia and anhedonia and consequently will eat more and enjoy it more; 2) the antidepressants themselves may excite the appetite centers of the subthalamic nuclei, causing a greater caloric intake; 3) an undefined metabolic change may occur which causes weight gain without appreciable excessive caloric intake.

Sexual side effects Occasionally patients report delayed ejaculation or inability to ejaculate. Impotence may also occasionally occur.

Other common side effects Excessive perspiration about the head and shoulders is transiently noted in many patients. A few of the tricyclic antidepressants have a tendency to cause nausea; an antacid is particularly useful for this complaint.

Adverse Reactions

Although far less common than side effects, adverse reactions requiring medical intervention and occasionally cessation or reduction of the medication may happen.

Psychiatric effects　All antidepressants have the potential to precipitate a manic episode in a patient with an underlying bipolar depressive disorder. The clinician should evaluate the patient periodically for the presence of racing thoughts, euphoria, hyperactivity, pressure of speech, and impaired judgment. The addition of lithium carbonate is appropriate at this time.

Precipitation of a schizophrenic episode has also very occasionally been noted, although at times this may be difficult to distinguish from a manic attack.

In recent years, attention has been drawn to the possible inducement of a psychosis by the tricyclics. This is related to their anticholinergic (atropine-like) effects. It is manifested by a confusional state, with disorientation, delirium, hallucinations, and elevated body temperature. This can be dramatically reversed by discontinuing the antidepressant and giving a small (0.5 to 1.0 mg) intramuscular dose of physostigmine.

Seizures　At higher dosages all antidepressants may cause seizures, generally of the grand mal type. Usually the addition of an anticonvulsant is sufficient to prevent recurrence. The patient should be evaluated to rule out coincidental underlying organic brain disease.

Glaucoma　Rarely, the anticholinergic properties of the antidepressants may precipitate an attack of narrow-angle glaucoma in patients predisposed to this disorder. In the case of a patient with pre-existing glaucoma, antidepressants may still be administered if ocular pressures are monitored.

Cardiovascular effects　Psychotropic drugs, including the antidepressants, commonly cause electrocardiographic changes, especially S-T and T wave changes. This, as well as occasional palpitations, are benign. Recent work has suggested, however, that some patients may experience more severe arrythmias, including ventricular tachycardia and asystole. These would require appropriate monitoring and medication and do not necessarily mean that the antidepressant has to be discontinued. Although antidepressants should not be used during the acute stage of a myocardial infarction, they may be used cautiously in the period following this if so indicated. They may be safely used in patients who have concurrent hypertension.

Other adverse effects　Rarely, the following additional adverse reactions are reported: allergic reactions, especially rashes; hematologic reactions; and liver toxicity.

ANTIDEPRESSANTS, THE PATIENT, AND THE FAMILY

In addition to the painful consequences of experiencing a depressive episode, the patient often has great difficulty dealing with family members, friends, and "important others." Patients are often told by these well-intentioned persons to "pull yourself together," to "lift yourself by your own bootstraps." They are told that they must help themselves, or that medicine can't do it all. The patient's self-esteem and ability to cope are already impaired; these pressures add to his self-blame and self-criticism. It is often useful for the therapist to intervene and explain to the family the nature of the illness and the counterproductive quality of such urgings. The family should be advised to let the patient do things at his own pace and not to push him into attempting activities which in reality won't make him feel better but rather will tend to aggravate the already existing pathologic elements of depressive illness.

An incidental question that frequently arises is whether the antidepressants are addictive. The therapist can state with absolute assurance that they are not.

MAO INHIBITORS

This class of antidepressants is greatly underutilized in the treatment of depressive illness. Because of liver toxicity and toxic interaction with certain foods when they were first introduced, they have acquired an undeserved bad name. Often a patient will be warned by persons only slightly familiar with MAO inhibitors that they are taking a toxic, dangerous drug. Liver toxicity was associated with one of the first MAO inhibitors, Marsilid, which was withdrawn from the market. Those currently on the market, in our experience, do not have any significant effect on the liver.

In our own experience, a significant minority of patients respond only to MAO inhibitors. We have found these drugs to be safe when appropriate dietary and drug restrictions are observed. Furthermore, on the whole their side effects are often less prominent and less distressing than those of the tricyclics.

The "Cheese Reaction"

When MAO inhibitors were first placed on the market, some patients experienced transient elevations of their blood pressure, sometimes to extreme levels. In several cases, patients experienced cerebral bleeding and died. It was soon discovered that these reactions occurred following the ingestion of aged cheeses. Further investigation revealed that this was related to the high levels of the bioamine tyramine which are present in aged cheeses. MAO inhibits the destruction of this monoamine, allowing it to accumulate and eventually act as a blood-pressure-elevating agent. Within minutes to hours after eating foods containing high levels of tyramine, the patient may experience a hypertensive crisis characterized by excruciating headache, chest pain, palpitations, and apprehension. The same reaction can occur with certain other foods containing large amounts of tyramine, including chicken livers, pickled herring, beer, and Chianti wine. Certain drugs, such as amphetamines and cold remedies containing decongestants, may also cause a hypertensive reaction (see Table 2 for a list of foods and substances to be avoided while on MAO inhibitors). For some as yet unexplained reason, the narcotic meperidine (Demerol) also has this effect,

Table 2
Foods and Substances Which May Cause Hypertensive Crises When Taken in Combination with MAO Inhibitors

Foods (contain high tyramine levels)*
    Cheese (especially aged cheeses)
    Wines (especially Chianti)
    Pickled herring
    Chicken liver
    Sour cream
    Beer
    Yeast extract
    Pods of broad beans (Fava beans)
    Soy sauce
    Canned figs
    Raisins
    Chocolate
    Excessive amounts of beverages containing caffeine

Substances
    Amphetamine and its derivatives (Dexedrine, Ritalin, Preludin, Tenuate, etc)
    Ephedrine[†]
    Pseudoephedrine
    Epinephrine[†]

*There is also some indication that high intake of cyclamates and monosodium glutamate may precipitate this reaction.
[†]Commonly contained in cold remedies.

although it is apparently unrelated to tyramine metabolism. With the patient properly instructed, this reaction will not occur, unless the patient inadvertently ingests one of the substances listed. In the event of hypertensive crisis, intravenous phentolamine (Regitine), a potent, rapid-acting hypotensive agent, is the appropriate treatment.

Patients with active asthma should not be placed on MAO inhibitors because of the need in these cases to use agents containing ephedrine. Neither should patients with pheochromocytoma, a rare tumor which causes hypertension, be placed on MAO inhibitors.

Side Effects of MAO Inhibitors

As noted previously, the side effects are generally less prominent than those of the tricyclics. Postural hypotension is the most common, but it usually diminishes with time. It is interesting that lowering of blood pressure is one of the basic actions of the MAO inhibitors. In fact, one of them (pargyline) is marketed for the treatment of hypertension.

Some patients experience mild anticholinergic side effects which include constipation, urinary hesitancy, blurred vision, and dry mouth. These effects are generally far less intense than those of the tricyclics.

Among other minor side effects, some patients report that they have difficulty getting to sleep. Taking the medication earlier in the day usually overcomes this insomnia. Excessive weight gain is sometimes experienced. Sexual dysfunction may also be reported by some patients; impotence and delayed ejaculation are the common complaints.

Other Drug Interactions

Synergism with the central nervous system depressant effects of alcohol, anesthetics, barbiturates, and other sedatives is a possibility with the use of MAO inhibitors, and patients must be cautioned to lower their intake of such substances and to report that they are taking MAO inhibitors prior to any surgery. Patients undergoing dental treatment should advise their dentists that they are taking MAO inhibitors, because the use of local anesthetics combined with epinephrine may elevate blood pressure.

COMBINATION THERAPY WITH MAO INHIBITORS AND TRICYCLICS

A small percentage of patients with depressive illness do not respond to the tricyclics, the MAO inhibitors, or to electroconvulsive therapy. In such patients the use of MAO inhibitors in combination with tricyclics has been found to be increasingly useful. Despite warnings on package inserts not to combine these two types of medication, a number of studies have demonstrated the combination to be safe. The original cases which formed the basis for prohibiting this combination have been found to have been either the results of toxic overdoses in suicide attempts or idiosyncratic reactions to either of the two medications, apart from their use in combination. When we give these medications in combination, we generally add small doses of tricyclics to the MAO inhibitor and gradually increase the tricyclic dosage.

CONCLUSION

The antidepressants have provided medicine with potent new tools for treating an illness that is painful and disabling. It should be noted that roughly one out of every eight persons will experience a depressive illness sometime in his or her life. The recognition and vigorous treatment of this disorder have been discussed in detail. To treat it effectively, an adequate trial of medication should be used. This trial demands: 1) a sufficient duration of treatment; 2) a high enough dosage; and 3) a systematic trial of all the antidepressants until one has been found which provides the appropriate therapeutic response.

REFERENCES

American Psychiatric Association: *Diagnostic and Statistical Manual of Mental Disorders.* 2d ed. Washington, D.C: American Psychiatric Association, 1968.

Ayd, F. J.: *Recognizing the Depressed Patient.* New York: Grune & Stratton, Inc., 1961.

Beck, A.T.: *Depression: Clinical, Experimental, and Theoretical Aspects.* New York: Harper & Row, Publishers, Inc., 1967.

Beck, A.T., Ward, C.H., Mendelson, M. et al: An inventory for measuring depression. *Arch Gen Psychiatr.* 4:561, 1961.

Chodoff, P.: The depressive personality: a critical review. *Arch Gen Psychiatr.* 27:666, 1972.

DiMascio, A. and Shader, R., eds: *The Clinical Handbook of Psychopharmacology*. New York: Science House, 1970.

Freedman, A.M. and Kaplan, J.I., eds: *Comprehensive Textbook of Psychiatry*. Baltimore: The Williams & Wilkins Co., 1975.

Gander, D.R.: Treatment of depressive illness with combined antidepressants. *Lancet* 1:107, 1965.

Gaylin, W., ed: *The Meaning of Despair*. New York: Science House, 1968.

Hollister, L.E.: *Clinical Use of Psychotherapeutic Drugs:* Springfield, Ill: Charles C Thomas, 1973.

Hussain, M.Z. and Chaudhry, Z.A.: Single vs divided doses of imipramine in the treatment of depressive illness. *Am J Psychiatr.* 130:1142, 1973.

Jacobsen, E.: *Depression: Comparative Studies of Normal, Neurotic, and Psychotic Conditions*. New York: International Universities Press, 1971.

Klein, D.F. and Davis, J: *Diagnosis and Drug Treatment of Psychiatric Disorders*. Baltimore: The Williams & Wilkins Co., 1976.

Klein, D.F. and Gittleman-Klein, R.: *Progress in Psychiatric Drug Treatment*. New York: Brunner/Mazel, Inc., 1975.

Saraf, K. and Klein, D.F.: The safety of a single daily dosage schedule of imipramine. *Am J Psychiatr.* 128:115, 1971.

Schuyler, D.: *The Depressive Spectrum*. New York: Jason Aronson, Inc., 1975.

Spiker, D. and Pugh, D.: Combining tricyclic and monoamine oxidase inhibitor antidepressants. *Arch Gen Psychiatr.* 34:828, 1976.

Zung, W.: From art to science: the diagnosis and treatment of depression. *Arch Gen Psychiatr.* 29:328, 1973.

8 Chemotherapy of Anxiety

Harry Zall, M.D.

DEFINITION OF ANXIETY

Anxiety refers to an apprehensive feeling tone which can become unbearably distressing, and to accompanying physical symptoms (eg, labored breathing, palpitations) which are the somatic manifestations of this state. In some persons the psychic aspect of anxiety is prominent, while in others somatic distress is the primary focus of concern. Anxiety feels quite similar to fear. Ordinarily, though, fear is defined as a response to a realistic, consciously recognized danger, whereas anxiety occurs as a reaction to vague, unclear dangers which are conjured up and magnified in the unconscious regions of the mind. Even when a realistic threat evokes a disproportionately excessive fear reaction, an element of anxiety is contained therein.

153

NORMAL ANXIETY IN DEVELOPMENT

Probably everyone experiences pangs of anxiety at some time during his life. In fact, normal anxiety is assigned an important role in fostering personality development. At every stage of development, the organism encounters opposing needs, which favor the status quo on one side and change on the other. Since both nature and society demand change, anxiety is aroused in response to the unknown which lies beyond change. This anxiety fuels the growing organism's need to use its resources to adjust to its biologic and psychic development. One reward of making a satisfactory adjustment at a new level of maturation is the alleviation of this anxiety. For example, an infant whose neurons have become myelinated will feel an urge to walk. However, walking may result in his moving too great a distance from the secure presence of mother, and this creates anxiety. The infant then hurries back to mother, and the anxiety is relieved. In normal development, the pleasure of learning the skill of walking, and finding that it results in no permanent loss of mother, overcomes the anxiety involved and leads to the acquisition of the motor function of walking. During adulthood, the need to make a decision which risks loss of a source of security, or an argument between marital partners which has similar risks, may arouse anxiety. If the anxiety is short-lived, is not disabling, and results in the mobilization of successful coping devices, it is not considered abnormal.

PATHOLOGIC ANXIETY

Pathologic anxiety is that which, because of its intensity, persistence, and/or recurrence, interferes with the performance of one's daily tasks. Also implied in this condition is the failure of the organism to take appropriate measures to relieve the anxiety. The distinction between usual, expected occurrences of anxiety and pathologic anxiety is not sharply delineated.

Some individuals can tolerate more subjective discomfort than others (as is true of tolerance for pain). Furthermore, a given individual will exhibit varying tolerances of anxiety at different times, depending upon his general internal sense of well-being, the amount of gratifying interactions with his environment, the subjective meaning of the stresses to which he is exposed, and the availability of flexible coping devices to manage stress. For example, a pregnant woman with no previous history of unmanageable anxiety may suffer this experience because of mounting pressures. Pressures from increasing physical discomfort in the third trimester of pregnancy, an irritable husband who is preoccupied with financial problems, worry about her ability to deliver a healthy baby because of a weight gain of over twenty pounds, and an inability to enjoy her usual, relaxing pastimes may combine to exceed her tolerance level for danger-evoking stimuli. Too much stress, too few gratifications, and limitations on her range of coping resources predispose her to an acute anxiety state. Implied in all instances of anxiety is a threat of future danger. The source of danger in anxiety states exists in the unconscious recesses of the mind, as opposed to the situation of fear, where the source of danger is external.

A stress (or stressor) is a stimulus, the threatening nature of which causes a heightened state of arousal in the central nervous system and activates the autonomic (especially the sympathetic) nervous system. Some stressors (such as an automobile accident) are universally acknowledged as unpleasant, but to certain anxiety-prone subjects the discomfort is exaggerated. Other stressors derive their identity as such only through their special meaning to the subject. For example, after learning that a much desired promotion had been granted him by his employer, a patient experienced anxiety because the promotion threatened him with separation from close friends whose goodwill had supported his sense of security and self-esteem in his former position.

Although it is common to think of unpleasant environmental events as sources of stress in themselves, it is actually the internal and unconscious, exaggerated sense of danger aroused by the environmental event which is more directly linked to anxiety. For example, a naval recruit who began living in confined quarters on board ship had an anxiety attack because the close proximity of the other sailors aroused latent, forbidden homosexual desires. Other unconscious sources of anxiety include hostile or dependency impulses, the expressions of which are threatening to the patient. Further sources are exaggerated fears of attack, physical harm, loss of prestige, competition, and losing a person who provides love and security. Any environmental event which implies one or more of these unconscious dangers can become a stressor for a vulnerable person and can precipitate an anxiety attack.

The term *conflict* refers to lack of harmony between what a subject can manage comfortably and the demands or pressures within him and/or from the environment. Conflict leads to a sense of danger and anxiety.

PSYCHOSOCIAL MODELS OF ANXIETY

Numerous theoretical models pertaining to the psychologic and social natures of anxiety have been constructed. Only a few will be referred to here. Sigmund Freud's theories (1936) view anxiety as an unpleasant psychologic state which is produced by the threat that an unconscious impulse, forbidden by society and/or personal conscience, will become consciously recognized and perhaps acted out. The anxiety serves as a signal for the mind to use defense mechanisms to ward off the impulse. If the defenses cannot keep the impulse under control, the threat of its eruption into consciousness can lead to intense anxiety, known clinically as an anxiety state (or anxiety neurosis). Freud emphasized what he considered to be the central role played by the forbidden, aggressive, and, especially, the sexual instincts in producing anxiety.

Harry Stack Sullivan's theories (1953) focus on the interpersonal rather than the instinctual sources of anxiety. He believes that the basis of most anxiety is a child's fear of mother's disapproval, and that this is later extended to a fear of disapproval from other important persons.

Erich Fromm (1941) speaks of anxiety as emanating from the intrinsic aspects of man's existence; of existential anxieties such as anxiety over death, physical damage, loneliness, and insignificance.

Carl Rogers (1951) has stated that anxiety occurs when an individual perceives a threat to his self-concept.

Sandor Rado (1956) has attempted to explain how inborn, biological reactions are integrated with psychosocial responses in man. He speaks of inborn emergency emotions, including fear (same as anxiety in his model), which are modified by social experiences during childhood development to produce higher stratifications of emotional reaction. For example, fear could be modified to guilty fear, a reaction which Rado believes is evoked to promote a maladaptive attempt at forcing forgiveness from others.

Klein and Davis (1969) refer to ethological studies which indicate the presence of innate fear responses. Young animals exhibit fear reactions upon being separated from parents (similar to separation anxiety in humans), and socially naive monkeys become fearful when shown photographs of aggressive males (similar, perhaps, to castration anxiety, a fear of having one's genitals mutilated). It appears likely that humans are born with some innate fear responses which can be modified by subsequent learning experiences. An innate predisposition to fear may facilitate learning to perceive danger.

NEUROPHYSIOLOGIC MODELS
OF ANXIETY

Mirsky (1960) defines anxiety as a complex, multidimensional response to any event, physical or symbolic, which threatens the physiologic, psychologic, or social integrity of the organism. Pathologic anxiety involves an intrapsychic threat from which there is no escape because the threat is not understood by the subject. Mirsky adds that the systems crucial to expressing anxiety are the brain's reticular system, the limbic system, and the hypothalamus. The reticular system is activated to establish an emotional background of danger; the limbic system provides further emotional coloring; the hypothalamus adds further coloring and also regulates the autonomic motor and hormonal responses associated with anxiety. The newborn infant reacts to noxious stimuli with a diffuse, reflexive, unpleasant feeling state. Later in development, unpleasant feeling states become more differentiated (fear, anxiety, anger, jealousy), and the child associates these with objects and situations. Memory traces of these early experiences are deposited in the brain. Later in life, stimuli with meanings similar to those of the childhood memories can evoke a latent anxiety state. Mirsky hypothesizes that some persons are more prone to anxiety than others due to genetic variations, different early object relationships, and different impacts of early learning experiences on the central nervous system.

Lehman and Ban (1973) note three components of anxiety: arousal, affect, and apperception. Arousal, a function of the brain's reticular activating system, accounts for the intensity of anxiety. Affect, which refers to feeling tone, somatic characteristics, and behavior associated with anxiety, is elaborated by the limbic system. (The limbic system refers to functionally related parts of the phylogenetically more primitive regions of the brain. These areas are buried anatomically by the neocortex, which grew over and around them in man.) Apperception, which refers to the cognitive aspects of a feeling experience, is a function of the brain's neocortex. Lehman and Ban believe that these three components are linked together in an integrated feedback network.

Lader (1972) has formulated a conceptual model of emotion which includes anxiety. He believes that stimuli, both external and intrapsychic (ie, drives, needs), are first evaluated cognitively. If a stress is perceived, either consciously or unconsciously, central nervous system arousal occurs which forms the background for the appropriate emotion. The particular emotion is determined by the interpretation of the cognitive data (eg, an imminent danger evokes anxiety). Arousal is produced by centers in the brain stem. Integration of the physiologic and behavioral aspects of the emotional response is a function of the limbic system and of the hypothalamus. The peripheral changes are mediated by the autonomic nervous system, especially by the beta-adrenergic system. Lader believes that chronic exposure to anxiety-evoking stimuli can produce such a heightened arousal state that arousal (and anxiety) can become autonomous—no longer dependent on specific stimuli.

NEUROCHEMICAL MODELS
OF ANXIETY

Obviously, knowledge of the biochemical correlates of anxiety would have important implications for drug treatment of this condition. However, due in part to the fact that complex chemical alterations take place throughout the body in anxiety, the primary causal factors continue to be elusive.

Neuroendocrine studies of anxious patients have often focused on adrenocortical activity. Stress and heightened anxiety frequently have been correlated with elevated levels of plasma and of urinary 17-hydroxycorticosteroids, the metabolic products of cortisol. Despite these elevations, the resultant levels of these metabolites are usually still within normal physiologic limits. Furthermore, it has been established that emotional arousal in other than anxiety states also exhibits increased secretion of cortisol by the adrenals. Therefore, it is possible that increased cortisol production is an expression of a relatively nonspecific state of arousal or distress rather than a specific manifestation of anxiety.

Warburton (1974) has hypothesized that stress is perceived

by the brain's neocortex and results in a signal to the hypothalamus, which in turn initiates the release of adrenocorticotropic hormone (ACTH) from the pituitary into the blood circulation. This results in increased secretion of corticosteroids into the circulation. Warburton believes that these hormones stimulate ascending neurochemical structures in the brain and cause heightened arousal and thereby contribute to anxiety.

Levi (1969) reports that the concentration of the catecholamines epinephrine and norepinephrine, both produced by the adrenal medulla, are increased in urine samples collected during stress situations. Other studies of catecholamine levels during stress show more equivocal findings. Basowitz (1956) infused epinephrine intravenously into subjects with histories of anxiety and evoked symptoms similar to those reported by the subjects at their initial interviews. Breggin's (1964) comment on Basowitz's work is skeptical. He notes that the anxiety symptoms which were evoked with epinephrine infusion might have been due to the stress of the experimental setting and to a learned response of anxiety to the heart palpitations caused by epinephrine rather than to a direct response to epinephrine per se. Elmadjian et al (1957) have reported that active, aggressive, emotional displays correlate with norepinephrine secretion, whereas tense, anxious, inhibited reactions correlate with increases in secretion of epinephrine.

Such findings may relate to the work of Gellhorn (1961). Gellhorn (1969) employs Hess' concept of two, opposing coping systems which normally operate to maintain the organism in an adaptive, homeostatic balance during its constant exposure to environmental and intrapsychic stimuli. These antagonistic systems are controlled by central nervous system mechanisms. One system, the ergotropic, is associated with heightened arousal and behavioral activity and with increased sympathetic nervous system responses (increases in blood pressure, heart rate, perspiration, respiratory rate, and muscle tone; slowing of gastrointestinal activity). Increased secretion of epinephrine, norepinephrine, corticosteroids, and thyroxin is also observed. The opposing system, the trophotropic, is characterized by relaxation, drowsiness, decreased behavioral activity, and a pronounced parasympathetic nervous system discharge (decreases in blood pressure, heart rate, perspiration, and skeletal muscle tone; increased gastrointestinal motility). Acetylcholine release and insulin levels are increased.

Normally, when one system is activated there follows a compensatory response of the opposing system to restore internal equilibrium. An acute fear response demonstrates this. At first there is a prominent trophotropic reaction (cardiac rate slows, blood pressure drops, muscle tone decreases, perhaps one faints), and this is followed by a compensatory increase in ergotropic activity.

Chronic anxiety states are believed to result from a repeated overactivation of the ergotropic system accompanied by a secondary overreaction of the trophotropic system. This results in a pathologic excitation of both systems simultaneously with no automatic return to an equilibrium. It is possible that an excess of the ergotropic hormone, norepinephrine, in the central nervous system may mediate many of the responses of anxiety.

Stein et al (1973) note that anxiety-relieving drugs (eg, the benzodiazepines, meprobamate) exhibit a disinhibitory effect on suppressed behaviors (eg, behaviors which have previously been punished). Antipsychotic drugs (eg, the phenothiazines) lack this property. From their data from animal studies, they conclude that the antianxiety effects of the benzodiazepines are probably not due to an inhibition of brain norepinephrine activity. Instead, their findings imply that the anxiolytic effects of these drugs result from suppression of a serotonin-mediated punishment system whose fibers originate in the lower brain stem and terminate in the diencephalon and midbrain. This antiserotonin (antianxiety) effect is a disinhibitory phenomenon. In contrast, they view the sedative and behavior-suppressing effects of high doses of the benzodiazepines as resulting from a direct, depressant action on a norepinephrine-mediated brain reward system.

Horovitz (1972) has suggested that anxiety may be related to cyclic adenosine monophosphate (AMP) activity in the brain, and that the antianxiety effects of drugs may be mediated by their impact on the cyclic AMP system. He has found that anxiety levels correlate with cyclic AMP phosphodiesterase activity, and that potent anxiolytic drugs depress this activity.

Other biochemical aspects of anxiety that are of particular interest are suggested in those findings which correlate increased thyroid activity with stress and anxiety, and in the observation that hyperthyroidism is often associated with heightened tension and anxiety. Plasma lipids are increased during stress and anxiety states.

Pitts and McClure (1967) report that intravenous infusions of sodium lactate in susceptible persons evoke anxiety symptoms very similar to the spontaneous anxiety attacks experienced by these patients. Their explanation for this phenomenon has been criticized. Nevertheless, there does appear to be a connection between lactate infusion and incidences of anxiety in some subjects. Since lactate stimulates release of epinephrine and norepinephrine from the adrenal medulla, perhaps this is further evidence that these catecholamines play a role in the genesis of anxiety. Pitts and McClure, however, believe that the mechanism of anxiety arousal caused by lactate concerns the complexing of ionized calcium on the surface of excitable membranes.

The James-Lange theory of emotions (1922) has generally not been well accepted. It postulates that the first step in producing emotion involves a change in visceromotor physiology. Then, due to a perception of these changes by the brain, an emotional feeling state is produced. Most researchers and clinicians believe that an emotional feeling tone is produced first, and that this then leads to physiologic changes.

However, Frohlich et al (1966) report that certain instances of cardiac palpitations lead to an anxious feeling state. They conclude that some persons possess overly sensitive beta-adrenergic receptor sites, and that when these cell sites in the heart are activated by epinephrine, tachycardia and palpitations are quickly produced. With time, these persons become noticeably overly sensitive to such changes and react with anxiety. The use of a blocker of the beta-adrenergic receptor site (propranolol) relieves tachycardia and anxiety in some anxious patients. This tends to confirm the belief that a peripheral mechanism (such as cardiac stimulation) may initiate an anxiety reaction in some patients. However, the possibility still exists that beta-adrenergic cell stimulation in the brain may better explain the origin of symptoms of anxiety, including palpitations. There is no conclusive evidence to date to establish the presence of a central nervous system beta-adrenergic cell receptor. (Beta-adrenergic activity in relation to anxiety will be mentioned later, in the drug treatment section.)

CLINICAL PRESENTATION OF ANXIETY

Psychologic Symptoms

Patients suffering from anxiety frequently report that they feel fearful, apprehensive, uptight, pressured, nervous, uneasy, constantly worried, confused, indecisive, or mixed up. There is a sense of insecurity, helplessness, and threat aroused by circumstances which offer no obvious dangers: work, social gatherings, the presence of particular personality types (eg, authoritarian figures, attractive members of the opposite sex). Obstacles which seem minor to the observer appear gigantic to the patient. The patient may express misgivings about his or her competency, despite a driving need to achieve. He or she is unable to relax, feels "like a bundle of nerves," and reveals marked timidity, dependence, and a need to be helped by another person. Along with the accompanying vague sense of apprehension, anxiety may become associated with particular situations, which are therefore avoided (eg, aloneness, crowds, animals, darkness, heights, open spaces). Such fears are termed *phobias*, and they often accompany nonspecific, free-floating anxiety. Temper outbursts, irritability, and a lowered tolerance for frustration are common. Patients report inability to concentrate well on work tasks, distractability, and memory lapses. Sleep is commonly disrupted by difficulty in falling asleep and/or awakenings during the night.

Physical Symptoms

To a greater or lesser extent, somatic complaints usually accompany psychic distress. Some patients will have predominant physical problems and relatively little psychic distress, and others will experience the opposite. Patterns of physical manifestations of anxiety vary from person to person. Some patients will exhibit symptoms of cardiovascular dysfunction, while others will complain of respiratory, gastrointestinal, musculoskeletal, or other somatic problems.

General, sensory, and musculoskeletal These symptoms may include excessive fatigue, often with difficulty in resting and sleeping; headache; pains in the neck, back, chest, or epigastrium; muscle tightness; a sense of pressure or other abnormal sensations inside the head; dizziness; light-headedness; weakness in the legs which interferes with walking; tension or tightness behind the ears; ringing or buzzing auditory sensations; grinding or clicking of the teeth; a heightened awareness of bodily processes.

Cardiovascular The patient may complain of palpitations, chest tightness or pain, excessive perspiration, or throbbing sensations in chest.

Respiratory Typical problems include hyperventilation (sometimes leading to light-headedness, faintness, and paresthesias), labored breathing, sighing, and sensations of choking or inability to swallow.

Gastrointestinal Patients may report dry mouth, nausea, vomiting, diarrhea, epigastric distress (sense of fullness, burning sensations, pain before or after meals), or bowel rumbling sounds.

Genitourinary Disorders include increased urinary frequency, irregular menstrual periods, decreased libido, impotence, and premature ejaculation.

Skin Complaints of facial flushing or pallor, or sensations of heat and/or chills may be made.

Objective Findings during Interview

There are numerous signs of anxiety which may become available to the scrutiny of the examining physician.The patient may assume tense, seemingly uncomfortable postures in his or her chair. He or she may sit far forward; have legs tightly crossed; alternately cross and uncross legs; or fidget from one position to another. Facial expression may appear intense and smiles forced or mechanical. Periodically, the patient may exhibit a wide-eyed stare accompanying an apprehensive facial expression. Pupils may be dilated, and perspiration—especially on the forehead, axillae, and palms—may be apparent. Facial muscles may twitch. Skin color may appear flushed or unusually pale. Vocal sounds may become shaky and hoarse, and frequent sighing is common. Hands may tremble, and frequent, repetitive movements of fingers, hands, or legs often occur.

Objective Measures of Anxiety

There are numerous physiologic changes which accompany anxiety. Their measurement has primarily concerned researchers; the practicing clinician relies largely on patients' reports of subjective discomfort. Examples of these physiologic changes, which can be monitored instrumentally, include increases in heart rate, perspiration, forearm blood flow, finger pulse volume, and electromyographic activity. An electroencephalogram may exhibit an alerting pattern of increased beta and decreased alpha rhythms. Other physiologic correlates of anxiety include a high mean skin conductance, increased fluctuation of spontaneous skin conductance, and decreased habituation of the galvanic skin response. None or several of these findings may be detected in a given instance of anxiety.

DIFFERENTIAL DIAGNOSIS
OF ANXIETY STATES

This chapter considers the nature and treatment of neurotic anxiety states which present clinically as the only (or at least as the overriding) symptom complex. This anxiety usually appears as vague, diffuse, and free-floating, or as anticipatory to some event. Less commonly, it appears as attacks of acute panic involving exquisitely intense symptoms.

In addition to producing these primary anxiety states, anxiety as a symptom can accompany other psychiatric disorders. It is commonly present in depressive illnesses, and when intense, it can mask the depressive component. Depression in middle-aged and older adults often masquerades as anxiety. A careful, probing interview is necessary to detect the underlying depressive disorder. Treatment of mixed anxious-depressive illnesses will be discussed later.

Phobias are anxiety states in which apprehension is connected to specific objects, animate or inanimate, or to certain situations (eg, crowds, enclosed spaces, heights). Often, phobic patients also suffer from nonspecific, free-floating anxiety and from anticipatory anxiety. When anxiety and phobias coexist, it may be difficult (sometimes impossible) to determine where one stops and the other begins. Phobic symptoms can sometimes be relieved by behavior modification techniques, especially systematic desensitization. Free-floating anxiety is not amenable to this technique, although the relaxation component of this treatment may attenuate the severity of the anxiety.

Anxiety can accompany other neuroses: conversion and dissociative reactions; obsessive-compulsive, hysterical, hypochondriacal, and depersonalization neuroses. Treatment of these disorders may be directed at relieving the prominent symptoms with behavior modification techniques or hypnotic suggestion, or at uncovering, by means of psychoanalysis or psychoanalytically oriented psychotherapy, the presumed, unconscious conflicts which give rise to the symptoms. If not severe, the accompanying anxiety may require no separate attention. However, if it causes significant discomfort, minor tranquilizers may be useful for symptomatic relief.

Schizophrenic patients frequently experience anxiety along with their more typically psychotic symptoms of illogical thinking, inappropriate emotional expression, and autistic withdrawal. Minor tranquilizers are usually of little benefit for this type of anxiety, and it is more effectively treated with antipsychotic drugs.

Anxiety is commonly encountered in patients suffering from organic brain syndromes. In part, it probably represents the patient's fear about the impairment of intellectual functioning which occurs in these conditions. Minor or major tranquilizers can be useful in relieving this anxiety.

Anxiety can occur during the aura or in the postictal phase of a seizure. In fact, temporal lobe seizures may sometimes present as brief anxiety attacks. In such cases, the phasic recurrences of anxiety along with other, ictal symptoms should raise a suspicion of a seizure problem and result in an electroencephalographic diagnostic study.

Sometimes anxiety can be confused with medical disorders. Hyperthyroidism also presents with nervousness, tremor, increased perspiration, tachycardia, and diarrhea. Anxiety which presents primarily as somatic complaints, with relatively little psychic distress, can mimic coronary artery disease, peptic ulcer, hypoglycemia, colitis, and bronchial asthma. Sometimes the physical symptoms of these disorders are relieved by treatment with antianxiety drugs alone. Such instances indicate a causal role by anxiety.

Pheochromocytoma is a rare condition which causes bouts of tension, diaphoresis, palpitations, cool extremities, and chest and abdominal pains. The outstanding feature is the severely elevated blood pressure which accompanies these episodes of acute symptoms.

The abstinence syndrome, which follows withdrawal from alcohol or sedative-hypnotic drugs, produces anxiety, tremors, sweating, and insomnia and, especially in mild to moderately severe cases, can be mistaken for an anxiety state. A thorough history, including interviews with friends and relatives, usually reveals the abuse problem.

Akathisia, an extrapyramidal system dysfunction usually associated with use of phenothiazines or other antipsychotic drugs, can also be mistaken for anxiety. The patient complains of tension, restlessness, sensations of shaking or quivering inside the abdomen, and an inability to sit quietly. Usually, subjective apprehension is not prominent. This involuntary state of motor overactivity can sometimes be relieved with antiparkinsonism drugs, antihistamines, or sedatives. Donlon (1973) reported that diazepam (5 mg three times per day) was useful in relieving akathisia even where the antiparkinsonism drug benztropine mesylate and the antihistamine diphenhydramine had failed.

DRUG TREATMENT
OF ANXIETY STATES

When the nature of anxiety was discussed earlier, it was noted that it is a stressful stimulus which contains in its subjective meaning to the patient a symbolic element of danger which initiates the events in the central and peripheral nervous systems which are associated with the state of anxiety. Those central mechanisms which are probably involved in this process include activation of the reticular formation and hypothalamus, and stimulation of parts of the limbic system. Presumably, effective drug treatment interferes with these events in the central nervous system. An exception may be the beta-adrenergic blocking agents, which may act primarily by interrupting the peripheral manifestations of anxiety.

Lader (1972) characterizes the drugs used in treating anxiety as palliative, not curative. They alleviate emotional and behavioral symptoms but do not alter the vulnerability of a patient in terms of constitutional factors, personality structure, or underlying psychic conflict. Rickels (1973) states that these drugs reduce the level of behavioral arousal, induce a sense of relaxation and well-being, increase responsiveness to environmental stimuli, disinhibit fear-inhibited behavior, and foster social approach behavior without impairing the sensorium, distorting judgments, or interfering with performance.

Those categories of drugs most commonly used in treating anxiety states are the barbiturates, the propanediols, the benzodiazepines, and diphenylmethane antihistamines. When employed primarily for relief of anxiety, these drugs are called antianxiety drugs, minor tranquilizers, anxiolytics, or sedative-hypnotics. These terms will be used interchangeably.

The drugs most commonly used in treating psychoses (the major tranquilizers, antipsychotic drugs, or neuroleptics) are sometimes helpful in relieving anxiety. Drugs usually indicated in the treatment of primary depressive disorders (tricyclic antidepressants, monoamine oxidase [MAO] inhibiting drugs) are on occasion also beneficial in alleviating anxiety symptoms.

BARBITURATES

Barbiturates were the uncontested drugs of choice for treating anxiety states until the 1950s, when the minor tranquilizers were introduced into clinical use in psychiatry. The more limited central nervous system depressant effects of the minor tranquilizers constituted an important reason for the change in preference. At comparable anxiety-relieving doses, barbiturates inhibit neocortical functions, whereas the minor tranquilizers do not; and the antianxiety:sedative dose ratio is greater with the latter. Consequently, the minor tranquilizers have a wider dose range in which anxiety relief occurs without drowsiness or notable loss of awareness and without impairment of reaction time, memory, social judgment, and intellectual functions.

A brief review of some pertinent pharmacologic characteristics of the barbiturates will be presented prior to a discussion of clinical usage. The central nervous system is quite sensitive to the depressant effects of these drugs at doses which have little impact on peripheral organs. Oswald and Priest (1965) observed that barbiturates alter the normal sleep pattern and in particular reduce the amount of rapid eye movement (REM) sleep. As tolerance to the drug develops, REM sleep returns to normal unless the dosage is progressively increased. When their use is discontinued, there may be a rebound effect, with increased time spent in REM sleep. Sleep during these nights is often restless and disturbed by unpleasant dreams.

Although the effects of the barbiturates are generalized in the brain, they have a particularly profoundly depressant effect on the reticular system, which accounts for the drowsiness which they commonly produce even at low doses. All barbiturates have anticonvulsant properties, but phenobarbital is the most widely beneficial in its selective antiseizure activity. At usual antianxiety dosages the barbiturates cause no significant impairment of respiratory or cardiac function. However, at higher dosages the neurogenic respiratory drive center is vulnerable to depression by these drugs.

Tolerance to the barbiturates develops rapidly when they are used at regular, frequent intervals. Two types of tolerance mechanisms are involved. One is the adaptation of central nervous system tissue to their effects. The second derives from their inducing synthesis of liver enzymes which are involved in their degradation. This effect shortens the active life of each molecule and results in a need for higher doses to produce a clinical effect.

The short- and intermediate-acting barbiturates which are commonly used for anxiety relief are metabolized by the liver before being excreted in the urine. Up to 50% of a dose of phenobarbital, a long-acting drug, may be eliminated unchanged by the kidneys. Phenobarbital has a biological half-life of 24 to 96 hours; amobarbital, of 14 to 42 hours.

Clinical Research Findings

There have been numerous reports in the literature to confirm that the barbiturates are effective in relieving anxiety and its somatic manifestations. Klein and Davis (1969) summarized the findings of controlled research investigations involving barbiturates, minor tranquilizers, and placebo. In 11 of 17 studies, barbiturates were significantly superior to placebo. Most of the reports indicated that the benzodiazepines were preferable to the barbiturates, although often not by a statistically significant margin.

Rickels et al (1959) found phenobarbital and placebo to produce significant relief of anxiety of six months' standing or less, but meprobamate and chlordiazepoxide were more effective for anxiety lasting longer than six months.

Lader and Marks (1971), after reviewing studies favoring phenobarbital and, especially, amobarbital over placebo for anxiety states, cautioned about the side effects of drowsiness and impaired psychologic functioning with the active drugs. Lader et al (1974), in a later publication which compared amobarbital, the benzodiazepines, and placebo in patients with chronic anxiety, found no improvement from pretreatment levels of anxiety in the placebo and phenobarbital groups, but the benzodiazepines were shown to be effective. A flexible dosage schedule was used, with a mean dosage of amobarbital of 140 mg/day (range: 60-300 mg); of chlordiazepoxide, 28 mg per day (range: 10-50 mg); and of diazepam, 11 mg per day (range: 2-20 mg).

In a controlled study using fixed dosage schedules (amobarbital, 60 mg three times per day and diazepam, 5 mg three times per day), McDowall et al (1966) found diazepam to be superior to amobarbital in relieving tension and anxiety. Jenner and Kerry (1967) reported similar results: diazepam (5 mg three times per day) was more effective than chlordiazepoxide (10 mg three times per day), and amobarbital (50 mg three times per day) was the least effective of the three. Lorr et al (1961) found that phenobarbital worsened the symptoms of chronically anxious male veterans.

Rickels et al (1970) reported that, after two weeks of treatment, chlordiazepoxide produced better global improvement of anxiety symptoms than did butabarbital. However, at four weeks, no significant differences between the two drugs were noted. Chlordiazepoxide was more effective for patients seen in private psychiatric practice, but amobarbital was preferred by anxious general practice patients. Stotsky (1972) reported better anxiety relief with butabarbital than with chlordiazepoxide in a mixed-age patient sample.

Wheatley (1973) found phenobarbital to be superior to placebo in relieving acute and chronic anxiety. However, chlordiazepoxide proved more effective than phenobarbital, especially after two to four weeks of use. In both trials, phenobarbital was much more useful in acute than in chronic anxiety.

Capstick (1965) compared diazepam (7.5 mg three times per day) and amobarbital (50 mg three times per day) with regard to anxiety-relieving benefits in two-week trials of each drug followed by the other. In all ratings of anxiety, depression, impaired work ability, and decreased appetite, diazepam was clearly superior to amobarbital in providing relief.

These several studies indicate that barbiturates are of greater value in relieving anxiety than are placebos, but that they are not as beneficial as the benzodiazepines. However, inadequate doses of barbiturates may have accounted for their relatively poor showing in some studies. Since they have demonstrated usefulness as anxiolytic drugs, the lesser cost of the barbiturates as compared to the benzodiazepines favors their use in the treatment of anxiety.

Tolerance, Addiction, and Withdrawal

In spite of the barbiturates' effectiveness and lower cost, their use for anxiety relief has declined markedly during the past 20 years. A major reason for this is the tolerance they induce (a patient who uses them regularly will require increasing doses to maintain an even clinical effect). Tolerance predisposes to physical addiction or a withdrawal syndrome if the drug is suddenly discontinued. The basis of barbiturate tolerance is a drug-induced modification of central nervous system tissue metabolism which results in a physiologic requirement for the drug in order to avoid withdrawal symptoms. A severe withdrawal reaction can occur, for example, when a dosage that is four times the usual is taken daily for at least three months and is then suddenly discontinued. An excellent description of the step-by-step evolution of this syndrome is provided by Isbell (1950). In its milder forms, withdrawal presents with anxiety, restlessness, weakness, trembling, and insomnia. In its more severe expressions, convulsions, a psychotic delirium, and death can ensue.

Chronic Intoxication and Overdosing

Because of their anxiety-relieving, euphoria-inducing effects, barbiturates—especially the short- and intermediate-acting compounds (secobarbital, amobarbital, and pentobarbital)— are subject to abuse. Addiction-prone individuals ingest higher than prescribed amounts and become chronically intoxicated. The cortical-depressing effects of this habit include muddled thinking, poor concentration, confusion, poor memory, somnolence, and impaired arithmetical calculating ability. There may also be cerebellar impairments such as a staggering gait, nystagmus, and slurred speech. Continued abuse leads to a loss of emotional control and episodic depressions, hostility, euphoric states, and exaggerated suspiciousness. The addict becomes increasingly preoccupied with achieving a desired state of mind; he disregards the feelings of others and loses interest in his work and in social conventions. A frequent compounding problem is the tendency of barbiturate addicts to abuse other central nervous system depressants, especially alcohol. The abuses can induce a severe clinical depression which may result in suicide through overdose. Ingesting more than ten times the usual hypnotic (sleep-inducing) dose of a barbiturate risks death. Furthermore, despite the development of a high tolerance to the euphoric effects of barbiturates, the required lethal dose may not be much increased. Blackwell (1975) noted the readiness of barbiturates to depress the neurogenic respiratory drive center in the reticular system. This represents an increased danger from even moderate overdosing for patients with bronchial asthma or other respiratory ailments and cardiac disease.

Although the short- and intermediate-acting barbiturates have a high potential for producing the abovementioned complications (habituation, tolerance, physical dependence, chronic intoxication, withdrawal syndromes, risks to life from overdosing), phenobarbital produces less tolerance in clinical practice. Its slow rate of absorption, prolonged activity, and delayed rate of disappearance from the body render it less prone to abuse.

Other Adverse Effects with Barbiturates

Among the numerous potential untoward effects of barbiturates, a drugged, hungover, or depressed feeling is particularly common. This reaction, as well as a paradoxical excitement, is reported most frequently with phenobarbital.

Dawson-Butterworth (1970) commented on the increase in toxic potential accompanying the use of barbiturates in the elderly. Oversedation, hypotension, neurologic symptoms, and excited, confused, delirious states were noted as problems of especial concern in this population.

Summary

In clinical usage, the barbiturates would appear to have a limited indication as primary choices for the treatment of anxiety. Although their anxiety-relieving properties rival those of the benzodiazepines and propanediols, their attendant liabilities (intoxication, dependence, overdosage, withdrawal syndromes) reduce the suitability of their use. Because its potential for addicting is less than that of the short-acting barbiturates, phenobarbital is a better choice of anxiety reliever from this group. However, since it often produces feelings of being drugged or depressed, it is not well accepted by some patients.

The average single dose of barbiturate employed for anxiety relief is one third or one fourth the hypnotic dose. Caution against using doses greater than four times the usual daily amount is necessary because of the risk of producing physical dependence. Parenteral use of amobarbital (200 to 300 mg intramuscularly) is often a rapid and effective means of controlling an acute panic reaction and of providing a patient with needed sleep.

BENZODIAZEPINES

In the late 1950s a new group of anxiolytic drugs, the benzodiazepines, was released for sale on the drug market. Along with meprobamate, they were called "minor tranquilizers" to distinguish them from the "major tranquilizers" (such as chlor-promazine), which are antipsychotic drugs. Unlike the major tranquilizers, the benzodiazepines give no relief from psychotic manifestations such as the distorted cognition and perceptions of schizophrenia and manic-depressive illness. However, like the barbiturates, the benzodiazepines do ameliorate anxiety and its somatic manifestations. Earlier in this chapter it was noted that the barbiturates had widespread depressant effects in both the cortical and subcortical regions of the brain. In contrast, the benzodiazepines have a distinctly subcortical predilection and thus cause less impairment of intellectual functioning at doses which reduce anxiety. Within subcortical structures they have a strong affinity for the limbic system, which is believed to be involved primarily in the modulation, integration, and expression of emotions. Unlike the barbiturates, the benzodiazepines exhibit only a low affinity for the reticular activating system and thus cause less impairment of alertness.

There are at least four benzodiazepines available for routine clinical use in treating anxiety states: chlordiazepoxide, diazepam, oxazepam, and clorazepate. Another benzodiazepine, flurazepam, is employed primarily at bedtime for its hypnotic effects. A brief survey of their pharmacologic properties will be presented prior to discussing the results of clinical research studies on their effectiveness.

Pharmacologic Properties

In addition to their anxiety-relieving effects, the benzodiazepines exhibit skeletal-muscle-relaxing and anticonvulsant properties. The muscle relaxation they cause may contribute to their anxiolytic potency. Anxiety can contribute to an increase in muscle tension, and awareness of this can magnify a person's anxiety and thus add further muscle tension. By interfering with this vicious cycle through muscle relaxation, the benzodiazepines may augment their more direct anxiolytic action. The muscle-relaxing effect is probably due to inhibition of the brain stem reticular formation, the extrapyramidal system, and spinal cord internuncial neurons.

In both animal and human basic research studies, the benzodiazepines released behaviors which had been suppressed by punishment prior to giving the drugs. Phenothiazines did not demonstrate this characteristic. Perhaps this property explains their usefulness for some phobic avoidance symptoms. Unlike the barbiturates, the benzodiazepines do not suppress REM sleep; but they do reduce stage four sleep. Since stage four sleep is reduced in some depressed patients, the mechanism involving its reduction by benzodiazepines may contribute to the side effect of depressed mood reported by some patients.

Their prominent effect on the electroencephalogram is to inhibit slower, alpha rhythms and to induce faster, beta activity and cause increased synchronization of electrical activity. These electroencephalographic changes are similar to those brought about by the barbiturates and meprobamate, but they differ from the slow-wave activity associated with the phenothiazines. The benzodiazepines have little or no effect on the electrocardiogram and cause minimal cardiovascular changes at usual doses.

Diazepam is rapidly absorbed from the gastrointestinal tract and reaches peak plasma concentration in one hour. Oxazepam requires four hours, and chlordiazepoxide, eight hours, to reach peak plasma concentrations. The biological half-lives of these three vary from several hours for oxazepam to approximately two days for chlordiazepoxide. Since diazepam and chlordiazepoxide have a relatively long persistence in the circulation (oxazepam is shorter acting), frequent dosing with these two drugs seems unnecessary. However, rather than use a once or twice per waking day dosage schedule, physicians commonly prescribe a three or four times per 24-hour day dosage schedule. Whether or not this is due more to the prescribing habit of the doctor than to a true drug effect associated with acceleration and deceleration of plasma drug concentrations is not certain. The long persistence of active drug and metabolites in the circulation renders the benzodiazepines less preferable as drugs for abuse (as with phenobarbital and in contrast to the shorter-acting barbiturates). Because of the long biological half-lives of chlordiazepoxide and diazepam, the onset of withdrawal symptoms may be delayed for up to one week in cases of drug abuse.

A large percentage of ingested diazepam is converted to its active metabolite, N-desmethyldiazepam. Dasberg et al (1974) have observed that steady-state plasma concentrations of diazepam cannot be achieved until at least the fifth treatment day, at which time the ratio of diazepam to its active metabolite may approach 1:1. They also note a possible correlation between positive clinical effects and a minimum plasma concentration of diazepam of 400 nanograms/ml. Plasma concentrations of its active metabolite, desmethyldiazepam, above 300 nanograms/ml may correspond to unfavorable responses of anxiety-related, autonomic nervous system symptoms (increased perspiration, tachycardia, increased urinary frequency).

Clinical Research Findings:
Benzodiazepines and Placebo

1. Chlordiazepoxide and placebo Jenner, in two early publications (1961a, b), reported that patients' reports showed chlordiazepoxide (20 mg three times per day) much superior to placebo and to amobarbital (60 mg three times per day). Patients preferred chlordiazepoxide to amobarbital on all parameters, except for the side effect of drowsiness, which was about equally disliked in both drugs. Bodi (1962) compared single, acute dosage trials of chlordiazepoxide and placebo in anxious neurotic outpatients. Thirteen of 14 patients given a single 10-mg dose of chlordiazepoxide exhibited at least a moderate response, as opposed to only 5 of 13 given placebo. In a controlled study involving 43 inpatients with a diagnosis of anxiety neurosis, Maggs and Neville (1964) found no advantages in chlordiazepoxide (10 mg three times per day) over inert placebo. After referring back to the Jenner et al study (1961a), in which chlordiazepoxide (20 mg three times per day) was clearly superior to placebo, Maggs and Neville concluded that the difference in dosages used in the two studies may have accounted for the disparity in clinical response. These conflicting findings are typical of the difficulties involved in assessing the value of drugs for treating anxiety. Neurotic symptoms are notoriously fickle and are responsive to a broad range of situational and interpersonal influences. For example, Rickels and Downing (1967) report that drug-placebo response differences are less notable in anxious clinic patients than in private practice patients.

2. Diazepam and placebo Jacobs et al (1966) found diazepam to be significantly superior to placebo for a group of anxious college students who were receiving psychotherapy. Gundlach et al (1966), in yet another controlled, double-blind study, which used diazepam at a maximum of 40 mg per day, found no differences between active drug and placebo in a group of neurotic outpatients. Dasberg and van Praag (1974) conducted an interesting study which compared diazepam and placebo in a group of inpatients in a crisis unit for a brief treatment period. Diazepam (20 mg per day) or placebo was given for five days. No significant differences were noted in relief of psychic tension or depression; diazepam was superior in relieving insomnia. Autonomic symptoms such as dry mouth, increased urinary frequency or urinary hesitancy, and heart throbbing improved more with placebo than with diazepam. However, respiratory complaints such as hyperventilation and chest tightness, and gastrointestinal problems such as anorexia and changes in eating habits responded better to diazepam than to placebo. This study also found that patients with high pretreatment levels of anxiety clearly responded better to diazepam than to placebo. In low-grade anxiety states no significant differences were observed. Menon and Badsha (1973), in a controlled study over a six-week period, found diazepam statistically superior to placebo for relief of anxious and depressive symptoms. Diazepam assisted patients in gaining confidence and in making a more satisfactory social adjustment.

3. Oxazepam and placebo Oxazepam (average dose: 45 mg per day) was clearly superior to placebo in the several clinical studies of Chesrow et al (1965), DiMascio and Barrett (1965), and Sanders (1965). McPherson (1965) used a crossover design in a double-blind evaluation of oxazepam at 10 mg three times per day, oxazepam at 15 mg three times per day, and placebo. Thirty-three patients with anxiety symptoms visited the hospital clinic for a week's trial of each drug. Both patient and physician ratings found oxazepam (at either dose) much better than placebo. The higher oxazepam dose caused more drowsiness. However, Janecek et al (1966) observed less impressive differences between oxazepam and placebo in another study of anxious outpatients over a short-term trial of one to two weeks.

4. Clorazepate and placebo Charalamporis et al (1973) found that, at doses ranging from 15 to 60 mg per day (mean: 31 mg), clorazepate was significantly superior to placebo in relieving anxiety symptoms. The mean duration of treatment was 21 days. Ricca (1972) reported a statistically superior anxiety-reducing effect of clorazepate to placebo over a 28-day trial period. Doses of clorazepate ranged from 22.5 to 45.0 mg per day.

Klein and Davis (1969) summarized the findings of controlled drug-placebo comparisons involving chlordiazepoxide, diazepam, and oxazepam. Each of the benzodiazepines was found to be statistically superior to placebo in the majority of trials. However, not all studies have favored the minor tranquilizers. For example, in drug research work with anxious U.S. Veterans Administration male patients, Lorr et al (1963) and Caffey et al (1970) found no significant advantage of benzodiazepines over placebo.

A preponderance of clinical research evidence strongly favors the benzodiazepines over placebo in chronic anxiety states. For acute anxiety precipitated by stress, studies still favor the active drugs over placebo, but nonspecific factors such as suggestion, patient expectation, and spontaneous remission tend to blur the advantages of the pharmacologic action in these cases.

Clinical Research Findings: Comparisons among Individual Benzodiazepines

Comparisons among individual members of the benzodiazepine group have, not surprisingly, produced inconsistent results. A few of the studies will be noted, and interdrug differences which offer potentially useful information for their clinical use will be emphasized. On a global basis, it appears that no one drug is far superior to the others.

Dureman and Norrman (1975) compared the effects of clorazepate, diazepam, and placebo in a patient group of anxious students. Both drugs were much superior to placebo. Each drug was given for one week: clorazepate at 10 mg three times per day; diazepam at 5 mg three times per day. Clorazepate was significantly better than diazepam in reducing anxiety and restlessness, muscular tension, and gastrointestinal disturbances. Both drugs were equally effective in managing fatigue, irritability, and sleep disturbances. In ratings by the patients, clorazepate was superior to diazepam in providing better sleep and in maintaining more alertness during the daytime. In a separate study by these same researchers which involved healthy volunteers, diazepam was given at 15 mg per day and clorazepate at 30 mg per day for three days. They were then each given as an additional, single dose shortly before a test of driving skill. There was no impairment of steering precision or brake reaction time with either drug as compared to placebo in these normal subjects. Clorazepate's superior anxiolytic effect in this study may have been due to its higher dosage, which was calculated on a molecular basis. In similar drug comparison studies in which anxiolytic benefits were about equal for both drugs, Wiersum (1972) and Kasich (1973) reported a lesser sedating effect for clorazepate versus diazepam.

Wittenborn (1966) reported that oxazepam was significantly more effective than chlordiazepoxide or placebo in relieving severe anxiety. This correlates with Warburton's finding (1974) that oxazepam was more effective in suppressing corticosteroids released during fear-inducing situations than was either chlordiazepoxide or diazepam. Warburton theorized that corticosteroids released by stress have an arousal effect on ascending neurochemical systems in the brain and that this arousal forms a basis for anxiety.

Tobin et al (1964) compared chlordiazepoxide (30 to 70 mg per day) with oxazepam (45 to 90 mg per day) in trials of two to eight weeks, using two patient study groups and no drug crossovers between groups. Oxazepam was significantly more effective in producing at least moderate global relief of anxiety.

Wheatley (1973) conducted a double-blind crossover evaluation of oxazepam (15 to 30 mg three times per day) and chlordiazepoxide (10 to 20 mg three times per day), with a two-week trial of each. When oxazepam was given first, chlordiazepoxide showed statistically significant superiority. When chlordiazepoxide was given first, it was rated better, but not significantly so statistically. These results show chlordiazepoxide preferable for relief of anxiety. It also caused slightly less drowsiness than oxazepam.

Shader (1970) stated that diazepam was preferable for the anxious, motor-retarded, inhibited patient; chlordiazepoxide was likely to be better for the anxious, hyperactive patient; and oxazepam was probably more suitable for the anxious patient prone to hostile outbursts. In normal volunteers, diazepam and chlordiazepoxide were associated with increased hostility; oxazepam was not. Hollister (1973) believed that the release of hostility by the benzodiazepines was a potentiality of little clinical importance.

In a double-blind, controlled study, Kerry and Jenner (1962) compared diazepam and chlordiazepoxide on the relief of manifestations of anxiety, and they found diazepam better. Both drugs were given in doses of 10 mg three times per day. Anxious neurotic outpatients received first one drug and then the other in two-week trials of each. Thirty-one of 75 patients preferred diazepam, while 16 preferred chlordiazepoxide. Twenty-five patients believed that the drugs were equally useful. Data on the remaining three patients was not available. According to Wittenborn (1966), diazepam has twice the milligram potency of chlordiazepoxide when given orally; therefore, Kerry and Jenner's study may have been biased in favor of diazepam. In separate studies, Aivazian (1964) and Daneman (1964) found diazepam preferable to chlordiazepoxide when given in usual clinical dosages to anxious outpatients.

Rickels (1973) tentatively concluded from statistics in his data bank that greater improvement would be expected for chlordiazepoxide used for higher levels of depression, hostility, and hypochondriasis, and for diazepam given for higher levels of somatization. Using a multiple-regression analytic technique, Rickels found that improvement with the benzodiazepines correlated with a favorable prognosis of the illness, with higher income or education, with the patient's ability to recognize his problems as emotional, and with a history of having received fewer drugs previously. Patients who were employed preferred diazepam or chlordiazepoxide, which are less sedating than hydroxyzine (400 mg per day) or phenobarbital (120 to 150 mg per day).

This sampling of studies would indicate that of the three older benzodiazepines, diazepam is usually superior to chlordiazepoxide for relief of anxiety, and that chlordiazepoxide and oxazepam are of approximately the same value in this respect. Clorazepate, a newer benzodiazepine, has not yet stood a sufficient test of time but shows evidence of being equal to or better than diazepam in its anxiety-reducing properties. However, the results of these and other studies find no one of these four drugs to be unquestionably preferable to the others for global relief of anxiety. The choice of one drug over another will probably depend on the individual clinician's experience with the drugs, on their side effects, and perhaps on certain target symptoms being more responsive to one drug than to another.

On the basis of the studies referred to above, diazepam would appear a good choice for anxiety accompanied by insomnia or gastrointestinal and respiratory complaints, but it would be less preferable when autonomic problems are prominent (eg, dry mouth, excessive perspiration, urinary frequency, heart pounding). Oxazepam would seem to be a rational first choice when irritability and anger accompany anxiety. Clorazepate, and to a lesser extent oxazepam, may be advantageous when daytime drowsiness must be kept at a minimum. Because oxazepam is metabolized more rapidly than the others (with a biological half-life of as short as three hours), it is less likely to accumulate in the body and therefore would be especially beneficial for elderly patients, who are more vulnerable to toxic drug effects. It may also cause less disinhibition in geriatric patients (ie, less agitation and irascibility). A research group of general practitioners (1975) found that clorazepate given in a single, nightly dose of 15 mg produced antianxiety effects throughout the day similar to those of diazepam at 5 mg three times per day.

Side Effects and Toxicity

Overall, the benzodiazepines are extremely safe, and in usual doses they cause only minor side effects. Their only absolute contraindications are a history of severe idiosyncratic or allergic reactions, shock, coma, and myasthenia gravis. Because of the long persistence of these drugs (especially diazepam and chlordiazepoxide) in the body, 5 to 10 days may be required for them to accumulate to the point of establishing a steady-state plasma level. Therefore, therapeutic and side effects may begin to appear only after five days.

The most common side effect is drowsiness, which is a dose-related phenomenon. Not as common, but related also to dose level, are ataxia and slurring of speech. Ataxia is more likely to occur in elderly and debilitated patients. A listing of other infrequently occurring side effects is presented below.

Psychiatric: paradoxical excitement; increased hostility (possibly less likely with oxazepam); euphoria; depersonalization; hallucinations and delusions; depressed feelings with suicidal ideas; rarely, a toxic delirium (more likely in the elderly)

Neurologic: headache; dizziness and vertigo; slurred speech; rarely, hyperkinesia, muscle tenderness, and paresthesias

Autonomic: hypertension; dry mouth; constipation; slow urination; decreased sex drive; increase or decrease in heart rate; weight gain; menstrual irregularities; various allergic rashes

Allergic, other: agranulocytosis and hepatic dysfunction

The benzodiazepines are frequently abused to the extent of causing psychologic dependence (ie, the user believes that the drug is required to ensure mental equanimity; but this does not imply an alteration of central nervous system physiology so as to produce an abstinence syndrome if the drug is withdrawn). Diazepam and chlordiazepoxide can be abused so as to produce physical dependence and an abstinence syndrome upon drug withdrawal. However, despite the widespread use of these drugs, Smith and Wesson (1970) estimate the incidence of these problems to be quite low. Physical dependence has not been reported with oxazepam or clorazepate. It is probable that oral dosages of 300 to 600 mg per day of chlordiazepoxide and of 80 to 120 mg per day of diazepam would have to be ingested for at least 40 to 60 days before physical dependence would develop. Hollister et al (1961) reported that 10 of 11 patients who received chlordiazepoxide at 100 to 600 mg per day for one to seven months developed withdrawal symptoms upon sudden cessation of the drug. Because of its long biological half-life (sometimes more than two days), there may be a delay of up to a week in the onset of withdrawal symptoms. The type of withdrawal syndrome mimics that of barbiturate abstinence. Corr (1973) noted that mild withdrawal occurred when chlordiazepoxide, 45 mg per day, was withdrawn after 20 (but not after 10) weeks. He believed that the long half-lives and active metabolites of chlordiazepoxide and diazepam helped to decrease the severity of withdrawal.

Another complication with the benzodiazepines is overdosing. Such abuse is probably common; however, because of the large margin of safety between therapeutic doses and lethal amounts, fatal incidents are extremely rare. At least 700 mg of chlordiazepoxide or diazepam taken acutely would be required for a fatal result (Jacobsen, 1971).

The benzodiazepines can potentiate, and can be potentiated by, other central nervous system depressants: alcohol, sedative-hypnotics, neuroleptics, tricyclic antidepressants. They can also produce a false elevation of the serum bilirubin, serum alkaline phosphatase, and serum glutamic oxide transaminase (SGOT).

Shader (1970) and Ayd (1962) observed that chlordiazepoxide and diazepam can produce increased hostility and attacks of anger in anxious patients. However, the author has observed this very uncommonly in actual clinical practice. Rickels and Downing (1974), in a double-blind, controlled study involving chlordiazepoxide and placebo, found that the active drug actually reduced irritability, hostility, and anger. However, there may exist a subgroup of anxious patients yet to be defined who do react with increased hostility to chlordiazepoxide and diazepam.

DiMascio and Barrett (1965) reported that oxazepam causes increases in anxiety when given to subjects with low-grade anxiety. This paradoxical effect did not occur when oxazepam was used for moderate to severe anxiety.

Driving skills are not notably impaired for most patients taking benzodiazepines or other tranquilizers in dosages prescribed by their physicians. However, Kielholz et al (1967) reported that using minor tranquilizers, even in recommended doses, along with alcohol can definitely impair judgment of distance, reaction time, motor coordination, and judgment of degree of danger. Alcohol is considered to be the major contributor to impaired skill in such cases.

Clinical Use

The minor tranquilizers are the most commonly prescribed psychotropic drugs in the United States (Parry et al, 1973). Diazepam and chlordiazepoxide are used more frequently than others in this category. Interestingly, these drugs are prescribed mostly by general practitioners and internists, and on over 50% of the occasions of their first being prescribed, the primary diagnosis is a physical disorder. However, the intent of the physician in most instances is to treat symptoms of, rather than a diagnosis of, psychic and emotional distress.

The benzodiazepines are believed to be at least as effective as the propanediols, the barbiturates, and the other sedative-hypnotic compounds in relieving symptoms of anxiety. Hollister (1973) summarized the additional advantages of the benzodiazepines in stating that there was a low risk of death from overdosing, low incidences of tolerance and dependence, a more sustained effect because of their long biological half-lives, and abstinence syndromes usually of only minor severity.

The benzodiazepines are considered the drugs of choice in the prevention and treatment of acute alcohol withdrawal syndrome. Diazepam and chlordiazepoxide, in both oral and parenteral forms, are the agents most frequently used. They do not produce the seizures or hypotension sometimes seen with the use of the phenothiazines. Also, the bad odor, injection site pain, and risk of toxic hepatitis which are associated with the use of paraldehyde are either absent or much lessened. More will be said about the treatment of this syndrome later in the chapter.

Chlordiazepoxide (25 to 50 mg) and diazepam (10 to 20 mg), given the night preceding and in the hours just prior to surgery, as well as postoperatively, can provide more significant calming, greater ease of inducing deep sleep with anesthetic agents, less postoperative nausea and vomiting, and a more cooperative attitude than does placebo (Corey, 1962; Brandt and Oakes, 1965).

A recent multivariate analysis (Cassano, 1973) of scores from a rating scale for depression gathered from patients with mixed anxious-depressive symptoms yielded the following results: the benzodiazepines' spectrum of application included insomnia, psychic and somatic anxiety, agitation, and somatic gastrointestinal symptoms. In anxious patients, a better response to treatment with benzodiazepines correlated with the presence of guilt, middle insomnia (awakening during the night), suicidal ideas, and loss of work capacity. The benzodiazepines were considered more valuable than the major tranquilizers for relief of anxiety in neurotic and in depressive-anxious patients because of their greater antianxiety properties and their fewer and less severe side effects.

PROPANEDIOLS

In 1955 meprobamate, the first of the minor tranquilizers, was released for sale on the drug market. Initially there was great enthusiasm in both medical and lay circles regarding the efficacy of this drug in relieving the discomfort of anxiety. Later, reports in the medical literature began to question its value, especially with respect to certain liabilities associated with its use. The most important of these liabilities concerned its potential for habituation, addiction, and death from overdosage. There are currently two propanediols available for use in the United States: meprobamate and tybamate.

Basic Pharmacology

Taken orally, meprobamate is rapidly absorbed from the gastrointestinal tract, reaches peak plasma levels in 2 hours, and has a biological half-life of 11 hours. Ninety percent of the dose is metabolized in the liver and excreted in the urine. Like the barbiturates, meprobamate induces synthesis of liver enzymes involved in its catabolism and thereby contributes to the development of drug tolerance. This, coupled with its relatively short biological half-life and its production of a mild euphoria in some users, has resulted in its frequent abuse.

Tybamate is less rapidly absorbed from the gastrointestinal tract, reaches peak plasma levels in 6 hours, and has a short biological half-life of 4 hours. Unlike meprobamate, it does not induce synthesis of liver enzymes. This characteristic, along with its short-lived systemic duration, results in lower drug tolerance and a lower potential for abuse. It is not likely to produce withdrawal symptoms.

Propanediols do not produce significant effects on the autonomic nervous system, but they do depress spinal cord internuncial neurons, thus impairing certain reflexes and inducing muscle relaxation. Similarly to the benzodiazepines, propanediols have relatively few direct effects on the neocortex or on the reticular system. Instead, they affect the thalamus and the structures in the limbic system, which are functionally associated with the modulation and expression of emotion.

Clinical Research Findings

Lorr et al (1961) compared meprobamate (1600 mg per day), chlorpromazine (100 mg per day), phenobarbital (2 grains per day), and placebo over an eight-week trial period in male patients attending Veterans Administration mental hygiene clinics. All patients received simultaneous weekly psychotherapy. Measures were taken of the drugs' effects on manifestations of anxiety and hostility. None of the active medications showed advantages over either placebo or psychotherapy alone in relieving anxiety. Paradoxically, all drugs were associated with increased amounts of verbal hostility.

In a later Veterans Administration study, McNair et al (1965) found that chlordiazepoxide was more effective than placebo in relieving anxiety, tension, and related criteria and was maximally helpful when used for a period of four to six weeks (average dosage: 10 mg four times per day). There was no evidence to suggest that meprobamate was superior to placebo.

Brill et al (1964) conducted a double-blind study which compared prochlorperazine, meprobamate, and phenobarbital, all in conjunction with brief visits (merely to report on symptom changes), in a group of 299 outpatients followed over several months. Controls included placebo or weekly psychotherapy groups. Patients in all groups improved, but the meprobamate and psychotherapy groups improved more than the others. However, even in these two, superiority did not reach statistical significance. Rickels' group (1959) reported in one study that meprobamate (1600 mg per day) was as effective as amobarbital (120 mg per day) and prochlorperazine (20 mg per day) in relieving anxiety symptoms in outpatients. Another study (Rickels and Snow, 1964), involving medical and psychiatric clinic patients, revealed that meprobamate (160 mg per day) was better than phenobarbital (60 mg per day) and placebo in mildly to moderately anxious patients; phenobarbital was more effective in severely anxious patients. A British study (West and daFonseca, 1965) using double-blind trials found meprobamate (1600 to 2000 mg per day) superior to placebo but approximately equal in effectiveness to amobarbital (260 to 325 mg per day).

Greenblatt and Shader reviewed the literature on controlled drug trials with meprobamate. They stated, "In only 5 of 26 studies was meprobamate clearly shown to be more effective in antianxiety action than a placebo in psychoneurotic patients, and in only 1 of 10 studies was meprobamate clearly more useful than a barbiturate. Thus the early enthusiasm over meprobamate has not been corroborated by more careful research." (1971)

Rickels group (1968) compared tybamate and placebo in a large group of anxious private practice patients. Only after four weeks did tybamate exhibit statistically superior benefits. These were most apparent in the more symptomatically distressed patients. Tybamate was more effective in relieving the somatic than the psychic manifestations of anxiety.

In another study (Vazuka and McLaughlin, 1965), tybamate (750 mg per day), meprobamate (120 mg per day), and chlordiazepoxide (30 mg per day) were each given for two weeks to 52 outpatients with anxiety. Placebo was given for a one-week washout prior to switching to a new trial drug. No significant benefits were reported for any drug, although tybamate was somewhat more effective than the other two. It also caused less drowsiness than did chlordiazepoxide or meprobamate.

Rickels et al (1964) reported on findings in a group of anxious neurotic medical clinic patients receiving tybamate and placebo in a controlled trial. Tybamate (500 mg four times per day) was clearly superior for these patients, especially for the more symptomatically ill, who had numerous somatic complaints.

In a study which employed flexible dosage schedules (Lader, 1969), tybamate was found to be significantly better than chlordiazepoxide. It was more beneficial for all symptoms, including agitation, anorexia, insomnia, somatic complaints, anxiety, poor concentration, crying, and headache. Tybamate also caused less drowsiness than chlordiazepoxide. In contrast, DiMascio et al (1965), in a study of the effects of tybamate in "high" and "low" anxious normal subjects, found this drug to have no significant anxiolytic effects.

Side Effects and Toxicity

Use of meprobamate can lead to physical dependence and drug withdrawal syndrome at dosages of as low as 3200 mg per day if it is suddenly discontinued after several weeks (Solow, 1971). The syndrome resembles that which occurs upon withdrawal of barbiturates. No withdrawal syndromes relating to tybamate have been reported (Mohr and Mead, 1958).

Overdoses with meprobamate are not uncommon. As little as 12 gm taken acutely has caused death. The average lethal dose in cases reported through 1969 was 28.1 gm, and the average overdose in less than fatal cases was 18.7 gm (Greenblatt and Shader, 1971). Therefore, as little as an average 10- or 12-day supply of this drug (at 1600 mg per day) in the possession of a suicidal patient poses the risk of a serious or fatal result.

Side effects associated with meprobamate are usually mild and infrequent, except for drowsiness.

Neuropsychiatric: drowsiness; feelings of unreality; panic, or confusion; ataxia (especially at high doses); impaired motor coordination (at high doses or at moderate doses when combined with other central nervous system depressants); seizures (reported when propanediols are given along with phenothiazines)

Allergic and idiosyncratic: urticaria; maculopapular pruritic rashes; bullous dermatitis; fever, chills; nausea, vomiting; hypotension; syncope; bronchial spasm; stomatitis; proctitis

Hematologic: rare reports of aplastic anemia, thrombocytopenia, leukopenia, and aplastic anemia

Other: headache; dizziness; vertigo; flushing and tachycardia (with tybamate)

Propanediols can potentiate and can be potentiated by central nervous system depressants, including alcohol, sedatives, neuroleptics, tricyclics, and monoamine oxidase inhibitors.

Propanediols, as well as barbiturates, can interfere with the anticoagulant effects of bishydroxycoumarin and can cause unpredictable shifts in urinary 17-hydroxy and 17-ketosteroid values.

Propanediols (and barbiturates) are contraindicated in patients with acute intermittent porphyria.

Clinical Use

In the sampling of drug trials noted above, tybamate appears to offer benefits for anxious patients, especially those with prominent somatic manifestations of anxiety. Unlike meprobamate, tybamate does not carry the risk of physical drug dependence. Despite these advantages, tybamate has enjoyed a very limited popularity in comparison to meprobamate. Whether this is due to a lack of true pharmacologic efficacy in clinical practice or to nonpharmacologic factors (eg, lack of strong promotion by the pharmaceutical industry; physicians' contentment with meprobamate) is not clear.

Meprobamate's usefulness as an anxiolytic has been questioned and its addiction and overdose liabilities emphasized. Because of these factors, it should rarely be the drug of first choice in treating anxiety states. A conservative, rational approach would be to limit its use to instances where the benzodiazepines and perhaps tybamate have failed to produce satisfactory results. It should be given only very cautiously to addiction-prone patients and for only a very limited time in such cases.

HYDROXYZINE

Hydroxyzine is a diphenylmethane derivative used in clinical medicine as an antihistamine and antiemetic. Although it reportedly has antianxiety properties, it has not received much attention in the psychiatric literature. In a double-blind crossover study, Breslow (1968) found hydroxyzine to be significantly superior to placebo in relieving anxiety, insomnia, hostility, depressed mood, overactivity, and assaultiveness.

Goldberg and Finnerty (1973) compared hydroxyzine and placebo in the treatment of 51 neurotic outpatients who had primary diagnoses of anxiety and, in many instances, accompanying depressive symptoms. Using a flexible dosage schedule (100 to 400 mg per day), they found no significantly superior advantage of hydroxyzine until the third treatment week. Hydroxyzine was beneficial for symptoms associated with anxiety but not with depression. Their evaluations were based on self-rating scales and on global ratings. The Hamilton Anxiety Scale (modified) did not demonstrate significant overall improvement until the fourth week. The authors noted that despite some benefits, the majority of self-rating scale items and Hamilton Scale items did not show significant improvement. Sleep disturbances were benefitted after one week. Consequently, hydroxyzine was concluded to be beneficial for anxiety, but its onset of action is delayed. Side effects were minimal, the most common being drowsiness and dizziness. More studies are needed to properly assess the value of this drug as an anxiolytic. An advantage to using an antihistamine such as hydroxyzine is the absence of the development of drug tolerance, physical dependence, and withdrawal syndromes.

NEUROLEPTICS (MAJOR TRANQUILIZERS, ANTIPSYCHOTIC DRUGS)

The neuroleptics (the phenothiazines, butyrophenones, thioxanthenes) are so named because of their usefulness in relieving psychotic symptoms such as illogical thinking, including delusions; distorted perceptions, including hallucinations; and major aberrations in conceptualizing reality. The minor tranquilizers do not exhibit antipsychotic properties. Since the neuroleptics do relieve the anxiety, agitation, and tension which frequently accompany psychotic episodes, the question naturally arises as to their value in reducing anxiety in mental disorders other than psychosis.

Klein and Davis (1969) stated emphatically that the phenothiazines were contraindicated for treating anxiety states because they are ineffective and often deleterious in such conditions. They added that their use may obscure an incipient psychosis, and that an incipient psychosis mistakenly viewed as an anxiety neurosis but treated with some success with phenothiazines may leave a patient unprepared for the serious consequences of a possible acute psychotic episode.

Rickels (1968), who has conducted numerous drug studies involving anxiety and depression, stated that treating anxiety with neuroleptics commonly produced feelings of discomfort. Patients often reported feeling doped up, strange, and detached. Furthermore, the piperazine group of phenothiazines (eg, perphenazine) frequently caused dystonic reactions in younger patients.

A California group (Yamamoto, 1973) compared the neuroleptic chlorpromazine and the benzodiazepine chlordiazepoxide for four weeks in a group of 81 anxious neurotic outpatients. Chlorpromazine was considered more effective in relieving hostility and emotional withdrawal, otherwise there were no significant differences in response to the two treatments in these patients. Consequently, this research group recommended chlordiazepoxide because of its greater freedom from adverse side effects and its efficacy comparable to that of chlorpromazine.

Rickels' group (1974) compared two neuroleptics, thiothixene and thioridazine, and placebo in treating 155 anxious neurotic outpatients during a six-week, double-blind, controlled study. Only at two weeks did the active drugs demonstrate any superiority over the placebo, and this was only minor. Thereafter, no differences were noted between drugs and placebo in relieving anxiety. The two neuroleptics did display antidepressant properties. The authors concluded that neuroleptics in anxious neurotics should be limited to those patients who have failed to respond to antianxiety agents.

Another study (Lord and Kidd, 1973) compared the neuroleptic haloperidol (1 mg per day), the benzodiazepine diazepam (15 mg per day), and placebo in a group of anxious neurotic outpatients. Each patient received each drug and placebo for one week. Both active drugs were significantly better than placebo. For patients who experienced anxiety without obvious precipitating factors, diazepam was better than haloperidol in eight areas: anxiety, tension, difficulty in concentrating, lack of initiative, asthenia, difficulty in falling asleep, decreased duration of sleep, and restlessness. The two drugs were of approximately equal benefit to patients who experienced anxiety with obvious precipitating factors.

This study confirmed the results of a previous one involving diazepam and haloperidol (1 mg per day) by Lord and Kidd (1973). However, it conflicted with another report on haloperidol (2 mg per day) in anxiety states which held that the frequent side effects of this drug ruled it out as a good treatment choice (Rickels, 1971). Perhaps the difference in dosage of haloperidol in the two studies might account for the contrasting conclusions.

Wheatley (1973) compared low doses of haloperidol (0.25 mg four times per day) and of chlordiazepoxide (10 mg four times per day) in a double-blind trial and found no significantly different results or side effects for the two drugs.

Other studies (Batterman et al, 1963; Smith and Chasson, 1964) found that low dosages of the neuroleptics fluphenazine, chlorpromazine, and trifluoperazine gave no advantages over the benzodiazepines diazepam and chlordiazepoxide in anxiety relief.

Lingl (1973) reported that the neuroleptics thioridazine and haloperidol were very useful in relieving anxiety symptoms in neurotic patients who had been unresponsive to minor tranquilizers. Haloperidol was better at reducing anxiety, agitation, and tension; thioridazine was better at relieving insomnia.

These representative studies confirm the impression that the benzodiazepines are at present the drugs of choice for treating neurotic anxiety states. Low dosages of the neuroleptics can be beneficial in individual cases where use of benzodiazepines and other minor tranquilizers has failed to produce satisfactory results or has caused serious toxic effects or has induced drug dependence (not a factor with the neuroleptics). Neuroleptics would also be appropriate when severe anxiety is accompanied by other symptoms which suggest incipient psychosis (eg, ideas of reference or fears of losing control and harming others). (The author acknowledges the concern voiced by Klein and Davis [1969] regarding the use of phenothiazines in incipient psychosis. However, one would hope that the attending physician would be aware of the psychotic potential of the patient and arrange for appropriate follow-up drug treatment and psychotherapy.) The anxiety, tension, and agitation of obsessive-compulsive neurotics may also be better relieved by neuroleptics than by minor tranquilizers.

The neuroleptics invariably produce some side effects (dry mouth, blurred vision, tachycardia, constipation, alterations in mental attitude), and these may increase the anxiety and irritation of an already uncomfortable patient.

PROPRANOLOL: BETA-ADRENERGIC BLOCKING DRUG

The sympathetic division of the autonomic nervous system contains receptor cells of two types, alpha and beta. Stimulation of the alpha sites causes vasoconstriction in cutaneous and in splanchnic vascular beds, mydriasis, sweating, piloerection, and constriction of the internal urethral sphincter. Beta-receptor-site stimulation leads to an increased heart rate, increased force of cardiac contraction, relaxation of bronchial muscles, a decrease in tone of blood vessels in skeletal muscles, decreased gastrointestinal motility, and relaxation of the urinary bladder smooth muscle.

In 1966, Granville-Grossman and Turner reported on the use of a beta-adrenergic blocking agent, propranolol, for patients suffering from neurotic anxiety states. Symptoms were evaluated in three categories: 1) mental: worry, fear, jumpiness, irritability; 2) physical symptoms related to the autonomic nervous system: palpitations, sweating, diarrhea; 3) all other physical symptoms: headache, tremulousness, unusual sensations. Propranolol (20 mg four times per day) improved anxiety primarily because of its significant reduction of autonomic symptoms. The investigators postulated that propranolol probably had a direct effect only on peripheral beta-adrenergic receptors, and that relief of mental anxiety was probably secondary to this action. They conceded that, although it is unlikely, propranolol might have direct central nervous system effects. Leszkovszky and Tardos (1965) reported that the use of subcutaneous propranolol in mice had central nervous system depressant (induced sleep) and anticonvulsive effects. Because the study was done with animals and employed high dosages, there is skepticism as to the applicability of these findings to man. Stone et al (1973) also favored the view that propranolol's antianxiety effects were due to its peripheral beta-adrenergic blocking action.

Wheatley (1969) reported findings with 105 patients suffering primarily from anxiety: 51 were treated with propranolol (30 mg three times per day), and 54 with chlordiazepoxide (10 mg three times per day) for six weeks. Improvement of anxiety was about equal. Depressive symptoms were better relieved with chlordiazepoxide, which also produced greater improvement in sleep disturbances. Tachycardia and tremor responded about equally to both drugs. The incidence of side effects was less with propranolol (27%) than with chlordiazepoxide (43%), and drowsiness was the most common side effect of both drugs.

Tyrer and Lader (1974) studied the effects of diazepam vs those of propranolol in 12 chronically anxious outpatients, 6 of whom complained primarily of somatic manifestations and 6 of whom were distressed mostly by psychic symptoms of anxiety. A flexible dosage schedule was used, and each patient received a week's trial each of the two drugs and of placebo. Diazepam (average dose: 9.6 mg per day) was clearly preferable to propranolol and placebo in relieving psychic anxiety. Propranolol (average dose: 120 mg per day) was better than placebo and almost as effective as diazepam in treating somatic symptoms. The authors concluded that propranolol was beneficial primarily for those anxious patients whose complaints were somatic, rather than psychic, manifestations of anxiety. Tachycardia, tremor, and associated psychic discomfort were especially responsive to treatment with propranolol.

Gallant et al (1973) reported that patients' rating scales showed no advantage of propranolol over placebo in treating chronic anxiety states in alcoholics, but that global ratings by a psychiatrist found propranolol to be significantly better.

Kellner et al (1974) used propranolol (median dose: 112 mg per day) in a group of anxious neurotic outpatients and found few significant short-term (one week) benefits for anxiety relative to placebo. However, there was a trend favoring propranolol for symptoms resulting from excessive beta-adrenergic cell stimulation.

Gottschalk et al (1974) reported that propranolol reduced basal anxiety scores in 12 subjects, but it did not relieve anxiety produced by a stress interview any better than did placebo. They concluded that baseline anxiety was maintained by peripheral afferent autonomic nervous system feedback and that this feedback (and the consequent anxiety) was reduced by beta-adrenergic blocking agents. On the other hand, because acute anxiety aroused by situational stress is believed to be a more direct manifestation of central nervous system activity, it was not much affected by propranolol.

Coleman (1975) reviewed the clinical indications for and contraindications to beta-adrenergic blocking drugs. He referred to studies which found promising effects of propranolol in relieving the anxiety, tremor, sweating, and tachycardia associated with the alcoholic withdrawal syndrome, thyrotoxicosis, and the withdrawal syndrome seen with sedative and hypnotic drugs.

These several studies suggest that propranolol can be useful in somatically preoccupied anxious patients whose complaints, especially those deriving from the cardiovascular system (tachycardia, palpitations, chest discomfort, sweating, and trembling), are psychogenic in origin. Because propranolol interrupts these physical symptoms, at least a fraction of the accompanying psychic apprehension is also reduced. The advantages to using propranolol rather than minor tranquilizers in anxiety states include its lack of drug dependence liability and its lesser sedative effects.

DRUG TREATMENT OF MIXED
ANXIETY-DEPRESSIVE SYNDROMES

It is almost axiomatic in clinical medicine and psychiatry that a pure depression is an uncommon entity. While an acute anxiety reaction without depressive features is encountered with moderate frequency, it is rare for a depressed patient not to acknowledge some elements of anxiety and tension. Furthermore, most instances of chronic anxiety are accompanied by some depressive symptoms. Patients who have been struggling unsuccessfully for years with the discomfort of anxiety become despondent and disillusioned about the unrelenting presence of their morbid apprehension.

There are numerous symptoms which are common to both anxiety and depressive states. Poor concentration, indecisiveness, helplessness, preoccupation with self, somatic complaints, disrupted sleep, altered eating habits, irritability, self-pity, and social withdrawal are but a few. Therefore, it is difficult—often impossible—to state whether a patient is primarily depressed or primarily anxious.

Sophisticated research efforts employing statistical and factorial analytic techniques have attempted to dissect the essence of anxiety illness from that of depressive illness but have not had notable success (Klerman, 1971; Mendels et al, 1972; Zung, 1971). Mendels et al (1971) administered six different self-rating scales to 100 inpatients aged 21 to 65 and were unable to isolate specific factors which distinguished anxiety from depression. They speculated that anxiety and depression may have different biologic substrates but similar mental content; or that anxiety and depression represent the same reaction to internal or external stress, but that a life-style which favors withdrawal, brooding, and apathy predisposes to depression while a life-style which tends toward vigilance, motor activity, and overt expression makes anxiety the more likely reaction to stress.

Downing and Rickels (1974) noted that many patients present with mixed symptoms of anxiety and depression. They opposed the practice of labelling this very heterogeneous patient population with the single, broad diagnosis of mixed anxiety and depression. Their multivariate analyses of data relating to these clinical problems and their associated treatments revealed that physicians were likely to prescribe an anxiolytic drug when the anxiety level was high relative to depression and an antidepressant when depressive symptoms were the more outstanding. The problems of establishing more clinically meaningful diagnostic categories and of prescribing predictably useful drugs for patients with varying mixtures of anxious and depressive symptoms have not been resolved. The findings of several studies in this area will be mentioned below not as an attempt to review the subject exhaustively but rather to present a glimpse of the divergent approaches to treatment which are being explored.

The studies of Overall et al (1964) and Hollister et al (1967) revealed subcategories of depressed patients: retarded, anxious, and anxious-hostile. The psychomotor-retarded depressed patients responded best to tricyclic antidepressants. The anxious-depressed patients responded best to the neuroleptics thioridazine and perphenazine or to a combination of perphenazine and amitriptyline (a tricyclic antidepressant drug).

Rickels et al (1970) compared the effects of chlordiazepoxide (40 mg per day) alone, amitriptyline (100 mg per day) alone, chlordiazepoxide plus amitriptyline, and placebo in treating both lower socioeconomic, clinic patients and middle-class, general practice patients who were neurotic and depressed. The greatest drug-vs-placebo response differences were seen in the general practice patients, who did well with active drugs and poorly with placebo. Patients were divided into four diagnostic groups: high depressed, low anxious; low depressed, high anxious; high depressed, high anxious; low depressed, low anxious. Amitriptyline used alone was best for high depressed (more psychomotor-retarded), low anxious patients. Chlordiazepoxide plus amitriptyline was best for high depressed, high anxious patients. Chlordiazepoxide used alone was best for low depressed, high anxious patients. Both drugs and placebo were equally effective for the low depressed, low anxious patients.

A double-blind study (Rosenthal, 1973) comparing thioridazine and diazepam in patients with chronic mixed anxious and depressive symptoms concluded that thioridazine was significantly superior to diazepam in relieving depressive symptoms such as suicidal ideas, psychomotor retardation, and feelings of helplessness, worthlessness, and guilt. In contrast, diazepam was significantly superior in alleviating somatic and psychic anxiety and difficulties in falling asleep. Another study comparing thioridazine and diazepam found thioridazine superior in a more global manner. Anxiety, depression, tension, cognitive impairment, and behavioral disturbances during the interview all responded better to thioridazine (Krivda et al, 1974). In a double-blind study using thioridazine (20 to 200 mg per day) and placebo, Fann et al (1974) found the active drug significantly better in mixed anxious-depressed states. They noted that an advantage of thioridazine over the benzodiazepines is the lesser tendency to drug dependence with the former.

Hollister (1971), who previously had upheld the advantages of the phenothiazines over the tricyclic antidepressants, compared acetophenazine (a phenothiazine) to diazepam (a benzodiazepine) in patients suffering from anxious depression. He used diazepam in dosages of up to 50 mg per day in his patient group. The two drugs were equally effective. Therefore, because of their fewer troublesome side effects, he recommended the benzodiazepines in preference to the phenothiazines for treatment of simple anxious depressions.

Rickels (1971) recommended that the use of combinations of tricyclic antidepressants and minor tranquilizers be avoided in mildly to moderately depressed, primarily anxious patients. He observed that these anxious patients reacted negatively to the sedative (and especially to the automomic) side effects of the tricyclic antidepressants. He advised a trial with a minor tranquilizer and, if that were not successful, the use of an antipsychotic drug as a second choice before resorting to a tricyclic. In an earlier paper, Rickels et al (1967) found that meprobamate (in average dosages) was as effective in relieving mixed anxious-depressed states as was protriptyline, a tricyclic antidepressant. Furthermore, those patients who experienced high levels of anxiety along with depression did better with meprobamate alone, or with meprobamate plus protriptyline, than with protriptyline alone.

Woodward et al (1975) made some interesting observations in a noncontrolled study of 458 anxious and depressed outpatients. Both minor and major tranquilizers were more effective in relieving depressive symptoms than in relieving anxiety. The more sedating tricyclic antidepressants (eg, amitriptyline) had a relatively greater effect on anxiety than on depression. Within each major category of psychotropic drugs (ie, minor tranquilizers, major tranquilizers, antidepressants), the more sedating members gave better anxiety relief, while the less sedating members were more useful in alleviating depression.

Certainly Woodward's findings contradict traditional concepts in drug treatment. That certain antidepressant medications may be more useful for anxiety and certain tranquilizers more beneficial for depression is vivid testimony to the very heterogeneous characteristics of mixed anxiety and depressive illnesses which are found in typical office-practice patients. It also emphasizes the importance of various nonspecific factors (placebo effects, doctor-patient relationships, patient and family expectations of treatment) which influence treatment outcome.

Rickels et al (1974) reported that the tricyclic antidepressant amitriptyline was superior to placebo in reducing anxiety and its accompanying somatic symptoms after two weeks and in alleviating depressed mood in four weeks. Patients complained about the sedative and autonomic side effects of amitriptyline, which were the major reasons for dose reduction and a high rate of dropout (45%) from the study. This confirmed Rickels' previous observation of low tolerance for the sedative side effects of drugs in middle-class, educated patients.

Covi et al (1974) compared the effects of imipramine (average dosage: 125 mg per day), diazepam (average dosage: 12.5 mg per day), and placebo in a group of chronically depressed, neurotic patients, most of whom also suffered significant anxiety. Analysis of results after 16 weeks of active drug treatment clearly favored the tricyclic antidepressant imipramine with regard to depression and anxiety. A follow-up maintenance study also favored imipramine. The authors acknowledged that these findings were in disagreement with other studies, which favored minor or major tranquilizers over the tricyclics in treating anxious depressions.

Raskin (1974) stated that depression was a self-limiting illness and that neurotic, depressed patients did as well or better with placebo as with any active drug treatment during two separate seven-week treatment studies involving Veterans Administration patients. He also found that minor tranquilizers, tricyclic antidepressants, and antipsychotic drugs relieved accompanying anxiety and sleep disturbances about equally.

Yet another approach to the treatment of mixed anxious-depressed states involves the use of monoamine oxidase (MAO) inhibiting antidepressant drugs. For many years British investigators considered the MAO inhibitors especially useful in so-called atypical depressions, wherein depressed mood is accompanied by anxiety, phobic avoidances, obsessional preoccupations, and hysterical symptoms. More recently, Johnson (1975) stated that the MAO inhibitors are the drugs of choice for atypical depressions associated with anxiety and with phobic and hysterical symptoms.

Robinson et al (1973) reported that patients with mixed anxiety-depressive syndromes responded significantly better to the MAO inhibitor phenelzine than to placebo. They noted a correlation between clinical improvement and dosages of phenelzine which produced at least 80% suppression of platelet MAO activity. Although this finding has useful implications, the risk of serious side effects when MAO inhibitors are used in the dosages which may be necessary to produce adequate platelet MAO suppression, and the unavailability of routine laboratory tests to measure platelet MAO activity, should serve to limit the use of high dosage schedules (ie, dosages higher than those approved by the Food and Drug Administration) to that by those physicians with a special interest and expertise in these drugs.

In general, MAO inhibitors, even at standard dosages, should be prescribed only for patients who are sufficiently intelligent and trustworthy to observe the dietary and medicinal restrictions required by their use.

CLINICAL APPROACH TO TREATMENT OF MIXED ANXIETY-DEPRESSIVE SYNDROMES

In light of these research findings, one might correctly conclude that opinion regarding treatment of anxious-depressed patients is as mixed as the syndrome itself. Despite the controversy, certain guidelines can be established.

Since the benzodiazepines (and perhaps the propanediols) are frequently effective in relieving depressive complaints which accompany the more overriding symptoms of anxiety, these drugs are considered a safe first choice for a majority of these mixed syndromes. If the benzodiazepines are not helpful, an antipsychotic drug should be tried next if the anxiety component is especially severe, or a tricyclic antidepressant if the depressive elements are very pronounced. If both components are intense and prominent, a tricyclic antidepressant given on a regular schedule, along with a minor tranquilizer on an as-needed basis two to four times per day, should be given a trial. If this regimen is not helpful, an antipsychotic drug can be substituted for the minor tranquilizer, but it should be given on a regular basis and in low dosage to avoid severe, additive anticholinergic and extrapyramidal side effects from the tricyclic and antipsychotic drugs being given together. An MAO inhibitor is appropriate for depressions with associated anxiety and for phobic avoidance symptoms occurring in primarily obsessional and hysterical personality types.

It should be clarified that the guidelines noted above apply to cases where depression is not profound, not debilitating to day-to-day functioning, not associated with prominent suicidal ideas or delusional thoughts of worthlessness or guilt, and not productive of somatic complaints (eg, anorexia, marked weight loss, early morning awakening, constipation). These latter accompany depressions which are believed to have a primarily biochemical cause. The drug treatment of choice in such cases is a tricyclic antidepressant.

USE OF ANTIDEPRESSANT DRUGS IN ANXIOUS-PHOBIC STATES

The British reported that they consider MAO inhibitors to be specifically indicated for the treatment of atypical depressions associated with anxious-phobic symptoms and for the treatment of a so-called anxiety-phobia-depersonalization syndrome. Kelly (1973) reported on the efficacy of phenelzine in relieving the intense anxiety in primary agoraphobia (fear of being outside on the street or of open spaces outside) and in school phobias. He speculated that the MAO inhibitors may have a direct blocking effect on panic attacks.

In the United States, Klein and Fink (1962) have described a group of patients who suffered from a sudden phobic reluctance to leave familiar, secure surroundings. Klein divided these patients into two groups. In one group, panics were brought on by separation or bereavement; in the other, panics were induced by physical illness which involved endocrine fluctuations. Minor and major tranquilizers and psychotherapy were not useful in alleviating these panic attacks, but the tricyclic imipramine was highly effective in eliminating them. Unfortunately, it was not useful in allaying the chronic, anticipatory anxiety which these patients continued to experience in advance of encountering what had previously evoked panic. Supportive psychotherapy and behavior modification techniques were found to be useful in managing this anticipatory anxiety. Howlett and Markoff (1975) also described four cases of panic episodes which responded excellently to surprisingly low dosages of imipramine (75 mg per day at bedtime) or amitriptyline (25 mg twice per day).

NONPHARMACOLOGIC FACTORS IN
DRUG TREATMENT RESPONSE

Exclusive of any drug treatment, anxiety states undergo apparently spontaneous improvements and worsenings and are subject to influence by a variety of situational (especially interpersonal) events. Because there is a multitude of variables which can affect symptoms, making an accurate appraisal of the unique pharmacologic benefits of a drug is extremely difficult. This is especially true for short-term drug trials in acute anxiety, where nonpharmacologic factors are quite influential. In chronic anxiety states, assessments of drug effects are more reliable, since a pattern of reaction to many nonspecific factors has been established against which the pharmacologic effects of a drug can be measured. Long-term drug trials in chronic anxiety provide more reliable information than do short-term trials. A brief survey of some drug/placebo phenomena and of some nonplacebo factors which invariably accompany the chemotherapy of anxiety states will be presented.

Wheatley (1972) found a positive response in 50% of anxious patients receiving placebo and in 75% of anxious patients receiving phenobarbital. He also observed a higher relapse rate in those patients treated with placebo as compared to those given phenobarbital.

Using a randomized crossover design, Schapira et al (1970) gave anxious patients different-colored preparations of oxazepam at 15 mg three times per day. A trend that favored green for anxiety and yellow for depression was not statistically significant. The only statistically significant finding was a superiority on the physician's rating scale of the green tablets for treating phobias.

Hussain (1972) compared the effects of chlordiazepoxide in tablet vs capsule form in treating anxiety states. Both forms produced significant improvement at 30 mg per day. No differences were noted by the rating physicians, but patients' self-assessments indicated a significant superiority of the capsules over the tablets with regard to relief of anxiety, irritability, phobias, and broken sleep.

Wheatley (1972) correlated certain sociodemographic factors with a positive response to drug treatment of anxiety. Patients who were unmarried, who had had fewer previous attacks of anxiety, and who had experienced symptoms for less than a year showed a much better response to drug treatment than did those patients with the opposite characteristics.

One of the numerous nondrug factors which influences response to drug treatment is the patient's attitude. Patients who are passive and compliant are more likely to accept the doctor and his drug and to report better drug effects than are more aggressive, suspicious patients and those who fear dependency. The latter will be prone to disregard prescription directions, report many adverse side effects, and give a negative assessment of the effects of drugs.

The patient's personality type will also affect his response to drug treatment. Extroverted, physically active persons frequently report negative side effects. They sometimes even report increased anxiety, as they believe the drugs are slowing them down. Such persons probably need activity and great alertness to bind their anxiety. Introverted, less active, intellectual "thinkers" respond more favorably to antianxiety drugs than do "doers."

Bonn (1972) observed that for patients on active drugs, important life-changes for the worse decreased chances of improvement, but changes for the better did not necessarily enhance improvement. Just the opposite was observed for patients on placebo: life-changes for the better increased chances of improvement, but changes for the worse did not impede improvement. Previous experiences with drugs will also often bias the effects of current medications, pro or con.

The doctor's personality and attitude play a definite role in the effect a drug has. Professional qualities which enhance the likelihood of successful treatment are: a positive regard for the patient, the doctor's display of his own positive self-esteem, a solid professional reputation in the community, and a high fee schedule.

The relationship between patient and physician and the physician's attitude toward drugs are very influential variables. Combined with a good patient-physician relationship, an attitude of optimism and confidence in drugs on the physician's part correlates with a better drug response. Drug response is not as good if the physician's attitude toward drugs is negative.

The atmosphere in which drugs are taken can also influence their effects. A patient taking drugs at home in the presence of family members who oppose drug use and upon whom the patient is dependent will be less likely to report benefits from the drug. However, a patient in a hospital environment, where use of drugs is routine and encouraged, will be more receptive and more likely to report a favorable drug response.

The placebo effect of drugs used in treating neurotic anxiety states lasts approximately two weeks. Patients who complain primarily of somatic problems and have little insight into their emotions generally are less responsive to the minor tranquilizers than are patients who can verbalize their anxiety. A truism often repeated in the drug treatment literature is that the more serious an illness is, and/or the more pharmacologically potent a drug is, the less likely it is that treatment outcome will be significantly influenced by nonspecific factors.

Knowledge of these nonpharmacologic factors will be less useful in predicting the future course of an illness than in helping to explain the causes of phasic ups and downs which occur during drug treatment. By taking such non-drug-specific factors into account, the physician will be less hasty in altering dosages or switching to other drugs.

CLINICAL APPROACH TO THE TREATMENT OF ANXIETY

According to the theoretical models surveyed earlier in this chapter, anxiety can be viewed as having two broadly defined sets of components: the psychosocial and the neurophysiosocial-biochemical. Instances of endogenous anxiety, in which symptoms are precipitated by shifts of biochemical elements independent of life experiences, are probably uncommon. It is presumed that in the majority of cases a symbolically significant stress has been encountered by the patient (although he may be unaware of it) and has initiated the anxiety reaction. For effective treatment, it is important that the physician attempt to identify at least "what" triggered the attack. He may or may not be able to ascertain "why" the "what" caused the anxiety, since the symbolic meaning of the "what" may be so subtle as to require a specifically trained psychiatrist to uncover it. Another view of this task is that, given some knowledge of the sources of anxiety to the unconscious mind (referred to earlier in the chapter), some awareness of the patient's personality, and an appreciation of stresses with which the patient has been contending (at work, with family, friends, finances, sex, etc), the physician can formulate an understanding of why the patient has become anxious. If this is even partially accomplished, the physician can then talk more meaningfully to the patient. This will foster the patient's confidence in accepting advice, suggestions, or other input offered by the physician. With a receptive patient attitude and with appropriate, "to-the-point" counseling by the physician, anxiety is often relieved and the propensity toward future recurrences of anxiety sometimes diminishes.

This approach suggests that drug treatment of anxiety should be considered adjunctive. Drugs relieve distressing, sometimes disabling, symptoms and facilitate better functioning and thereby enhance personal fulfillment. However, antianxiety drugs which have the potential for abuse are believed to alter effects, not causes. Since anxiety reactions commonly recur, an effort to reduce the likelihood of recurrence should be made by dealing with the psychologic causes. Even if a precise understanding of the causes is not achieved, the attempt at understanding may itself, over the short-term, reduce the anxiety as well as a drug would. This may result from the supportive, helping influence of the physician as well as from the clarification of personal problems which had not previously been obvious to the patient. Such clarification could lead to better coping.

Through clinical practice the family doctor will become astute in diagnosing an anxiety state if he or she is actively considering this disorder as a cause for physical complaints. If the physician is too prone to make only physical diagnoses, he or she will miss opportunities to provide appropriate treatment. Furthermore, he or she may even unwittingly perpetuate a patient's tendency to somatize his or her anxiety because of all the concern and interest the physical complaints attract. After making a diagnosis of anxiety reaction, and following the initial interview and physical examination, the physician will often order laboratory and radiologic examinations to ascertain whether there is coexisting tissue pathology. The discovery of an organic disorder (eg, peptic ulcer) in no way excludes the presence of an anxiety state. Only if the severity of the anxiety is such as to interfere with the patient's essential daily routine (working, eating, sleeping) should medication be prescribed.

A second interview should be arranged which allows extra time, perhaps half an hour, to assess the degree of impairment of functioning caused by the anxiety, to gain a better appreciation of what precipitated the symptoms, and to consider with the patient a better means of coping with the stress confronting him or her.

Thereafter, periodic visits of 20 to 30 minutes, spaced in accordance with the patient's progress (usually once or twice per week), should be arranged over a minimum three- to four-week follow-up treatment period. It is often helpful to speak to someone well acquainted with the patient in order to enhance one's understanding of factors which contributed to the onset of symptoms, to assess more accurately the functional impairment caused by the anxiety, and to consider what measures of support and assistance family members and friends can offer to the patient. These contacts should be approved by the patient in advance. Often a patient will confide to a family member or friend information which he is embarrassed to reveal directly to a physician but about which he would not object to the doctor's knowing.

In order to make maximum use of time spent with a patient, the doctor should be acquainted with the common sources of stress for patients in different age groups. This awareness will allow the doctor to ask pointed questions covering potentially sensitive areas, and it may facilitate a patient's "opening up" and talking about relevant personal issues. Questions about the context(s) in which the symptoms began will often provide clues as to the identity of the stress factors. The patient should be assured of the confidential nature of the material discussed during an interview.

Common sources of stress for an adolescent or young adult are conflicts with parents, teachers, boyfriends or girlfriends; pressures to compete or be more independent when confidence is lacking; illicit drug experimentation; fears about sexual matters; pressures to make decisions about or commitments to school, work, or personal relationships before feeling ready to do so.

From the mid-twenties through the thirties, stress and resultant anxiety often derive from marital friction; conflict and uncertainty about role assignments: pregnancy, motherhood, choices between career and family, husband adjusting to presence of children who rival him for wife's attention; financial problems; pressures at work; relocating family; divorce; illness in parents.

In middle-aged and older persons, stress more commonly presents as situations representing loss, disappointment, and disillusionment (eg, loss of health, family, friends, vigor, attractiveness, employment security). It is not surprising that anxiety states in this age group are often expressions of masked, underlying depressions.

Psychotherapy refers to any of a variety of techniques in which the influence of one person (the therapist) is used to alter the feelings, behavior, and thinking of another or others exclusive of the direct application of a physical device (drug, any mechanical instrument). Some form of psychotherapy which enables the patient to experience relief of his symptoms, along with a sense of having relied largely upon his own resources (ie, ingenuity, intellect, physical strength, perceptiveness, sensitivity, self-discipline, education, religious conviction, insights) in overcoming the problem, is potentially the most effective treatment for anxiety. The role of the physician is to foster this recovery by helping the patient to mobilize coping devices which the anxiety state has undermined.

An example of a patient who might experience significant anxiety is a businessman in his late middle-age who has suffered a myocardial infarction and has emerged from the acute episode without somatic complication but has had to alter a previously chaotic, highly pressured life-style. There are many potential sources of anxiety. The illness undermines his sense of indestructibility: he is human and fallible. Repressed childhood fears of being hurt and damaged are aroused; consequently, some childish behaviors like excessive complaining, pouting, whining, and requests for reassurance may surface. He confronts the reality of dying or of being chronically disabled. If such matters are highly sensitive to the patient, he may become preoccupied with worries about dying and may find his attention riveted to sensations in his chest. An itch, a brief sigh, a palpitation, indigestion, or a cough may all become stimuli which arouse exaggerated anxiety. He may fear that an end to his career is imminent. This leads to worries about financial security. If his marriage had been troubled previously, he may entertain fears that his wife will withdraw her support of a "sick" man. His insatiable need for constant activity, late hours, hard work, and hard play will be compromised. Since this constant activity had in part been a defense against anxiety and insecurity throughout his life, restrictions now threaten him with the emergence of that anxiety. Fears of losing in competition may be aroused, for he now envisions himself as a loser. He may think of these and other matters and fear that he is not capable of adjusting or of making the necessary changes in his life-style.

Psychotherapy for this patient does not require probing into childhood memories, interpreting the hidden meanings of dreams, or encouraging the patient to become conscious of repressed incestuous desires for his mother. The patient should be given a truthful explanation of his medical problem, but with an emphasis on the hopeful, encouraging, and optimistic aspects. The physician should display a genuine interest in the patient as a total human being with many assets who has encountered a crisis. The patient needs to be given time to express his fears and worries and to have his questions answered forthrightly. In responding to the patient, the doctor's attitude should convey understanding, empathy, and a high regard for the patient's dignity. The patient's distorted conceptions of his condition should be corrected without criticism, and in their place the physician should offer his own, more realistic and objective perceptions. If the patient overlooks or denies certain harsh implications of his condition, and if the consequences of such denials seem not especially dangerous, the doctor need not bother to correct the patient. Such denials (eg, a cooperative patient follows medical advice and his medical condition is stable, but he denies that his illness could have fatal consequences) indicate that the patient's anxiety relative to such matters is too great for him to confront. For the present, those sleeping dogs should be left lying. Later, when his anxiety has diminished, the patient may not need to overlook and bypass the facts.

The physician should repeatedly allude to the patient's resourcefulness and should repeatedly express confidence in the patient's coping abilities. He should consult with the patient on modification of business hours and recreational pursuits. Using his own common sense and experience in life and his knowledge as to the patient's strengths and weaknesses, the physician can help to turn the patient's attention from morbid preoccupations to constructive plans for the future. The patient's role as an active participant in this process, with the support of a respected professional, has built-in anxiety-relieving value.

This type of approach toward alleviating anxiety, called supportive psychotherapy, encourages the patient to use his ego strengths to buttress him against his anxieties. It also includes intervening in the patient's environment to reduce excessive stress. In a survey of family practitioners, Fisher et al (1975) discovered that physicians who graduated from medical school after 1950 routinely employed some form of counseling psychotherapy and were more reluctant to use psychotropic medications as frequently as did pre-1950 graduates. This phenomenon is ascribed in part to better post-1950 medical school training in the management of psychologic problems.

Supportive psychotherapy is the treatment of choice for acute episodes of anxiety. Unfortunately, there are many patients who do not receive this treatment, because it requires more time and patience than some physicians are willing to offer. Some patients do not respond sufficiently well to psychotherapy alone and therefore require the assistance of adjunctive drugs. If supportive psychotherapy and drugs have not produced satisfactory results after one or two months, a patient should be referred to a psychiatric specialist.

Lesse (1970) described two phases in the treatment of an acute anxiety state. The first involves reducing anxiety to a level at which the patient feels comfortable enough to carry out necessary daily tasks. The doctor-patient relationship, which provides reassurance and encouragement to the patient, is a powerful force in accomplishing this. The placebo effects of a drug, together with its pharmacologic actions, are additionally helpful. (Lesse, however, opposes the routine use of anxiolytic drugs for mild to moderate cases of anxiety.) Lesse terms the second phase of treatment *re-educational*. It involves the patient's learning about himself, his expectations, and his patterns of interaction with his environment. The patient is encouraged to gain a better understanding of the limits of his adaptive capacities and to decline participating in situations which reach beyond these.

AN OVERVIEW OF DRUG TREATMENT OF ANXIETY STATES

The benzodiazepines are generally regarded as the drugs most suitable for the treatment of anxiety. They have a lesser potential for addictive abuse than do the barbiturates and meprobamate, but since they are not free of abuse potential, the Food and Drug Administration has placed some restrictions on their prescription. Similar restrictions had already been imposed on the barbiturates and meprobamate. The benzodiazepines are less likely to cause the unpleasant mental, neurologic, and autonomic side effects experienced with neuroleptics—effects which often prompt patients to discontinue their use. Rickels (1971) observed that clinic patients from the lower social classes were not disturbed by the sedative effects of minor tranquilizers but that they strongly objected to the autonomic and extrapyramidal side effects of antipsychotic drugs. In contrast, middle-class, private practice patients objected to the drowsiness, or the sense of being slowed down, which accompanies the minor tranquilizers.

Greenblatt and Shader (1976) stated that there was no consistent evidence that tricyclic antidepressants, antipsychotic drugs, or a combination of these were any better than the ben-zodiazepines in the drug treatment of neurotic anxiety. Neverthe-less, treatment must always remain flexible and individualized. For some anxious patients, especially those of middle age or older in whom depressive symptoms are either manifest or suspected because of the nature of the precipitating stress, an antidepres-sant drug with sedative effects will often produce more satisfac-tory results than will the minor tranquilizers. Doxepin has been publicized as such an agent, as has the standard tricyclic, ami-triptyline. A minority of patients with mild to moderate anxiety will do well with a neuroleptic given at low dosages. The physi-cian might prefer to use an antipsychotic drug or a sedating antihistamine (eg, hydroxyzine) in treating an anxious patient known to abuse drugs.

For certain patients with high levels of both psychic and somatic anxiety, a benzodiazepine may not provide adequate re-lief. In these cases, the addition of propranolol to the ben-zodiazepine may be useful, especially for alleviation of symptoms of autonomic overactivity. Lader (1974) suggested that the com-bination of a lower than usual dosage of diazepam along with propranolol seems useful for patients who primarily show soma-tic expression of their anxiety.

Although research has attempted to correlate relief of specific patterns of anxiety symptoms with individual drugs, there is still no solid consensus favoring one benzodiazepine over another, or even one category of minor tranquilizer over another, for relief of target symptoms. This is unfortunate, since global measurements of improvement are too nonspecific.

Blackwell's summary (1975) of the results of a survey of general practitioners revealed the following frequencies of use for diazepam. The conditions listed represent those categories of primary diagnoses in which emotional factors were felt to play a causal role. In 64% of the cases, other drugs were used along with diazepam.

Mental disorders	30%
Musculoskeletal	17%
Circulatory	16%
Geriatric	8%
Medical, surgical aftercare	7%
Gastrointestinal	6%
Central nervous system	6%
Genitourinary	3%
Other	7%

Studies which have suggested the use of particular drugs for certain target symptoms require confirmation. As noted previously, some controlled studies have found that chlordiazepoxide seemed preferable to diazepam for anxious patients with higher levels of accompanying depression, hostility, and hypochondriacal worries, whereas diazepam was superior for patients with higher levels of somatization. Another study found diazepam to display especially favorable effects in anxiety states with prominent insomnia and cardiac and respiratory complaints. However, it adversely influenced autonomic nervous system symptoms. Better responses to benzodiazepines and other drugs are repeatedly observed with higher initial levels of anxiety. Although Gardos and Shader (1968) reported increases in hostility with chlordiazepoxide, Rickels et al (1974) observed this drug to be significantly superior to placebo in relieving clinical hostility according to physician and patient ratings. Whether or not oxazepam causes fewer problems with elevations of hostility than the other benzodiazepines in actual clinical practice is unclear. Its short biological half-life makes drug accumulation unlikely and the drug therefore useful for treating geriatric patients. It has also been useful in relieving somatic complaints in lower socioeconomic level patients. Clorazepate seems to be effective in anxiety relief, and it may have lesser sedative effects than the other benzodiazepines. If response to the benzodiazepines is unsatisfactory, tybamate is a more sensible alternative than meprobamate, as tybamate does not produce liver enzyme induction, induce significant tolerance, or have much chance of evoking a withdrawal syndrome. It's short biological half-life recommends it for anxious geriatric patients.

Hollister (1973) has wisely referred to the varying levels of tolerance to given dosages of benzodiazepines (as is true of other drugs with sedative effects) in different patients. He recommended giving the initial doses of these drugs in the evening, when the patient is at home (weekends would also be appropriate), to avoid the inconvenience of initial excessive sedation while at work. He noted the relatively long biological half-lives of these drugs and suggested a twice per day dosage schedule that gives most of the day's total dose at night. Such a routine capitalizes on the drugs' hypnotic action to assist with nighttime sleep and leaves only a mild, residual sedation which is beneficial for anxiety relief during the day.

The higher the dosages of antianxiety drugs employed and the longer they are used, the greater are the risks of drug tolerance and dependence. It is better to reduce the dosage and then discontinue the drug altogether following the relief of anxiety than to maintain the patient on medication indefinitely. Such limits placed on the length of time of drug use minimize the patient's tendency to overvalue the drug's effects and allow his confidence in his own coping devices to depreciate. Obviously, if anxiety symptoms recur, medication can be reinstated. While the most important criterion of progress is to be found in the patient's report about his feelings, more objective measures—such as those reflected in his functioning at work and with friends, family, and the doctor—should be considered as indices which confirm or dispute the patient's subjective appraisal.

In his discussion of oxazepam in clinical practice, Ayd (1975) made some observations which hold true for all minor tranquilizers. He noted that oxazepam was most effective in patients with previously stable personalities whose illnesses were of recent origin and who had had little previous exposure to drugs and/or alcohol. Conversely, the more immature the personality, the more chronic will be the disorder; and the greater the prior consumption of drugs or alcohol, the less favorable will be the outcome with oxazepam (or any other minor tranquilizer).

Patients suffering from anxiety usually have problems with disrupted sleep. In contrast to sedative-hypnotic drugs, the benzodiazepines have been shown to cause only a minimal disruption of the normal sleep pattern. Hollister (1973) and Kales and Scharf (1973) concluded that all benzodiazepines cause improvements in sleep induction and sleep maintenance. They found that chlordiazepoxide was less effective than diazepam for short-term use. Flurazepam, a benzodiazepine used almost exclusively as a hypnotic, was the most effective benzodiazepine for sleep induction and sleep maintenance, as well as for persistence of desired effect over weeks. Kales and Scharf also noted that all benzodiazepines suppress stage four (deep) sleep but leave other sleep stages intact when given at usual therapeutic dosages.

Psychotropic drugs (antidepressants, minor tranquilizers, neuroleptics, sedative-hypnotics) are all too often given injudiciously in combination with each other. Such polypharmacy has been criticized for many valid reasons. Ayd stated the case strongly, saying, "Admittedly some combinations are desirable and fill a true need. Most, however, are of very limited usefulness, are potentially dangerous and injudiciously conceived. Such multiple drug therapy is a costly victimization of patients who are overmedicated, underdosed and exposed to the side effects hazard

of each drug as well as to the risks of their adverse interaction."
(1972) Of course, there are more than a few instances in clinical
practice, especially in severe mental disorders such as schizophrenia and manic-depressive psychoses, where use of more than a
single drug offers advantages. However, in treating most cases of
anxiety, even when they are accompanied by depressive and
somatic complaints, a single psychotropic drug should be satisfactory. No advantage is observed in giving two or more minor
tranquilizers at the same time, but these drugs can be given
safely with other medications being used for a concurrent medical
problem.

Some psychotropic drugs can alter the plasma concentrations
of other psychotropics: barbiturates, chloral hydrate, lithium, and
oral contraceptives lower plasma tricyclic levels; methylphenidate and phenothiazines increase plasma tricyclic concentrations.
The benzodiazepines do not appear to produce such effects (Ayd,
1973).

With the exception of lithium carbonate, routine measurements of the plasma concentrations of psychotropic drugs are not
carried out. In light of the wide variations in plasma concentrations of anxiolytic drugs in different patients receiving the same
dosages (eg, threefold in patients receiving meprobamate and
eightfold in patients on diazepam), individual drug dosage requirements will obviously vary (Hollister, 1973). Bianchi et al
(1974) reported that the plasma concentration of diazepam two
hours after a single pretreatment dose of this drug correlated
with the steady-state plasma level of diazepam measured after
one week of treatment. A low two-hour plasma level after a single
dose correlated strongly with improvement after the first week of
treatment. A high two-hour plasma level after a single dose
correlated with reports of excessive tiredness throughout a
three-week treatment period with the drug. In all likelihood,
laboratory determinations of plasma concentrations of antianxiety drugs will become routine in the future as a guide to proper
dosage schedules.

DRUG TREATMENT OF
PSYCHOSOMATIC DISORDERS

Antianxiety agents clearly have a place in treating anxious
and depressive symptoms which accompany medical disorders.
More controversial is the place of minor tranquilizers in treating

the physical symptoms of psychosomatic illnesses in which anxiety or depression is believed to be the underlying cause. However, the controversy is largely based on theoretical rather than practical, clinical grounds, since these drugs are commonly prescribed for essential hypertension, peptic ulcer, bronchial asthma, migraine headaches, coronary insufficiency, colitis, and dermatologic and other disorders.

Marino (1973) reviewed his experience with a combination of amitriptyline and chlordiazepoxide for patients with anorexia nervosa. All of the patients involved had been unresponsive to other pharmacologic treatments and to psychotherapy. This drug combination was associated with striking improvement of somatic (anorexia, weight loss) and psychologic symptoms. It was also useful in spastic gastrointestinal disorders and essential hypertension.

Wheatley (1973) compared an anticholinergic drug, a minor tranquilizer, and a combination of both drugs with regard to improvement of symptoms of peptic ulcer disease (pain, heartburn, nausea, vomiting, flatulence, anorexia). He found that the minor tranquilizer alone was at least as effective as the other two approaches and produced fewer troublesome side effects. Minor and major tranquilizers and tricyclic antidepressants have been prescribed for various gastrointestinal disorders, including anorexia, obesity, peptic ulcer, colitis, diarrhea, and constipation. These drugs are used for their sedative, anxiety-relieving, antidepressant, or autonomic-stabilizing effects. In separate studies, hydroxyzine (Heurich, 1972), oxazepam (Kaunn, 1968), imipramine (Spiegelberg, 1968), and chlorpromazine (Baum, 1957) were found to be beneficial for bronchial asthma. Imipramine (Spiegelberg, 1968) was helpful in relieving symptoms of ulcerative colitis, as was lithium carbonate (Zibrook, 1972). The presumption was that an underlying depressive process contributing to the colitis was relieved by these agents.

Minor tranquilizers are commonly used in patients with coronary insufficiency for relief of accompanying overt anxiety and of underlying anxiety which may be a factor in the pathophysiology. Ishikowa et al (1971) reported on the importance of emotions (especially anxiety and hostility) in inducing attacks of angina pectoris, and they distinguished between emotionally and physically caused attacks. Bishop and Reichert (1971) emphasized the importance of stabilizing emotions in the management of patients with both acute and chronic congestive heart failure. Daniell (1975) found that intravenous diazepam and chlordiazepoxide caused an increase in coronary blood flow and cardiac output and a decrease in myocardial oxygen consumption in animals. Therefore, it is possible that these drugs may benefit a patient with angina pectoris not only by relieving anxiety but also by their direct cardiovascular effects.

Wheatley (1974) reported on a study by a general practitioners' research group which found that an antianxiety drug given along with antihypertensive medication not only relieved anxiety but also probably reduced the medical complications of hypertension.

Minor tranquilizers also have skeletal muscle relaxing properties. Consequently, these drugs have been used in many disorders in which exaggerated muscle tone and muscle spasm are believed to be factors. Martin (1972) stated that for headaches resulting from muscle contraction, minor tranquilizers are helpful but rarely permanently beneficial. He recommended psychotherapy and adjunctive drug treatment for tension headaches. He further recommended combining non-narcotic analgesics with sedative-hypnotics for treating such headaches. Another controlled, double-blind study (Gilbert and Koepke, 1973) found aspirin useful for relieving the pain of musculoskeletal disorders, but not for reducing emotional distress. Meprobamate relieved emotional symptoms, but it was not very effective against pain. The combination of aspirin and meprobamate was preferred for treating severe musculoskeletal symptoms associated with anxiety.

Okasha et al (1973) reported that doxepin (30 to 90 mg per day) was superior to diazepam (6 to 18 mg per day), amitriptyline (30 to 90 mg per day), and placebo in relieving the pain of psychogenic headaches. The headaches were vascular, muscular contraction, or combined types and developed after periods of anxiety and/or depression, which persisted after the headache developed. Improvement of the headache correlated with a lessening of anxiety and depression.

Medansky (1971) commented on the benefits of chlordiazepoxide and of a combination of amitriptyline and perphenazine in dermatologic disorders in which anxiety played an important, aggravating (and possibly precipitating) role. In an open study (Boueri, 1971), oxazepam was found to be effective in relieving various allergic disorders which had strong emotional components. A complete remission of allergy symptoms (including asthma, skin disorders, rhinitis, bronchitis) occurred in approximately 50% of the cases.

The above studies are but a sampling of the numerous reports in the literature which recommend minor tranquilizers for the relief of anxiety as well as of somatic symptoms accompanying certain medical problems. Lesse (1970) noted that patients with various psychosomatic disorders usually pass through a period of mounting anxiety before manifesting physical symptoms. He recommended that severe anxiety first be relieved with antipsychotic drugs (or a minor tranquilizer if the anxiety is only moderate), and that psychotherapy be undertaken only after the anxiety is reduced.

A careful interview with the patient with a psychosomatic illness will often uncover emotional components. If the past medical history reveals recurrent depressions, and if a depressive mood is associated with the current physical problem, a tricyclic antidepressant drug should be given a trial. If the interview reveals anxiety as the prominent emotional factor, a minor tranquilizer should be given. Often a patient will speak of anxiety or depression as a consequence of a physical ailment. However, a thorough interview will frequently reveal that these affects actually preceded the somatic dysfunction. Middle-aged and older persons often suffer from masked depressions. Their complaints are primarily physical and thereby obscure the mood disorder. A history of a previous depressive illness, of depressive symptoms accompanying the physical disorder, or of an overly pessimistic outlook are but a few indicators of the real, underlying problem.

Whether or not anxiolytic drugs truly benefit patients with psychosomatic disorders when there is little or no accompanying overt anxiety is not clear. However, many clinical reports have indicated that the anxiolytics are often useful for bronchial asthma, dermatologic disorders, essential hypertension, coronary insufficiency, peptic ulcer, allergies, colitis, migraine headaches, muscle tension headaches, and other ailments.

DRUG TREATMENT OF ACUTE ALCOHOLIC WITHDRAWAL SYNDROME AND OF THE ABSTINENT ALCOHOLIC

In its earliest phase, abstinence from heavy alcohol consumption can resemble a functional anxiety state. Mild to moderate anxiety, tension, tremulousness, and insomnia are prominent. As abstinence is prolonged, visual and auditory hallucinations appear, without significant disorientation. In the more advanced, delirious stage, terrifying visual and tactile hallucinations, great agitation, and severe disorientation are present. Convulsions can occur at any time.

Although paraldehyde and barbiturates treat this withdrawal syndrome successfully, use of the benzodiazepines is preferable, as noted earlier in the chapter. During the most severe phase of withdrawal, intramuscular dosages of up to 50 to 100 mg of chlordiazepoxide, or of 5 to 20 mg of diazepam, every 1 or 2 hours for 12 to 24 hours can achieve the steadying, quieting effect desired. Thereafter, use of oral preparations is indicated, since absorption of drug from intramuscular sites is irregular, slow, and often incomplete. After initial quieting occurs, 50 mg of oral chlordiazepoxide three or four times per day is usually effective in maintaining symptom control.

Chlordiazepoxide and diazepam have anxiety-relieving, sedative, and muscle-relaxing properties and do not carry great risks of severe hypotension. These qualities represent advantages over other drugs, especially the phenothiazines, which can cause marked hypotension and lower the seizure threshold. Kessen and Gross (1970) found paraldehyde better for relieving hallucinations, and chlordiazepoxide preferable for preventing seizures. Oxazepam can be used, but it is not available in parenteral forms.

Treatment of the alcoholic who is no longer drinking is a complex, challenging task requiring a multimodality treatment program of drug therapy, individual counseling or psychotherapy, group therapy, attendance at Alcoholics Anonymous meetings, marital and family therapy, vocational rehabilitation, and other approaches. Psychotropic medications relieve the feelings of anxiety, depression, and hostility which previously motivated the use of alcohol. Whether a minor tranquilizer, an antipsychotic, or an antidepressant drug should be used depends upon the individual patient. A risk in using the minor tranquilizers involves their potential for abuse which can lead to serious drug dependence. Fortunately, their margin of safety is wide: at least eight times the average daily dosage of chlordiazepoxide would have to be taken over several weeks before a withdrawal syndrome would become a significant threat. A problem arising more frequently is that of the patient combining tranquilizers and alcohol; this leads to severe intoxication. For patients at risk to abuse alcohol and drugs, an antipsychotic drug would be preferable to a minor tranquilizer since the former is not associated with abuse.

MINOR TRANQUILIZERS IN
PSYCHIATRIC DISORDERS OTHER
THAN ANXIETY STATES

The primary symptoms of neurotic disorders other than anxiety states are not as responsive to anxiolytic medication. Hysterical neuroses, conversion or dissociative type, ordinarily require psychotherapy, hypnotic techniques, or an amytal interview. Anxiolytic drugs provide a calming effect when required. Obsessive-compulsive neuroses are not responsive to these drugs except for relief of associated anxiety. Shader (1971) stated that anxious obsessional patients with vivid imaginations and poor reality testing respond better to the phenothiazines than to the minor tranquilizers. For phobic disorders, minor tranquilizers may relieve anticipatory anxiety but usually do not in themselves do away with phobic avoidance behavior.

Anxiety accompanying schizophrenia is treated with antipsychotic drugs. Occasionally anxiety will persist or develop when psychotic manifestations have cleared, despite adequate dosing with antipsychotic drugs. A trial with a minor tranquilizer added to the antipsychotic drug may then be useful.

Minor tranquilizers are also helpful in relieving anxiety associated with organic brain syndromes. Because of their short biological half-lives, tybamate and oxazepam are especially useful. This property minimizes drug accumulation and consequent untoward effects. If a brain syndrome presents clinically with psychotic symptoms as well as anxiety, an antipsychotic drug is indicated, specifically, one with fewer autonomic side effects than chlorpromazine. In general, psychotropic drugs are not tolerated well by elderly patients. Also, minor tranquilizers given in excessive doses and/or for prolonged periods can increase these patients' depression and confusion.

REFERENCES

Aivazian, G.H.: Clinical evaluation of diazepam. *Dis Nerv System* 25:491, 1964.

Aklquist, R.P.: A study of the adrenotropic receptors. *Am J Physiol.* 153:586, 1948.

Alexander, F. et al: Experimental studies of emotional stress. 1. Hyperthyroidism. *Psychosom Med.* 23:104, 1961.

Appleton, W.S.: Third psychoactive drug usage guide. *Dis Nerv System* 37(1):39, 1976.

Ayd, F.J.: A critical appraisal of chlordiazepoxide. *J Neuropsychiatr.* 3:177, 1962.

Ayd, F.J.: Oxazepam: an overview. *Dis Nerv System* 36[5(2)]:14, 1975.

Ayd, F.J.: Once-a-day neuroleptic and tricyclic antidepressant therapy. *Int Drug Ther Newsletter* 7(9,10), 1972.

Ayd, F.J.: Interaction of barbiturate and non-barbiturate hypnotics and benzodiazepines with tricyclic antidepressants. *Int Drug Ther Newsletter* 8(4), 1973.

Basowitz, H. et al: Anxiety and performance changes with a minimal dose of epinephrine. *Arch Neurol & Psychiatr.* 76:98, 1956.

Batterman, R.C., Mouratoff, G.J., and Kaufman, J.E.: Comparative treatment of the psychoneurotic reactive type anxiety states with fluphenazine and chlordiazepoxide. *J New Drugs* 3:297, 1963.

Baum, G.L. et al: The role of chlorpromazine in the treatment of bronchial asthma and chronic pulmonary emphysema. *Dis Chest* 32:574, 1957.

Beaubren, J. et al: Doxepin in the treatment of psychoneurotic patients. *Curr Ther Res.* 12:192, 1970.

Bianchi, G.N. et al: Plasma levels of diazepam as a therapeutic predictor in anxiety states. *Psychopharmacologia* 35:113, 1974.

Bishop, L.F. and Reichert, D.: Emotions and heart failure. *Psychosomatics* 12:412, 1971.

Blackwell, B.: Minor tranquilizers: use, misuse or overuse. *Psychosomatics* 16:28, 1975.

Blackwell, B.: A critical review of oxazepam: efficacy and specificity. *Dis Nerv System* 36[5(2)]:17, 1975.

Bliss, E.L. et al: Reaction of the adrenal cortex to emotional stress. *Psychosom Med.* 18:56, 1956.

Bodi, T.: Clinical use of benzendopyrine and two analogs. In *The First Hahnemann Symposium of Psychotropic Medicine,* edited by J.H. Iodine and J.H. Moyer, p. 543. Philadelphia: Lea & Febiger, 1962.

Bonn, J.A.: Some recent advances in the management of anxiety. *Postgrad Med J.* 48 (September suppl): 24, 1972.

Boueri-Atem, S., Brahim, D., and Curi, J.O.: Oxazepam in allergic conditions. *Psychosomatics* 12:46, 1971.

Brandt, A.L. and Oakes, F.O.: Preanesthesia medication: a double-blind study of a new drug, diazepam. *Anesth Analg.* 44:125, 1965.

Breggin, P.R.: The psychophysiology of anxiety with a review of the literature concerning adrenalin. *J Nerv & Mental Dis.* 139:558, 1964.

Breslow, I.: Evaluation of hydroxyzine pamoate concentration as an ataractic. *Curr Ther Res.* 9:10, 1968.

Brill, N.Q. et al: Controlled study of psychiatric outpatient treatment. *Arch Gen Psychiatr.* 10:581, 1964.

Byck, R.: Drugs in the treatment of psychiatric disorders. In *The Pharmacological Basis of Therapeutics,* edited by L.S. Goodman and A. Gilman. New York: Macmillan Publishing Company, 1975.

Caffey, E.M. et al: Veterans Administration (VA) cooperative studies in psychiatry. In *Principles of Psychopharmacology,* edited by W.G. Clark and J. del Guidice. New York: Academic Press, Inc., 1970.

216

Caffey, E.M. et al: Drug treatment in psychiatry. *Int J Psychiatr.* 9:432, 1970-71.

Capstick, N.S. et al: A comparative trial of diazepam (Valium) and amylobarbitone. *Br J Psychiatr.* 111:517, 1965.

Cassano, G.B., Castrogiovanni, P., and Conti, L.: Drug responses in different anxiety states under benzodiazepine treatment. Some multivariate analyses for the evaluation of 'rating scale for depression' scores. In *The Benzodiazepines,* edited by S. Garattini, E. Mussini, and L.O. Randall, p. 379. New York: Raven Press, 1973.

Charalamporis, K.D., Tooley, W., and Yates, C.: Clorazepate dipotassium: A new benzodiazepine antianxiety agent. *J Clin Pharm & New Drugs* 13:114, 1973.

Chesrow, E.J. et al: Blind study of oxazepam in the management of geriatric patients with behavioral problems. *Clin Med.* 72:1001, 1965.

Coleman, J.H.: Concepts in beta blockade. *Dis Nerv System* 36(1):46, 1975.

Coleman, J.H. and Evans, W.E.: Pharmacotherapy of the acute alcoholic withdrawal syndrome. *Dis Nerv System* 36(4):151, 1975.

Corey, P.J., Deaver, J.M., and Haupt, G.J.: The use of Librium for surgical patients. *Penn Med J.* 65:1053, 1962.

Corr, L. et al: Length of treatment with anxiolytic sedatives and response to their sudden withdrawal. *Acta Psychiatr Scand.* 49:51, 1973.

Covi, L. et al: Drugs and group psychotherapy in neurotic depression. *Am J Psychiatr.* 131:191, 1974.

Daneman, E.A.: Double-blind study with diazepam, chlordiazepoxide, and placebo in the treatment of psychoneurotic anxiety. *J Med Assoc Georgia* 53:55, 1964.

Daniell, H.B.: Cardiovascular effects of diazepam and chlordiazepoxide. *Eur J Pharmacol.* 32(1):58, 1975.

Dasberg, H.H. et al: Plasma concentrations of diazepam and of its metabolite, N-desmethyl diazepam, in relation to anxiolytic effect. *Clin Pharmacol Ther.* 15:473, 1974.

Dasberg, H.H. and van Praag, H.M.: The therapeutic effect of short-term oral diazepam treatment on acute clinical anxiety in a crisis center. *Acta Psychiatr Scand.* 50:326, 1974.

Dawson-Butterworth, K.: Chemotherapeutics of geriatric sedation. *J Am Geriatr Soc.* 18:97, 1970.

DiMascio, A. and Barrett, J.: Comparative effects of oxazepam in 'high' and 'low' anxious student volunteers. *Psychosomatics* 6:298, 1965.

DiMascio, A. et al: Tybamate: an examination of its actions in high and low anxious normals. *Dis Nerv System* 30:758, 1969.

Donlon, P.T.: Diazepam for akathisia. *Psychosomatics* 14:222, 1973.

Dureman, I. and Norrman, B.: Clinical and experimental comparison of diazepam, clorazepate and placebo. *Psychopharmacologia* (Berlin) 40:279, 1975.

Elmadjian, F.: Excretion of epinephrine and norepinephrine in various emotional states. *J Clin Endocrinol.* 17:608, 1957.

Fann, W.E., Lake, C.R., and Majors, L.F.: Thioridazine in neurotic anxious and depressed patients. *Psychosomatics* 15:117, 1974.

Fisher, J.V., Mason, R.L., and Fisher, J.C.: Emotional illness and the family physician. 2. Management and treatment. *Psychosomatics* 16:107, 1975.

Freud, S.: *The Problem of Anxiety*. New York: W.W. Norton & Co., 1936.

Frohlich, E.D., Dustan, H.P., and Page, I.H.: Hyperdynamic beta-adrenergic circulatory state. *Arch Intern Med.* 117:614, 1966.

Fromm, E.: *Escape From Freedom*. New York: Farrar and Rinehart, 1941.

Gallant, D.M. et al: A controlled evaluation of propranolol in chronic alcoholic patients presenting the symptomatology of anxiety and tension. *J Clin Pharmacol.* 13:41, 1973.

Gardos, G. et al: Differential actions of chlordiazepoxide and oxazepam on hostility. *Arch Gen Psychiatr.* 18:757, 1968.

Gellhorn, E.: Prolegomena to a theory of the emotions. *Perspect Biol & Med.* 4:403, 1961.

Gellhorn, E.: Further studies on the physiology and pathophysiology of the tuning of the central nervous system. *Psychosomatics* 10:94, 1969.

Gilbert, M.M. and Koepke, H.H.: Relief of musculoskeletal and associated psychopathological symptoms with meprobamate and aspirin: a controlled study. *Curr Ther Res.* 15:820, 1973.

Goldberg, H.L.: Doxepin in a single, bedtime dose in psychoneurotic outpatients. *Arch Gen Psychiatr.* 31:513, 1974.

Goldberg, H.L. and Finnerty, R.J.: The use of doxepin in the treatment of symptoms of anxiety neurosis and accompanying depression: a collaborative controlled study. *Am J Psychiatr.* 129:74, 1972.

Goldberg, H.L. and Finnerty, R.J.: The use of hydroxyzine (Vistaril) in the treatment of anxiety neurosis. *Psychosomatics* 14:38, 1973.

Goldstein, B.J. and Brauser, B.: Pharmacologic considerations in the treatment of anxiety and depression in medical practice. *Med Clin North Am* 55(2):485, 1971.

Gottschalk, L.A. et al: Studies of relationships of emotions to plasma lipids. *Psychosom Med.* 27:102, 1965.

Gottschalk, L.A., Stone, W.N., and Gleser, G.C.: Peripheral versus central mechanisms accounting for antianxiety effects of propranolol. *Psychosom Med.* 36(1):47, 1974.

Granville-Grossman, K.L.: Propranolol, anxiety, and the central nervous system. *Br J Clin Pharmacol.* 1:361, 1974.

Granville-Grossman, K.L. and Turner, P.: The effect of propranolol on anxiety. *Lancet* 1:788, 1966.

Greenblatt, D.J. and Shader, R.I.: Meprobamate: a study of irrational drug use. *Am J Psychiatr.* 127:1297, 1971.

Greenblatt, D.J. and Shader, R.I.: Anxious states: drug therapy. In *Progress in Psychiatric Drug Treatment*, Vol. 2, edited by D.F. Klein and R. Gittelman-Klein, p. 596. New York: Brunner/Mazel Inc., 1976.

Grosz, H.J. and Farmer, B.B.: Blood lactate in the development of anxiety symptoms. A critical examination of Pitts' and McClure's hypothesis and experimental study. *Arch Gen Psychiatr.* 21:611, 1969.

Gundlach, R. et al: A double-blind outpatient study of diazepam (Valium) and placebo. *Psychopharmacologia* 9:81, 1966.

Harvey, S.C.: Hypnotics and sedatives: the barbiturates. In *The Pharmacological Basis of Therapeutics,* edited by L.S. Goodman and A. Gilman, p. 102. New York: Macmillan Publishing Company, 1975.

Heurich, A.M. et al: Bronchodilator effects of hydroxyzine hydrochloride. *Respiration* 29:135, 1972.

Hollister, L.E.: Antianxiety drugs in clinical practice. In *The Benzodiazepines,* edited by S. Garattini, E. Mussini, and L.O. Randall, p. 367. New York: Raven Press, 1973.

Hollister, L.E.: *Clinical Use of Psychotherapeutic Drugs.* Springfield, Ill: Charles C Thomas, 1973.

Hollister, L.E.: Uses of psychotherapeutic drugs. *Ann Intern Med.* 79:88, 1973.

Hollister, L.E., Motzenbecker, F.P., and Degan, R.O.: Withdrawal reactions from chlordiazepoxide (Librium). *Psychopharmacologia* 2:63, 1961.

Hollister, L.E. et al: Drug therapy of depression: amitriptyline, perphenazine, and their combination in different syndromes. *Arch Gen Psychiatr.* 17:486, 1967.

Hollister, L.E. et al: Acetophenazine and diazepam in anxious depressions. *Arch Gen Psychiatr.* 24:273, 1971.

Horovitz, Z.P. et al: Cyclic AMP and anxiety. *Psychosomatics* 13:85, 1972.

Howlett, L. and Markoff, R.A.: Clinical experiences with antidepressant drugs in the treatment of anxious-phobic patients. *Comp. Psychiatr.* 16(5):461, 1975.

Hussain, M.Z.: Effect of shape of medication in treatment of anxiety states. *Br J Psychiatr.* 120:507, 1972.

Isbell, H.: Manifestations and treatment of addiction to narcotic drugs and barbiturates. *Med Clin North Am.* 34:425, 1950.

Ishikowa, H. et al: Psychosomatic study of angina pectoris. *Psychosomatics* 12:390, 1971.

Jacobs, M.A., Globus, G., and Heim, E.: Reduction in symptomatology in ambulatory patients. The combined effects of a tranquilizer and psychotherapy. *Arch Gen Psychiatr.* 15:45, 1966.

Jacobsen, E.: Properties of psychotropic drugs. In *Modern Psychiatric Treatment,* edited by T.P. Detri and H.G. Jarecki, p. 617. Philadelphia: J.B. Lippincott Co., 1971.

James, W. and Lange, C.G.: *The Emotions.* Baltimore: The Williams & Wilkins Co., 1922.

Janecek, J. et al: Oxazepam in the treatment of anxiety states. A controlled study. *J Psychiatr Res.* 4:199, 1966.

Jenner, F.A. and Kerry, R.J.: Comparison of diazepam, chlordiazepoxide and amylobarbitone (a multidose, double-blind, crossover study). *Dis Nerv System* 28:245, 1967.

Jenner, F.A., Kerry, R.J., and Parkin, D.: A controlled trial of methaminodiazepoxide (Librium) in the treatment of anxiety in neurotic patients. *J Ment Sci.* 107:575, 1961a.

Jenner, F.A., Kerry, R.J., and Parkin, D.: A controlled comparison of methaminodiazepoxide (Librium) and amylobarbitone in the treatment of anxiety in neurotic patients. *J Ment Sci.* 107:583, 1961b.

Johnson, W.C.: A neglected modality in psychiatric treatment—the monoamine oxidase inhibitors. *Dis Nerv System* 36:521, 1975.

Kales, A. and Sharf, M.B.: Sleep laboratory and clinical studies of the effects of benzodiazepines on sleep: flurazepam, diazepam, chlordiazepoxide, and RO5-4200. In *The Benzodiazepines*, edited by S. Garattini, E. Mussini, and L.O. Randall, p. 577. New York: Raven Press, 1973.

Kasich, A.M.: Clorazepate dipotassium in the treatment of anxiety associated with chronic gastrointestinal disease. *Curr Ther Res.* 15:83, 1973.

Kaunn, J. and Jokl, H.: Treatment of asthmatic dyspnea. *Med Klin.* 63:1814, 1968.

Kellner, R. et al: The short-term antianxiety effects of propranolol. *J Clin Pharmacol.* 14(5,6):301, 1974.

Kelly, D.: Antidepressant drugs for treating anxiety states. *Proc R Soc Med.* 66:5, March, 1973.

Kerry, R.J. and Jenner, F.A.: A double-blind crossover comparison of diazepam with chlordiazepoxide in the treatment of neurotic anxiety. *Psychopharmacologia* (Berlin) 3:302, 1962.

Kessen, B. and Gross, M.M.: Drug therapy in alcoholism. *Curr Psychiatr Ther.* 10:135, 1970.

Kielholz, P. et al: Circulation routieri tranquillisants et alcohol. *Hyg Ment.* 2:39, 1967.

Klein, D.F. and Davis, J.M.: *Diagnosis and Drug Treatment of Psychiatric Disorders.* Baltimore: The Williams & Wilkins Co., 1969.

Klein, D.F. and Fink, M.: Psychiatric reaction patterns to imipramine. *Am J Psychiatr.* 119:432, 1962.

Klerman, G.L.: Clinical research in depression. *Arch Gen Psychiatr.* 24:305, 1971.

Krivda, J.F.: Major or minor tranquilizers for relief of common symptoms of psychoneurosis. *J Psychiatr Nursing & Ment Health Services* 12(4):28, 1974.

Lader, M.H.: The effect of anxiety on response to treatment. *Austr & NZ J Psychiatr.* 3:288, 1969.

Lader, M.H.: The nature of anxiety. *Br J Psychiatr.* 121:481, 1972.

Lader, M.H.: The peripheral and central role of catecholamines in the mechanisms of anxiety. *Int Pharmacopsychiatr.* 9:125, 1974.

Lader, M.H. and Marks, I.: *Clinical Anxiety.* New York: Grune & Stratton, 1971.

Lehman, H.E. and Ban, T.A.: Pharmacotherapy of tension and anxiety. In *Handbook of Psychiatric Therapies*, edited by J. Masserman, p. 251. New York: Jason Aronson Inc., 1973.

Lesse, S.: *Anxiety: Its Components, Development, and Treatment.* New York: Grune & Stratton, 1970.

Leszkovsky, G. and Tardos, L.: Some effects of propranolol on the central nervous system. *J Pharm Pharmacol.* 17:518, 1965.

Levi, L.: Neuroendocrinology of anxiety. In *Studies of Anxiety*, edited by M.H. Lader. London: Royal Medico-Psychological Association, 1969.

Lingl, F.H.: Double-blind comparison of haloperidol and thioridazine in treatment resistant psychoneurotic outpatients. *Psychosomatics* 14:235, 1973.

Lord, D.J. and Kidd, C.B.: Haloperidol versus diazepam: a double-blind crossover clinical trial. *Med J Austr.* 1:586, 1973.

Lorr, M., McNair, D.M., and Weinstein, J.: Early effects of chlordiazepoxide (Librium) used with psychotherapy. *J Psychiatr Res.* 1:257, 1963.

Lorr, M. et al: Meprobamate and chlorpromazine in psychotherapy. *Arch Gen Psychiatr.* 4:381, 1961.

Maggs, R. and Neville, R.: Chlordiazepoxide (Librium): A clinical trial of its use in controlling symptoms of anxiety. *Br J Psychiatr.* 110:540, 1964.

Marino, A.: Behavioral and psychosomatic effects of benzodiazepines: interactions with other drugs. In *The Benzodiazepines*, edited by S. Garattini, E. Mussini, and L.O. Randall, p. 631. New York: Raven Press, 1973.

Martin, M.J.: Muscle contraction headache. *Psychosomatics* 13:16, 1972.

McDowall, A., Owen, S., and Robin, A.A.: A controlled comparison of diazepam and amylobarbitone in anxiety states. *Br J Psychiatr.* 112:629, 1966.

McNair, D.M. et al: Some effects of chlordiazepoxide and meprobamate with psychiatric outpatients. *Psychopharmacologia* 7:256, 1965.

McPherson, F.M. and LeGassicke, J.: A single-patient, self-controlled and self-recorded trial of Wy3498 (oxazepam). *Br J Psychiatr.* 111:149, 1965.

Medansky, R.S.: Emotion and skin. A double-blind evaluation of psychotropic drugs. *Psychosomatics* 12:326, 1971.

Mendels, J., Weinstein, N., and Cochrane, C.: The relationship between depression and anxiety. *Arch Gen Psychiatr.* 27:649, 1972.

Mendelson, M., Hirsch, S., and Webber, C.S.: A critical examination of some recent theoretical models in psychosomatic medicine. *Psychosom Med.* 18:363, 1956.

Menon, M.S. and Badsha, H.: A controlled clinical trial with diazepam. *Antiseptic* 70(3):171, 1973.

Miner, G.D.: Evidence of genetic components in the neuroses, a review. *Arch Gen Psychiatr.* 29:111, 1973.

Mirsky, I.A.: Psychophysiological basis of anxiety. *Psychosomatics* 1:1, 1960.

Mohr, R.C. and Mead, B.T.: Meprobamate addiction. *N Engl J Med.* 259:865, 1958.

Okasha, A., Ghaleb, H.A., and Sadek, B.: Double-blind trial for clinical management of psychogenic headache. *Br J Psychiatr.* 122:181, 1973.

Oswald, I. and Priest, R.G.: Five weeks to escape the sleeping pill habit. *Br Med J.* 2:1093, 1965.

Overall, J.E. et al: Imipramine and thioridazine in depressed and schizophrenic patients: are there specific antidepressant drugs? *JAMA.* 189:605, 1964.

Parry, J.H. et al: National patterns of psychotherapeutic drug use. *Arch Gen Psychiatr.* 28:769, 1973.

Persky, H. et al: Relation of emotional responses and changes in plasma hydrocortisone after a stressful interview. *Arch Neurol & Psychiatr.* 79:434, 1958.

Pitts, F.N. and McClure, J.N.: Lactate metabolism in anxiety neurosis. *N Engl J Med*. 277:1329, 1967.

Raab, E., Rickels, K., and Moore, E.: A double-blind evaluation of tybamate in anxious neurotic medical clinic patients. *Am J Psychiatr*. 120:1005, 1964.

Rado, S.: *Psychoanalysis of Behavior*, Vol. 1. New York: Grune & Stratton, Inc., 1956.

Raper, C. and McCullough, M.W.: Adrenoreceptor classification. *Med J Austr*. 2:1331, 1971.

Raskin, A.: A guide for drug use in depressive disorders. *Am J Psychiatr*. 131:181, 1974.

Ricca, J.: Clorazepate dipotassium in anxiety: a clinical trial with diazepam and placebo controls. *J Clin Pharm & New Drugs* 12(7):286, 1972.

Rickels, K.: Drug combination therapy in neurotic depression: its advantages and disadvantages. *Pharmakopsychiatric Neuropsychopharmakologie* 4(6):308, 1971.

Rickels, K.: Predictors of response to benzodiazepines in anxious outpatients. In *The Benzodiazepines*, edited by S. Garattini, E. Mussini, and L.O. Randall, p. 391. New York: Raven Press, 1973.

Rickels, K. and Downing, R.W.: Drug- and placebo-treated neurotic outpatients. *Arch Gen Psychiatr*. 16:369, 1967.

Rickels, K. and Downing, R.W.: Chlordiazepoxide and hostility in anxious outpatients. *Am J Psychiatr*. 131:442, 1974.

Rickels, K., Hesbacher, P., and Downing, R.W.: Differential drug effects in neurotic depression. *Dis Nerv System* 31:468, 1970.

Rickels, K. and Snow, L.: Meprobamate and phenobarbital sodium in anxious neurotic psychiatric and medical clinic outpatients. *Psychopharmacologia* 5:339, 1964.

Rickels, K. et al: Evaluation of tranquilizing drugs in medical outpatients (meprobamate, prochlorperazine, amobarbital sodium, and placebo). *JAMA*. 171:1649, 1959.

Rickels, K. et al: Drug treatment in depression: antidepressant or tranquilizer? *JAMA*. 201:675, 1967.

Rickels, K. et al: Tybamate—a perplexing drug. *Am J Psychiatr*. 125:320, 1968.

Rickels, K. et al: Differential effects of chlordiazepoxide and fluphenazine in two anxious patient populations. *Psychopharmacologia* 12:181, 1968.

Rickels, K. et al: Butabarbital sodium and chlordiazepoxide in anxious neurotic outpatients: a collaborative controlled study. *Clin Pharmacol Ther*. 11:538, 1970.

Rickels, K. et al: Haloperidol in anxiety. *J Clin Pharmacol*. 11:440, 1971.

Rickels, K. et al: Thiothixene and thioridazine in anxiety. *Br J Psychiatr*. 125:79, 1974.

Rickels, K. et al: Amitriptyline in anxious-depressed outpatients. *Am J Psychiatr*. 131:1, 1974.

Robinson, D.S. et al: Controlled clinical trial of the MAO inhibitor phenelzine in the treatment of depressive-anxiety states. *Arch Gen Psychiatr*. 29:407, 1973.

Rogers, C.R.: *Client Centered Therapy.* Boston: Houghton Mifflin Co., 1951.

Rosenthal, S.H. and Bowden, C.L.: A double-blind comparison of thioridazine versus diazepam in patients with chronic mixed anxiety and depressive symptoms. *Curr Ther Res.* 15:261, 1973.

Roth, M.: The phobic-anxiety-depersonalization syndrome and some general etiological problems in psychiatry. *J. Neuropsychiatr.* 1:293, 1960.

Sanders, J.F.: Evaluation of oxazepam and placebo in emotionally disturbed aged patients. *Geriatrics* 20:739, 1965.

Sargant, W.: The treatment of anxiety states and atypical depressions by the monoamine oxidase inhibitor drugs. *J Neuropsychiatr.* 3(Suppl):96, 1962.

Sargant, W.: Drugs in the treatment of depressive disorders. *Am J Psychiatr.* 131:181, 1974.

Schapira, K. et al: Study on the effects of tablet color in the treatment of anxiety states. *Br Med J.* 2:446, 1970.

Shader, R.I.: Antianxiety agents: a clinical perspective. In *Clinical Handbook of Psychopharmacology,* edited by A. DiMascio and R.I. Shader. New York: Science House, 1970.

Shader, R.I.: Drugs in the management of anxiety. *Curr Psychiatr Ther.* 11:81, 1971.

Shapiro, A.K.: Rational use of psychopharmaceutic agents. *NY J Med.* 64:1084, 1964.

Shelton, J. and Hollister, L.E.: Simulated abuse of tybamate in men. *JAMA.* 100:116, 1967.

A single-dose antianxiety drug. Report from the General Practitioner Research Group. *Practitioner,* 215(1285):98, 1975.

Slater, E. and Shields, J.: Genetic aspects of anxiety. In *Studies in Anxiety,* edited by M.H. Lader, p. 62. London: Royal Medico-Psychological Association, 1969.

Smith, D.E. and Wesson, D.R.: A new method for treatment of barbiturate dependence. *JAMA.* 213:294, 1970.

Smith, M.E. and Chasson, J.B.: Comparison of diazepam, chlorpromazine, and trifluoperazine in a double-blind clinical investigation. *J Neuropsychiatr.* 5:593, 1964.

Solow, C.: Drug therapy of mental illness: tranquilizers and other depressant drugs. In *An Introduction to Psychopharmacology,* edited by R.E. Rech and K.E. Moore, p. 289. New York: Raven Press, 1971.

Spiegelberg, U.: Pharmacotherapy and psychosomatics. *Int Pharmacopsychiatr.* 1:87, 1968.

Stein, L., Wise, C.D., and Berger, B.D.: Antianxiety action of benzodiazepines: decrease in activity of serotonin neurons in the punishment system. In *The Benzodiazepines,* edited by S. Garattini, E. Mussini, and L.O. Randall, p. 299. New York: Raven Press, 1973.

Sterlin, C. et al: A comparative study of doxepin and chlordiazepoxide in the treatment of psychoneurotic outpatients. *Curr Ther Res.* 12:195, 1970.

Stone, W.W., Gleser, G.C., and Gottschalk, L.A.: Anxiety and beta-adrenergic blockade. *Arch Gen Psychiatr.* 29:620, 1973.

Stotsky, B.A.: Sodium butabarbital for emotional disorders and insomnia. *Dis Nerv System* 33:798, 1972.

Stotsky, B.A. and Borozne, J.: Butisol sodium vs Librium among geriatric and younger outpatients, and nursing home patients. *Dis Nerv System* 33:254, 1972.

Sullivan, H.S.: *The Interpersonal Theory of Psychiatry.* New York: W.W. Norton, 1953.

Tobin, J.M. et al: Clinical evaluation of oxazepam for the management of anxiety. *Dis Nerv System* 25:689, 1964.

Tyrer, P.J. and Lader, M.H.: Response to propranolol and diazepam in somatic and psychic anxiety. *Br J Med.* 2:14, 1974.

Vazuka, F.A. and McLaughlin, B.E.: Chemotherapy of symptoms of chronic anxiety states and other neurotic disorders. *Psychosomatics* 6:73, 1965.

Warburton, D.M.: Modern biochemical concepts of anxiety. *Int Pharmacopsychiatr.* 9:189, 1974.

West, E.D. and daFonseca, A.F.: Controlled trial of meprobamate. *Br Med J.* 2:1206, 1965.

Wheatley, D.: Comparative effects of propranolol and chlordiazepoxide in anxiety states. *Br J Psychiatr.* 115:1411, 1969.

Wheatley, D.: Evaluation of psychotropic drugs in general practice. *Proc R Soc Med.* 65:317, April, 1972.

Wheatley, D.: *Psychopharmacology in Family Practice.* London: Heinemann Medical Books, Ltd., 1973.

Wheatley, D.: Psychiatric aspects of hypertension. *Psychopharmacol Bull.* 10(2):4, 1974.

Wiersum, J.: Clorazepate dipotassium in anxiety: a double-blind trial with diazepam controls. *Curr Ther Res.* 14:442, 1972.

Wittenborn, J.R.: *The Clinical Psychopharmacology of Anxiety.* Springfield, Ill: Charles C Thomas, 1966.

Wolpe, J.: The experimental foundations of some new psychotherapeutic methods. In *Experimental Foundations of Clinical Psychology,* edited by A. Bachrach, p. 554. New York: Basic Books, 1962.

Woodward, J., Henry, B.W., and Overall, J.E.: Patterns of symptom change in anxious-depressed outpatients treated with different drugs. *Dis Nerv System* 36(3):125, 1975.

Yamamoto, J., Kline, F.M., and Burgoyne, R.W.: The treatment of severe anxiety in outpatients: a controlled study comparing chlordiazepoxide and chlorpromazine. *Psychosomatics* 14:46, 1973.

Zibrook, S.: Ulcerative colitis: case responding to treatment with lithium carbonate. *JAMA.* 219:755, 1972.

Zung, W.W.K.: The differentiation of anxiety and depressive disorders. A biometric approach. *Psychosomatics* 12:380, 1971.

9 Antipsychotic Drugs

Burton J. Goldstein, M.D.

INTRODUCTION

It is difficult for a psychiatrist who received his or her psychiatric training after 1956 to fully appreciate the impact of the serendipitous discovery of chlorpromazine in 1952 (Swazey, 1974) on altering treatment of mental disorders. Prior to the introduction of the antipsychotic drugs (neuroleptics and major tranquilizers), the treatment of the psychotic patient, especially the schizophrenic, included all modalities of treatment, some rational and some not. Included were psychotherapy, wet packs, insulin coma, and various drugs ranging from pineal gland extracts to vitamin injections.

Schizophrenia is a widespread illness; it has been estimated that between 1% and 3% of the adult population will experience a schizophrenic episode at some point in their lives (Klerman, 1974). The disease is manifested most frequently in individuals under the age of 35—in 1962, 65% of all patients diagnosed as schizophrenic who were admitted to state and county hospitals for the first time were under the age of 35 (PHS, 1974).

It is difficult to measure precisely the full impact of the discovery and wide usage of the antipsychotic drugs. One can say with a fair degree of accuracy that without these agents the majority of patients entering mental hospitals would most likely remain there for most of their lives. Figure 1 lists the number of resident patients in state and county mental hospitals in the United States between the years 1946 and 1975 (PHS, 1976c). In 1955 there were approximately 551,000 patients hospitalized for mental illness in the United States, compared to 193,436 at the end of June, 1975 (PHS, 1975a; 1976a).

Over this 19-year period, the decrease in the resident population has been 64%. The 10.3% decrease in the resident patient population between 1974 and 1975 represents the nineteenth year the patient population has decreased. A combination of factors has led to a shift in the primary setting of treatment from in-hospital to outpatient facilities. During 1973 there were 5,475,000 patient care episodes, which are defined as the number of residents in an inpatient facility at the beginning of the fiscal year (or the number of persons on the rolls of non-inpatient facilities), including the patients admitted or readmitted to a facility during a fiscal year. In 1973, 31% of patients were treated as inpatients and 65% as outpatients. Figure 2 illustrates the shift in locale of patient care episodes that has taken place since 1955; at that time, 77% of the patients were hospitalized and only 23% were treated as outpatients (PHS, 1976c). Between 1955 and 1973 the rate of admission and readmissions to mental health facilities rose from 1032 to 2522 per 100,000 population (PHS, 1976c). It would appear that, while the population of inpatient facilities declined, the volume of both inpatient and ambulatory visits increased, with the greatest increase occurring among hospitalized patients. The "revolving door syndrome" is becoming more common, with more patients being discharged and readmitted. Yet the total amount of time a patient spends in the hospital is decreasing (PHS, 1975b).

The cost of mental illness in the United States, measured conservatively, was $36,786,000,000 in 1974 (PHS, 1976c). Of this amount, the cost of direct care alone amounted to $14,506,000,000, or roughly 15% of all direct health expenditures in the United States, and represented 1% of the gross national product. The remainder of the cost of mental illness was allocated

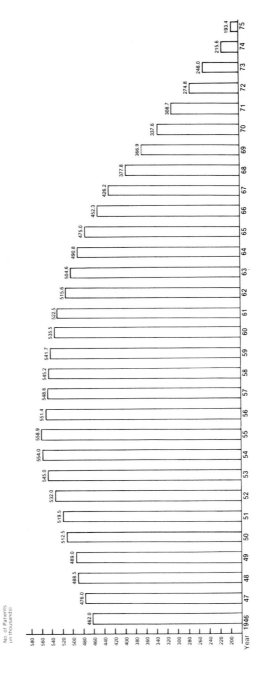

Figure 1. Number of resident patients in state, local, and government mental hospitals in the United States, 1946–1975. (Note: Phenothiazines introduced in 1956—64% decline in resident populations between 1956 and 1975.)

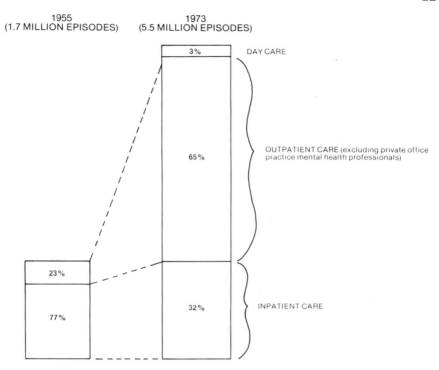

Figure 2. Percent distribution of patient care episodes (number of admissions and readmissions) by modality in mental health facilities (exclusive of federal facilities other than those operated by the Veterans Administration): United States, 1955 and 1973.

to supportive activities (research, training and fellowships, facilities development, etc) for all direct care expenditures and indirect costs in 1974. Figure 3 gives a breakdown of the $36,786,000,000 and shows the proportionate distribution of the total cost by cost sources. Costs for direct care constituted almost 40% of the total; indirect costs accounted for 54%; and the remainder derived from supporting activities. Nursing homes, together with public mental hospitals, accounted for slightly over 50% of the expenditures.

In 1955 there were 551,000 patients hospitalized, and it was projected that in 1966 this number would rise to over 700,000. In 1966, ten years after the introduction and widespread use of the phenothiazines, the resident population had decreased to 452,300.

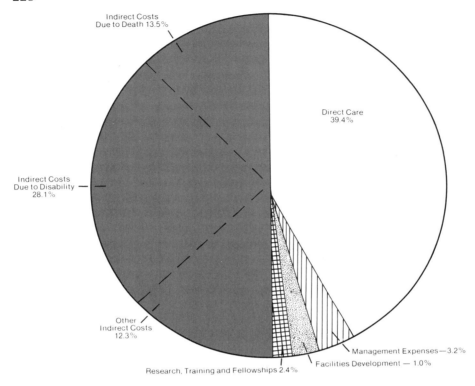

Total Cost in 000's		$36,785,827
Direct Care		14,506,028
Research		607,003
Training and Fellowships		284,842
Facilities Development		385,230
Management Expenses		1,167,298
Unallocated Expenditures of NIMH		22,658
Indirect Costs		19,812,768
Due to Death		4,942,320
Due to Disability		10,345,951
Due to Patient Care Activities		4,524,497

Figure 3. The cost of mental illness, 1974.

The actual magnitude of the decrease is greater than the 21% figure or the sheer numerals would indicate, as during this period the birth rate had been increasing and the death rate decreasing.

Other factors have contributed to the population dynamics of mental hospitals. These factors operate to a greater or lesser degree in every state and include the following: an increased availability and utilization of alternate care facilities for the aged; increased availability and utilization of outpatient and aftercare facilities; and a reduction in the length of hospitalization. The approximate duration of hospitalization for a schizophrenic patient in 1953 was between one and two years; in 1971, the mean duration of hospitalization for psychiatric inpatients was less than four weeks (PHS, 1973). Patients 65 years and older generally have longer hospital stays than do patients among the younger age groups.

The purpose of providing "health statistical data" in the opening remarks of this chapter is to provide the reader with some perspective on the following facts: (1) there has been a decrease in the resident population of hospitals since 1956; (2) the majority of first-admission patients to mental hospitals are diagnosed as schizophrenic; (3) there has been a shift in the locale of treatment from hospitals to outpatient ambulatory facilities; (4) the number of readmissions has increased and the revolving door syndrome has emerged; (5) the cost of mental illness reflects itself not only in human misery but also in large expenditures of funds.

While the title of this chapter is "Antipsychotic Drugs," the reader often hears the terms *neuroleptic, tranquilizer*, and *antipsychotic* drugs used synonymously. Although this nomenclature is widely accepted and understood in 1976, this was not always the case. Shortly after the discovery of chlorpromazine in 1952, a controversy arose among investigators over the classification of this group of drugs. The French psychiatrists differentiated between the terms neuroleptic and tranquilizer according to the properties attributed to the neuroleptic agents. (1) These drugs, by virtue of their action on the reticular activating system, the limbic system, and the hypothalamus, reduce psychotic symptoms. (2) Their pharmacologic activity upon the structures of the basal ganglia may evoke extrapyramidal side effects (Levitt, 1975).

The term tranquilizer was introduced by Benjamin Rush in 1810 to describe a wooden chair with restraining straps which he designed and named "The Tranquilizer." The pharmacologist F. Yonkman first used the term *tranquilization* in 1954 to describe the pharmacologic effects of reserpine: "Unlike barbiturate or other standard sedatives, reserpine does not produce grogginess or a lack of coordination; patients appear to be relaxed, quiet and tranquil" (Bein, 1970). Later investigators added to the confusion in nomenclature by describing meprobamate as a tranquilizer, and the terms *major* and *minor* tranquilizers were introduced (Bradley, 1967). The obvious pitfalls of a major/minor dichotomy resulted and have persisted since that time (Jacobsen, 1959b; 1963). The term *antipsychotic* drug implies that the drug is used to treat psychoses, just as drugs classified as antianxiety or antidepressant are used to treat anxiety or depression. The term neuroleptic was adopted in 1970 by the International Drug Reference Center (WHO-NIMH), which recommended that it replace the terms major tranquilizer (Leeds and Levine, 1970) and antipsychotic (Labhardt, 1959). In practice, however, this recommendation was never fully carried out, and the three terms—neuroleptic, major tranquilizer, and antipsychotic—are used interchangeably today (Bobon, 1973).

CHEMICAL STRUCTURE–ACTIVITY RELATIONSHIPS

The major focus of this section will be on neuroleptic drugs available by physician's prescription in the United States today. It has been estimated that at least 160 antipsychotic drugs have been studied in preclinical or clinical trials (Hollister, 1973).

There were five distinct chemical classes of neuroleptics available in 1976, not including reserpine, which is seldom used today in mental illness. While there are differences in structure among the classes of drugs, there are also certain similarities, and these appear to account for the similarity of their clinical effects. Figure 4 gives the prototype structure of the phenothiazine drugs. The various substitutions in the phenothiazine nucleus at positions 2 and 10 yield 13 individual drugs. At the 10 position, substitution may be by an aliphatic, piperazine, or piperidine group. The particular group occupying position 10 determines qualitative properties of the drug: substitution with an aliphatic or piperidine side chain results in more sedation, a higher degree of anticholinergic activity, and a lower incidence of extrapyramidal side effects; with the piperazine side chain, the reverse is observed. Substituting a trifluorinated carbon (CF_3) of the piperazine phenothiazines for a chlorine grouping (Cl) at position 2 increases the potency of the drug. Thus, fluphenazine (CF_3) is used in a dosage range of 2 to 20 mg daily, and perphenazine (Cl) in a dosage range of 8 to 64 mg daily.

The chemical difference between the phenothiazines and the thioxanthenes is shown in the structural formulas in Figure 5. In

Classification

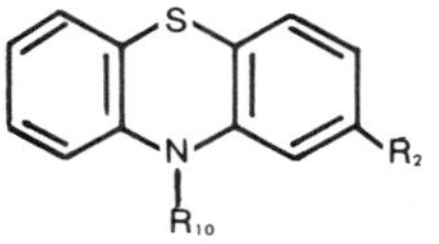

Phenothiazine nucleus 13 phenothiazine drugs made by substitutions at R_{10} and R_2

● *Aliphatics* (R_{10} = $CH_2CH_2CH_2N$ $\langle$ CH_3 / CH_3 $\rangle$)

chlorpromazine   (Thorazine®)

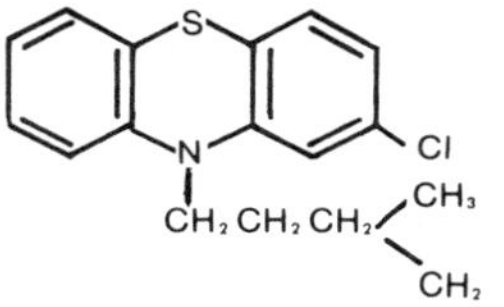

triflupromazine   (Vesprin®)

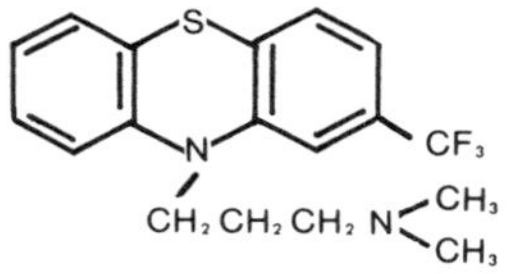

● *Piperazines* (R_{10} = $CH_2CH_2CH_2N$ ⟨ ⟩ N-CH_2CH_2OH; R_2 = $COCH_3$ [acetophenazine])

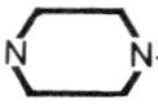

     acetophenazine (Tindal®)
     fluphenazine (Permitil, Prolixin®)
     perphenazine (Trilafon®)
     prochlorperazine (Compazine®)
     carphenazine (Proketazine®)
     trifluoperazine (Stelazine®)
     thiopropazate (Dartal®)
     butaperazine (Repoise®)

● *Piperidines* (R_{10} = CH_2CH_2-⟨N-CH_3⟩ ; R_2 = $COCH_3$ [piperacetazine])

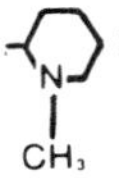

     thioridazine (Mellaril®)
     piperacetazine (Quide®)
     mesoridazine (Serentil®)

Figure 4. Chemical structures of the phenothiazines.

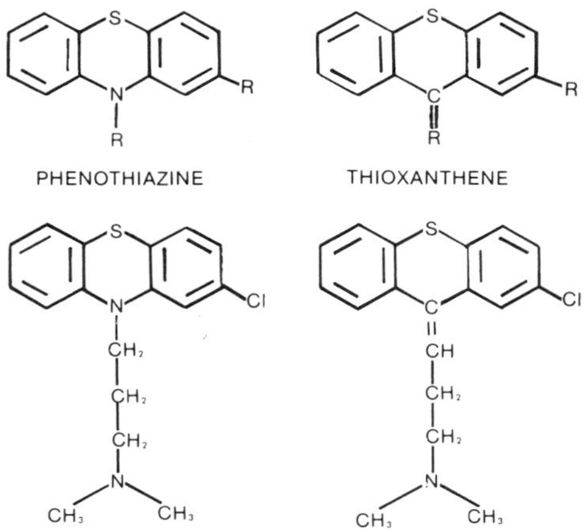

Figure 5. Structural formulas of phenothiazines and thioxanthenes. *Top*, general formulas; *bottom*, specific drug formulas.

the thioxanthenes, a nitrogen atom replaces the carbon atom of the phenothiazine nucleus. Structural differences between two derivatives of the above classes of compounds, chlorpromazine and chlorprothixene, are shown in the bottom portion of Figure 5. The specific difference here is in the attachment of the side chain to the tricyclic nucleus. In the case of chlorpromazine, the side chain is attached to the nitrogen by a single bond and allows for the chain configurational changes. The side chain of chlorprothixene is attached to the nucleus by a double bond that prohibits any rotation of the first carbon in the chain (Madsen and Ravn, 1959; Petersen et al, 1958; Møller et al, 1962; Itil et al, 1974).

The butyrophenones were the first group of neuroleptic drugs not to possess a phenothiazine ring structure (Janssen, 1970a). Haloperidol is the only neuroleptic drug of this class available in the United States at this time, although there are several other butyrophenones currently under investigation. (Haloperidol is highly specific for a rare disease of children, Gilles de la Tourette's syndrome, which is characterized by motor tics, loud outcries, and outbursts of expletives [Challas and Brauer, 1963].)

The dihydroindolone compound, molindone, is structurally similar to the indole chain of the rauwolfia alkaloids (Davis, 1976). Molindone resembles the piperazine phenothiazines in dosage requirements and side effects. It does not inhibit the norepinephrine uptake pump; therefore, unlike chlorpromazine, it does not interfere with the hypotensive action of guanethidine. Nor has molindone been reported to cause weight gain.

Of the dibenzoxazepine class, loxapine was released in 1975 (Davis, 1976). This newest class of drugs is chemically interesting as the center ring of the tricyclic structure is a 7-atom structure also seen in the tricyclic antidepressants. The drug possesses antipsychotic activity equal to that of the neuroleptic drugs currently on the market. The drug is presently approved by the Food and Drug Administration for the treatment of schizophrenia. One study has reported its efficacy in the treatment of mixed anxiety and depression in nonpsychotic patients (Goldstein et al, 1974). Figure 6 shows the structural formulae of these drugs.

A BUTYROPHENONE:

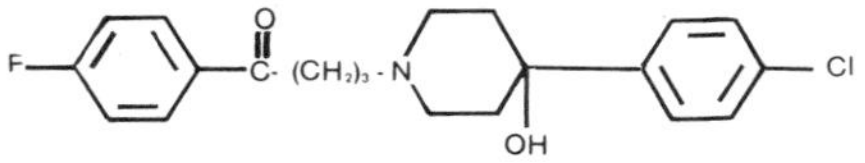

HALOPERIDOL

A DIHYDROINDOLONE COMPOUND:

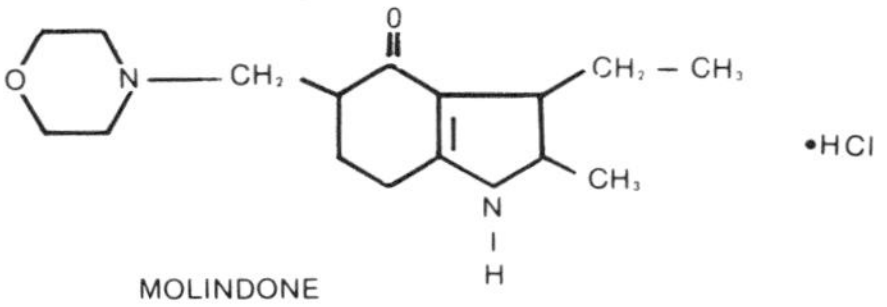

MOLINDONE

DIBENZOXAZEPINES:

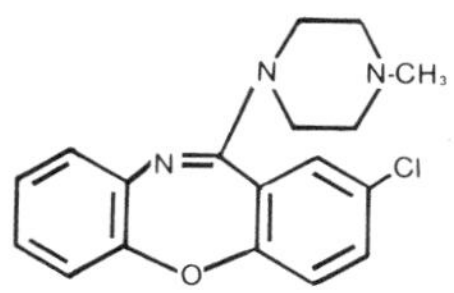

LOXAPINE

Figure 6. Chemical structures of commercially available butyrophenone, dihydroindolone, and dibenzoxazepine neuroleptics.

For historical purposes, the rauwolfia alkaloid reserpine (Ayd, 1957) should be mentioned, although it is not used as a neuroleptic today. It was introduced at about the same time as chlorpromazine was, but it was soon learned that approximately 10% to 15% of patients receiving reserpine developed severe depression. Its major use today is in the treatment of hypertension.

It appears that the side chains of the phenothiazines, the thioxanthenes, and the butyrophenones possess a 3- or 4-carbon bridge connected to a nitrogen atom of a phenolic ring, R-C-C-C-N-R or R-C-C-C-C-N-R (Janssen, 1970b; Stach and Poldinger, 1966), which is believed to be essential for antipsychotic activity. Pharmacologically, it is believed that the antipsychotic properties of the neuroleptic drugs are, in part, related to their ability to block the action of the neurotransmitter dopamine. The phenothiazine drugs appear to block dopamine by virtue of their stereotypic similarities to dopamine in the spatial configuration of the phenothiazine ring and side chain at the dopamine receptor site (Horn and Snyder, 1971). Molindone, an indole derivative, and loxapine, a dibenzoxazepine, are not structurally similar to the phenothiazine drugs, nor do they contain the carbon-nitrogen bridges of the butyrophenones and thioxanthenes. Although all the neuroleptics possess the ability to block dopamine transmission, the mechanism of this action is not fully known.

Still, the most popular theory explaining the therapeutic action of the neuroleptic drugs in the treatment of schizophrenia has been related to this ability to block dopamine receptors in the brain (Matthysse, 1973; Snyder et al, 1974). The cell bodies of the dopamine tracts lie within the substantia nigra, and the terminals in the caudate nucleus and in the putamen of the corpus striatum (basal ganglia). In Parkinson's disease, the nigrostriatal dopamine pathway, located in the basal ganglia, degenerates, and this appears to be related to a deficiency of dopamine. Thus, administration of L-dopa, the precursor of dopamine, results in a dramatic reduction in the symptoms of parkinsonism. The neuroleptic drugs may induce parkinsonism and other extrapyramidal symptoms due to their ability to cause a depletion of dopamine at receptor sites of the structures located within the basal ganglia (caudate nucleus, putamen, corpus striatum).

Dopamine tracts are also located in the areas of the brain believed to be associated with emotion: those structures comprising and associated with the limbic system. It is postulated that the blockade of the postsynaptic dopamine receptor sites in the limbic system and other subcortical areas of the brain produces a dopamine deficiency, which results in amelioration of psychotic symptoms.

It would appear that these two properties of the neuroleptic drugs, reduction of psychotic symptoms and production of extrapyramidal side effects, may be explained on the basis of dopamine blockade. If the neuroleptic drugs all produce dopamine blockade by similar mechanisms, then theoretically all the neuroleptic drugs, when given in doses sufficient to ameliorate schizophrenic symptomatology, should also produce extrapyramidal symptoms. All of the neuroleptic drugs marketed in the United States today do produce extrapyramidal side effects, but with individual variations in frequency. The piperazine phenothiazine drugs are associated with a higher incidence of extrapyramidal side effects than is chlorpromazine, a member of the aliphatic group of phenothiazines. Thioridazine rarely produces extrapyramidal side effects, and the investigational drug clozapine appears to elicit few or no extrapyramidal side effects. Such variations would indicate that the "dopamine hypothesis" is an oversimplification.

The neuroleptic drugs are also anticholinergic. Within the brain the acetylcholine receptors are muscarinic in nature; that is, they mimic the alkaloid muscarine. Other acetylcholine receptors are nicotinic, so named because of their pharmacologic effects on skeletal muscles. It would appear that within the basal ganglia there is a balance between the neurotransmitters dopamine and acetylcholine (Snyder et al, 1974). When a drug such as haloperidol, a potent dopamine-blocking agent, is administered, an imbalance results between the two neurotransmitters. It is postulated that those neuroleptics which are the most potent dopamine blockers produce the greatest frequency of extrapyramidal side effects. Conversely, the more potent their anticholinergic properties, the fewer extrapyramidal side effects they would produce. Thioridazine is a potent anticholinergic neuroleptic. It produces a high incidence of side effects such as dryness of the mouth, constipation, and blurred vision. These side effects are also often observed in patients receiving atropine, a blocker of muscarinic acetylcholine receptors. Thus, the greater the anticholinergic activity, the fewer the extrapyramidal side effects, but the greater the frequency of atropine-like effects. A hypothetical dose-response curve for antidopaminergic and anticholinergic action is presented in Figure 7 to explain this phenomenon (Hollister, 1975).

> A possible explanation for the paradoxical disappearance of extrapyramidal symptoms of high doses of antipsychotic drugs is suggested by hypothetical dose-response curves for antidopaminergic and anticholinergic actions. The balance is most disturbed between dopaminergic and cholinergic function in the middle range of the dose-response curve. Extrapyramidal symptoms do not emerge at low doses of antipsychotic drug. At very high doses the antidopaminergic and anticholinergic effects become close, so extrapyramidal symptoms disappear. (Hollister, 1975)

It is not surprising that the early practice of the French psychiatrists was to use dosages high enough to produce extrapyramidal side effects, for they felt that without extrapyramidal side effects no antipsychotic activity could occur (Hasse and Janssen, 1965). This practice derived from the observation that neuroleptics both produce extrapyramidal side effects and reduce antipsychotic symptoms. The belief was that the therapeutic activity could not occur without the production of extrapyramidal symptoms.

The Americans felt that eliciting extrapyramidal side effects was not a prerequisite for producing antipsychotic activity. Now, 20 years later, it would appear that both viewpoints were partially correct.

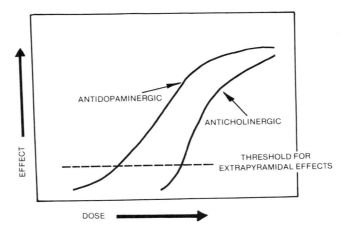

Figure 7. Antidopaminergic-anticholinergic dose-response curve. At higher doses, the anticholinergic effects of the neuroleptics tend to bring the ratio between antidopaminergic and anticholinergic concentrations into balance.

The practice of using extremely high doses of neuroleptics to control extrapyramidal side effects is understandable in terms of effect but questionable in terms of safety. As an example, if extrapyramidal side effects were observed with haloperidol at 10 mg, doubling the dose or raising it eightfold would eliminate the extrapyramidal side effects. However, taking these measures to gain the temporary balance achieved by blocking both dopamine and acetylcholine receptor sites may be potentially dangerous, since no one knows at this time the long-range effects of the indirect manipulation of dopamine and acetylcholine levels.

Another physiologic approach to the indirect estimation of brain dopaminergic activity is the study of prolactin secretion (Buckman and Peake, 1976). Pituitary prolactin secretion is largely under the control of the hypothalamic neurohumor prolactin inhibiting factor (PIF), which in turn is sensitive to dopaminergic activity in the tuberoinfundibular system. In man, the dopamine precursor L-dopa suppresses prolactin secretion, while chlorpromazine and other neuroleptics stimulate its secretion. That thioridazine, a potent anticholinergic antipsychotic agent, also stimulates prolactin secretion was evidenced in studies by Sachar et al (1975), who demonstrated increased prolactin levels following the administration of thioridazine, even though this drug shows few extrapyramidal side effects.

Other postulated bases of antipsychotic activity include: (1) interaction with norepinepherine transmission; (2) biophysical considerations which involve alterations in membrane kinetics; (3) metabolic inhibition of oxidative phosphorylation which results in decreased neuronal excitability.

The neuroleptic drugs affect the functioning of the three major integrating systems of the brain: the reticular activating system, the limbic system, and the hypothalamus. One might speculate that these drugs possibly reduce extraneous or distracting sensory information, reduce the affective charge of all sensations, and reduce the somatic responses. However, no one theory or combination of theories yet developed explains the action of the neuroleptic drugs.

EVALUATION OF EFFICACY OF NEUROLEPTIC DRUGS

One major problem affecting all drug efficacy studies is making sure the patients studied are all suffering from the same disease. Clinicians differ greatly on diagnosing schizophrenia. Therefore, the "target symptoms" approach is often used (NIMH, 1964).

In order to quantify the magnitude of change prior to, during, and after drug treatment, rating scales have been developed to evaluate the symptoms which characterize the disease. The target symptoms include those symptoms associated with the various types of schizophrenia, and also Bleuler's primary and accessory symptoms. The major advantage of utilizing a target symptom rating scale is that it enables the clinician to evaluate the initial severity of the patient's symptoms and the changes in these symptoms over time. Schizophrenia is viewed as a group of disorders manifested by characteristic disturbances in thinking, mood, and behavior. Some examples of the target symptoms which reflect disturbances of thinking, affect, and behavior in acute and chronic schizophrenic patients are listed below:

1. Thinking or speech disturbance
2. Catatonic motor behavior
3. Paranoid ideation
4. Hallucinations
5. Delusional thinking other than paranoid
6. Blunted or inappropriate emotion
7. Disturbance of social behavior and interpersonal relations.

Comparative Efficacy

The first major study undertaken to evaluate the efficacy of the neuroleptic agents was sponsored by the National Institute of Mental Health in 1961 (NIMH, 1964). This study was a collaborative one carried out in nine hospital settings. Newly admitted acute schizophrenic patients were randomly assigned to placebo, chlorpromazine, thioridazine, or fluphenazine and were treated for six weeks. The results of this study are widely known. In summary: (1) no differences could be detected among the three neuroleptic agents in respect to overall efficacy or in respect to the specificity of symptom reduction; (2) all three drugs were superior to placebo; (3) the side effect profiles for the three drugs differed (NIMH, 1964). More than 90% of the drug-treated patients responded favorably; only 1 in 10 did not show any improvement, and no patients worsened. Seventy-five percent of the drug-treated patients showed moderate to marked improvement. Twenty-five percent of the placebo-treated patients improved; the remaining placebo-treated patients either failed to improve or became worse (see Figure 8).

While much time and effort has been devoted over the years to finding "the right drug for the right patient," this has not yet happened. Perhaps Hollister et al (1974) best summarize the questions of differential efficacy: "Past difficulty in replicating the specific indications for antipsychotic drugs, as well as the few differences found in this study, force the clinicians to choose

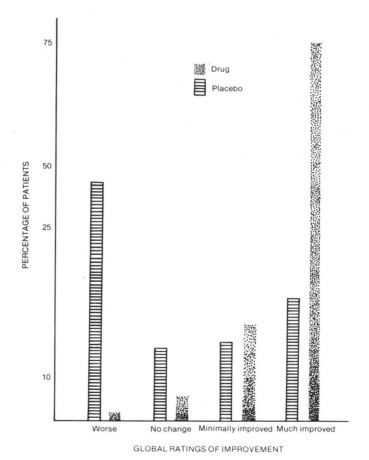

Figure 8. Doctors' rating of global improvement in patients after treatment with phenothiazines or placebo.

empirically. Differing reactions of individual patients to various drugs are more likely due to differences in 'drug genetics' than to any important pharmacological differences."

Davis (1975) reviewed the comparative efficacy of neuroleptic drugs as used in well-controlled studies, and his results are listed in Table 1.

Molindone (Davis, 1976) has been evaluated in six controlled studies involving approximately 200 patients. It was slightly superior in one study, equal in three, and slightly inferior in two. The empirical data suggest molindone to be equally effective as reference neuroleptics (Davis, 1976).

Loxapine has been evaluated in 15 studies. Twelve studies found loxapine to be essentially equal to reference compounds; 1 study found it more effective; another found it less effective. In a study in which the drug was compared to thiothixene, it showed more effective in older patients but less effective in younger ones (Davis, 1976). In the series of 15 studies, over 600 patients were evaluated under controlled conditions, and the consensus is that

Table 1
Drug-Placebo Comparisons
in Controlled Studies of Schizophrenia

Drug		Number of Studies in Which Drug Was	
		More Effective than	*Equal to*
Generic Name	*Trade Name*	*Placebo*	*Placebo*
Chlorpromazine	Thorazine	54	11
Reserpine	Serpasil	20	9
Triflupromazine	Vesprin	9	1
Perphenazine	Trilafon	5	0
Prochlorperazine	Compazine	7	2
Trifluoperazine	Stelazine	16	2
Fluphenazine	Prolixin	15	0
Butaperazine	Repoise	4	0
Thioridazine	Mellaril	7	0
Mesoridazine	Serentil	3	0
Mepazine	Pacatal	2	3
Carphenazine	Proketazine	2	0
Promazine	Sparine	3	4
Phenobarbital	Luminal	0	3
Chlorprothixene	Taractan	4	0
Thiothixene	Navane	2	0
Haloperidol	Haldol	*	*

*References unavailable at this time.

loxapine is as efficacious as reference neuroleptics in the treatment of schizophrenia. (The side effect profiles of these drugs will be discussed later.)

CLINICAL PRACTICE

Choice of Neuroleptics

Given the large number of neuroleptic drugs available today—18 drugs from five chemical classes—and given the results of both large-scale, collaborative studies and individual investigational trials, which conclude that all of the drugs are efficacious (no statistical differences in either relief of global severity or in reduction of target symptoms), the clinician cannot but be in a dilemma (Ban, 1972; Cole and Davis, 1975; Klein and Davis, 1969; Lasky et al, 1962; Michaux et al, 1964). Some clinical misconceptions which warrant mentioning have crept into clinical practice. Some believe that the agitated, hostile, belligerent psychotic patient would respond best to sedating neuroleptics, and that an apathetic, withdrawn, socially isolated patient would respond well to a low-milligram phenothiazine or to a thioxanthene or butyrophenone. Data obtained from numerous studies indicates that such generalized conclusions are invalid. Both types of patients have responded well to neuroleptic drugs of all chemical classes.

Some very agitated patients tolerate the sedative effects of neuroleptics poorly. It is postulated that such patients require a constant input of sensory stimuli; a sedative neuroleptic drug blunts incoming stimuli (Sussex, 1976), and the patients appear more agitated. In such cases, the less sedative neuroleptics would be indicated, as they calm with little sedation. Conversely, the apathetic patient is not stimulated by the "stimulating" neuroleptics. Generally these compounds have a higher incidence of akathisia and it is this which is reported as stimulation.

There seem to be two fairly objective criteria for choosing a neuroleptic drug: (1) a patient's previous response to a drug in respect to both therapeutic and adverse effects; and (2) differences in the side effect profile of the drug. With a newly admitted patient with no history of neuroleptic treatment, the choice of initial medication should be based upon clinical experience. The patient who is readmitted to the hospital or treated in an outpatient setting should continue on his previous drug if his experience with it was beneficial. A patient who responds well to medication but who develops side effects which do not remit in one to two weeks should be switched to another drug with a different side effect profile. It is recommended that the clinician become familiar with at least one drug from each of the currently known chemical classes; this would be seven drugs.

Obtaining a thorough drug history is vital. Since the overall readmission rate is 50% to 60%, such a history should be available from the patient, from his relatives, or from his medical record. The clinician should heed the patient's wishes in regard to choice of drug whenever possible since the patient knows which drug he responded to best. This author recently had the opportunity to evaluate a patient in another institution. The patient was doing poorly (because of side effects) on the three drugs he had been prescribed. In the course of obtaining a drug history, the patient revealed the drug he "tolerated best." Yet his physicians had never asked any questions which would have given them this information. The medication was changed (to the medication the patient requested), and in two weeks he was markedly improved. He still did experience side effects, but these were tolerable to him. This case illustrates two points: (1) obtain a drug history; (2) the patient often knows what drug he responds to best. Side effects which may be of concern to the physician, such as blurred vision or constipation, may not be of as much concern to the patient. If the side effects are potentially dangerous, then the physician must exercise his best clinical judgment. However, if the side effects are not dangerous and are not objected to by the patient, he should heed the patient's wishes. The clinician should balance his personal experience with prescribing a certain drug with the patient's desires and with the data reported in the scientific literature.

Dosage

The initial dosage of medication should be given either parenterally or in a liquid concentrate form. The rationale behind this suggestion is that these methods ensure that the patient receives the medication. Very often the clinician increases the dosage of medication because the patient shows no response. The physician believes the medication may not be working when in fact the patient may not be taking the medication. This is especially true with paranoid patients.

In the treatment of acute schizophrenic conditions, a dosage of 300 to 1000 mg per day of chlorpromazine (Thorazine) or its equivalent is indicated, as shown in Table 2. Smaller doses may be effective, but the majority of acute schizophrenics will require daily amounts of at least 400 mg. Two of the most common errors committed in the neuroleptic treatment of schizophrenia are the use of inadequate doses of and too rapid changes of medication. If the physician changes the drug he is prescribing every two weeks because he is not satisfied with the therapeutic results, he might never discover the proper drug, dosage, and time required to produce improvement. A good rule to follow is that of not changing to another drug or treatment until the drug that was originally chosen has been given, at gradually increasing doses, for a period of six to eight weeks without any noticeable

Table 2
Dosage Relationships among Antipsychotic Drugs

Drug Group	Generic Name	Trade Name	Potency Mg Equivalents to 100 mg Chlorpromazine	Total Daily Dose in Milligrams Outpatient Range	Hospital Range
Phenothiazines					
Aliphatic	Chlorpromazine	Thorazine	100	50–400	200–1600
	Triflupromazine	Vesprin	25	50–150	75–200
Piperidine	Thioridazine	Mellaril	100	50–400	200–800
	Mesoridazine	Serentil	50	25–200	100–400
	Piperacetazine	Quide	10	10–40	20–160
Piperazine	Carphenazine	Proketazine	25	25–100	50–400
	Acetophenazine	Tindal	20	40–60	60–80
	Prochlorperazine	Compazine	15	15–60	30–150
	Thiopropazate	Dartal	10	10–30	30–150
	Perphenazine	Trilafon	10	8–24	12–64
	Butaperazine	Repoise	10	10–30	10–100
	Trifluoperazine	Stelazine	5	4–10	6–30
	Fluphenazine	Prolixin	2	1–3	2–20
Thioxanthenes	Chlorprothixene	Taractan	100	30–60	95–600
	Thiothixine	Navane	4	6–15	10–60
Butyrophenones	Haloperidol	Haldol	2	2–6	4–15
Dihydroindolone	Molindone	Moban	20	15–60	30–150
Dibenzoxazepine	Loxapine	Loxitane	4	25–125	50–250

improvement. In the early stages of treating schizophrenia, it is better to exceed the minimal required dosage than to remain below it. Since the acute toxicity of most neuroleptics is amazingly low, there is very little risk involved in raising the dosage rapidly to achieve maximum control of motor activity and agitation within a day or two. The treatment-resistant patient will be discussed later in this chapter.

It may take several weeks or months before all acute symptoms disappear. In the meantime, how does the physician know that he is treating his schizophrenic patient with an adequate dosage? Dosage requirements of neuroleptic drugs often vary widely among individuals. Recent work indicates that these different requirements reflect differences in the way various individuals metabolize the drugs. Genetic-constitutional differences of enzymatic breakdown mechanisms and protein binding are probably responsible for the fact that identical doses of neuroleptic drugs may produce greatly divergent plasma levels in different individuals (Curry et al, 1970). Other factors which influence response include age, body size, and previous and concurrent drug usage. Plasma levels of a drug cannot be used to calculate what dosage an individual patient should receive. The determination of plasma levels of neuroleptic drugs is technically difficult and is rarely available to most practicing clinicians. Also, no strict correlation between drug plasma levels of neuroleptics and their therapeutic effects has been established so far, although trends in this direction have been shown to exist and a definite correlation of drug plasma levels and the occurrence of side effects has been reported (Curry et al, 1970; Green and Forrest, 1966; Rivera-Calimlim et al, 1973).

Lehman (1966) has described the importance of length of time of drug treatment in relation to observing a response, and this description can be used as a guide in evaluating a patient's individual drug requirements and in developing realistic treatment goals. *Arousal symptoms* (psychomotor excitement, restlessness, irritability, aggressiveness, insomnia) are the first to be controlled, usually within 48 to 72 hours after medication has been started. *Affective symptoms* (quality of interpersonal relationships, social withdrawal, anxiety, depression) are the next group controlled, at 2 to 5 weeks into treatment. As a rule, *symptoms related to perceptual and cognitive functions* (hallucinations, delusions, and thinking disorders) disappear last—in many cases only after 5 to 8 weeks (and sometimes only after up to 26 weeks) of treatment.

Evaluation according to this "timetable" of therapeutic response to neuroleptic treatment often enables the clinician to determine whether the dosage of a drug he is prescribing is adequate for a given patient. As an example, if after two weeks of treatment a patient is still restless, agitated, and sleepless, or if after five weeks he is still isolated and withdrawn, pays little attention to self-care, and refuses to leave his room, there may well be a need to increase the daily dosage of the neuroleptic he is receiving. On the other hand, if after four weeks of therapy the patient is quiet, sociable, and cooperative, the dosage may be adequate even though the patient is still hallucinating and delusional. These latter symptoms may not respond to treatment for another few weeks.

Figures 9 and 10 show the average improvement rates of acute schizophrenic patients. There is wide variability of response; some patients improve rapidly, while others require several months to show the same amount of improvement. Improvement in socialization and interpersonal relationships and elimination of accessory symptoms (hallucinations, delusions, etc) are seldom clearly defined.

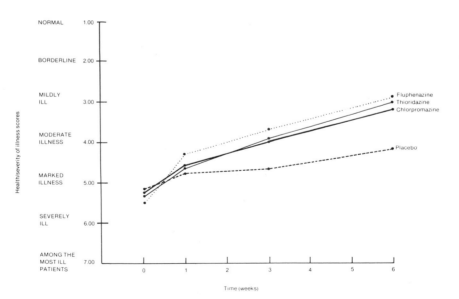

Figure 9. Severity of illness over time in patients being treated with phenothiazines or placebo (NIMH-PSC, 1964).

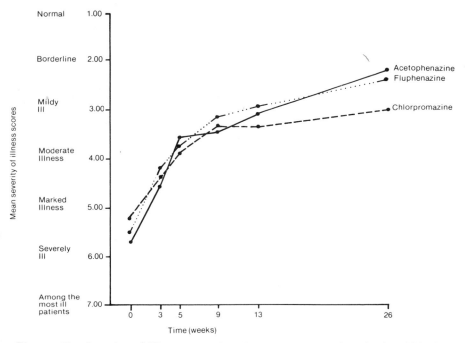

Figure 10. Severity of illness over time in patients treated with phenothiazines (NIMH-PSC, 1964).

Today patients seldom remain in the hospital for as long as six to eight weeks. The average hospital stay for acute schizophrenic patients is 16 to 30 days (PHS, 1976). It would appear from the data on the time required for symptom reduction, as evidenced by the results of collaborative studies, that the majority of patients leave the hospital shortly after showing improvement in socialization, self-care, and interpersonal relationships. Yet the accessory symptoms might still be present. This is probably the case with most schizophrenic patients: they leave the hospital less agitated, less belligerent, less socially isolated, and caring more about their personal appearance, although the symptoms of thought disorder manifested by delusions or hallucinations may be present to some degree. If community resources (outpatient clinics, halfway houses, day hospitals, and community mental health centers) are available, if the patient will utilize them, and if the patient has a home to return to and a family that is willing to accept him, then prolonged hospitalization seems not to be indicated.

Unfortunately, the availability of community resources is limited, and when they are available, the patient may not take advantage of them. In addition, the family support system is often lacking. The lack of family support generally results in an increase in the number of readmissions to the hospital. Therefore, the issue of whether or not prolonged hospitalization is less effective than rapid discharge is debatable.

Treatment-Resistant Patients and Use of High Dosages

Prien and Cole (1968) studied chronically hospitalized schizophrenic patients who were administered 2000 mg of chlorpromazine or its equivalent per day over a six-month period. Results of the study indicate that dosages of 2000 mg daily may enhance improvement in some chronic patients, especially those under 40 years of age who have been hospitalized for less than 10 years.

High-Dosage Treatment (Megadoses)

Itil et al (1970) and Rifkin et al (1971) performed exploratory studies using massive dosages (300 to 1200 mg per day) of fluphenazine and found that both chronic and acute treatment-resistant schizophrenics showed good to excellent responses. They noted that at low dosages the predominant side effects were extrapyramidal ones, but that at higher dosages the predominant side effect was sedation. These promising results led Rifkin's group to perform a double-blind study which compared fluphenazine at a dosage of 30 mg per day to fluphenazine at a dosage of 1200 mg per day. There was little difference in the therapeutic outcomes of the two groups.

A differentiation must be made between the use of moderately high dosages—such as double the normal dosage, as Prien and Cole used—and the megadose strategy which Rifkin et al used, which employs 60 times the normal dosage. The controlled study tends to caution against undue optimism that megadose antipsychotic drug treatment may cure many drug-resistant schizophrenic patients. Doubling or quadrupling the normal, recommended dosage may benefit some acute or subacute patients, and perhaps a significant number of patients may be helped by increases greater than this. The increment in the number of patients being helped as one goes from increments of 3 times the normal dosage to 30 times the normal dosage remains to be determined, since much of the critical evidence on this question is as yet unknown.

The drug treatment of every chronic schizophrenic patient who has reached a "steady state" of functioning and whose condition has not changed for months should be interrupted at regular intervals—at least once a year—to observe his response to discontinuation of the drugs. Those who manifest an intensification of their symptoms within a short time (up to 12 weeks) should resume their pharmacotherapy immediately. A number of patients may temporarily improve when the neuroleptic medication is stopped. They may become more active and less apathetic. After 2 to 4 weeks, however, many of these temporarily improved who are off medication will relapse and manifest their old symptoms. There will be other chronic patients who, after discontinuation of their medication, will either improve permanently or, at least, be no worse than they were while receiving neuroleptics. These patients should not be continued indefinitely on drug treatment, since there is no obvious advantage in doing so. Some patients should also be tried on reduced dosages (about 25% of their previous dosage) to see whether the reduced dosage might be sufficient to stabilize their condition. Every 4 to 6 weeks the dosage should be further decreased (usually by 25%), until the minimal dosage that brings about the greatest improvement has been found.

One should consider using neuroleptics from the other chemical classes should a patient be refactory to the neuroleptic he has received in sufficient dosage for an adequate period—if it has been established that he has been taking the medication. (One study [Blackwell, 1973], carried out in an inpatient psychiatric unit, found that approximately 20% of the patients there did not take their medication.) If a patient is not responsive to phenothiazines, then the butyrophenones, the thioxanthenes, the indole derivatives, or a dibenzoxazepine should be considered. Some patients may absorb and metabolize different neuroleptic drugs in such a way that the drug never reaches the central nervous system because of genetic or chemical factors (Curry et al, 1970). Thus, one should be prepared to use a drug from another class when a favorable drug response does not occur after a reasonable trial.

Maintenance Therapy

Several studies have established that the relapse rate among schizophrenic outpatients who do not continue to receive neuroleptic drug treatment is between 40% and 60% (Gardos and Cole, 1976). The clinician must address himself to several issues concerning maintenance treatment. One of these is distinguishing between those patients who do and those who do not require maintenance neuroleptic treatment. Possibly 50% of the patients on maintenance treatment do not need to take their medication and would not relapse without it (Gardos and Cole, 1976). Unfortunately, there is no way to predict which patients would remain well without treatment. The clinician has to make the decision to either begin a patient on a maintenance regimen of indefinite duration or risk (in 50% of his patients) an exacerbation of the patient's illness by not instituting maintenance therapy.

Schizophrenic patients tend to deteriorate a little more after each acute episode, particularly after they have had three or four relapses. Even if they again become free of symptoms, they usually lose some of their social skills and begin to go down on the socioeconomic and occupational indices. There are good reasons for taking every reasonable precaution against a recurrence of an acute schizophrenic attack, and there are also some reasons for not continuing medication. The clinician must determine the benefit-to-risk ratio.

Neuroleptic drugs in the prevention of relapses and rehospitalization Other major studies of maintenance phenothiazine treatment were reported by Engelhardt and Freedman (1965) and by Engelhardt et al (1967) (see Figure 11). These investigations concluded that phenothiazines definitely produced better adjustment in the community and decreased the number of relapses and the total amount of time spent in the hospital. Neuroleptic drugs are not curative, but they do alter the course of the disease by reducing exacerbation of the illness and subsequent rehospitalization. For 12 months Goldstein (1969) studied ambulatory chronic schizophrenic patients who were being treated with thiothixene. His results were similar to those reported in the Engelhardt studies.

Effects of social, vocational therapy and neuroleptic drugs in prevention of relapse Recently, Hogarty and Goldberg (1973) conducted an important study on maintenance treatment. In the study, 374 schizophrenic patients were

250

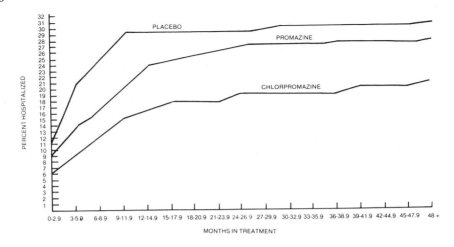

Figure 11. Prevalence of hospitalization for successive 3-month periods of treatment exposure (up to 48 months).

discharged from state hospitals upon recovery. After a stabilization period on maintenance phenothiazine, half of these patients were assigned to placebo. Half of each group (drug and placebo) received psychotherapeutic sessions consisting of individual casework and vocational rehabilitation counseling. At the end of a year, 73% of the placebo patients not undergoing psychotherapy had relapsed, and 63% of the patients receiving placebo plus psychotherapy had also relapsed. Thirty-three percent of the group receiving maintenance drug therapy plus psychotherapy relapsed. Thus, there is a substantial drug-placebo difference: a total of 31% of the drug-treated group relapsed, while a total of 68% of the placebo group relapsed. This study demonstrates very dramatically the fact that maintenance phenothiazines are necessary to prevent relapse in most schizophrenic patients. Also, at the end of the 12-month period, both groups who had participated in psychotherapy had done somewhat better than had the other patients. Patients receiving psychotherapy plus drug therapy did slightly better (by about 7%) than did those patients receiving drug therapy alone, and patients receiving both psychotherapy and placebo did better (with a 10% lower relapse rate) than did those patients receiving only placebo (see Figure 12).

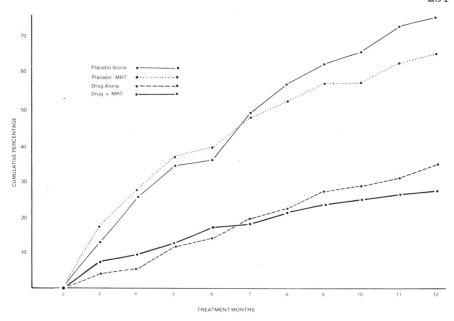

Figure 12. Major role therapy (MRT): cumulative relapse rates.

Duration of maintenance drug therapy There are only educated guesses as to how long maintenance drug therapy should continue. Following the first schizophrenic attack, it appears best to continue treatment for at least 12 to 18 months; after the second attack, for 3 to 5 years; and after three or more relapses, treatment should be continued indefinitely, possibly for the patient's lifetime (Hogarty and Goldberg, 1973; Prien and Klett, 1972; Hughes and Little, 1967).

Potential risks of long-term therapy The disadvantages of maintenance treatment, besides the inconvenience and cost associated with any long-term therapy, lie mainly in the uncomfortable side effects which the drugs often elicit. In one survey of hospitalized, chronically mentally ill patients, 36% were diagnosed as suffering from tardive dyskinesia (Fann et al, 1972). No treatment is completely effective in managing this disorder. Other complications (discussed under Side Effects) of long-term neuroleptic treatment must also be considered.

In summary, the evidence available would indicate that the decision of whether or not to implement maintenance neuroleptic therapy should be made for each patient individually. In general, after a documented schizophrenic episode, neuroleptic treatment should be undertaken for at least one year. The risk of tardive dyskinesia is of genuine concern. The dosage of the neuroleptic should therefore be the minimal dosage necessary to control symptoms. This dosage can be arrived at by reducing the initial, higher dosage by decrements of 25% every three to four months.

Drug Holidays

This practice originated as an effort to meet staff shortages in hospitals on Saturdays, Sundays, and holidays which made it difficult to make sure all patients received medication. A Veterans Administration collaborative study (Caffey et al, 1964; Prien et al, 1973) was undertaken in which 250 chronic schizophrenic patients on stabilized dosages of antipsychotic drugs had placebo substituted for active medication for two or three days a week for four months. Only 7% of the patients relapsed. This finding is supported by other studies, which show a low relapse rate for two- or three-day withdrawal schedules. Elimination of medication for more than two or three days a week results in a significantly higher relapse rate. There are several advantages of drug holidays to the patient. There is less medication to be taken, less expense, and possibly a lower incidence of side effects. On a somewhat more negative note, patients who find that they do not need medication for up to three days per week may feel that they do not need medication at all and may discontinue their medication completely. The physician has to weigh the positive and negative aspects of drug holidays in regard to the patient's acceptance of an "intermittent" dosage regimen. There are obvious advantages for the staff as there is a reduction in workload for the institution. There is also a reduction in cost, since the total amount of medication a patient will take during his hospitalization will be less.

Frequency of Daily Doses

After a patient becomes "stabilized," neuroleptic drugs may be administered on a once or twice per day schedule. The practice of administering psychotropic drugs to stabilized patients in three or four equally divided doses per day has been questioned. Studies comparing different daily dose frequencies in chronic schizophrenics have shown no major undesirable consequences arising from the once- or twice-daily schedules (Ayd, 1973; Stewart and Cluff, 1972).

The goal of treating patients over long periods should be to achieve a dosage schedule of once- or twice-daily drug administration. Drugs with a high sedative profile should be given primarily in the evening, and drugs with less sedative action should be given in the morning. If a twice per day schedule is selected, one third of the drug can be given in the morning and two thirds in the evening, or the reverse. (Elderly patients, those patients who are chronically or acutely physically ill, and those patients who are small in stature may require smaller doses given more frequently.)

In maintenance treatment programs, the fewer the doses of drugs required per day, the better the compliance (Blackwell, 1973a). Thus, a patient is more likely to adhere to a dosage schedule of one or two doses of medication per day than to a regimen which requires taking three or four doses. In addition, there is less chance of a medication error when fewer doses are taken per day.

ANTIPARKINSONISM MEDICATION

These drugs should be administered only to control extrapyramidal symptoms. The practice of using them prophylactically is not advised, as the potential for increased anticholinergic side effects increases because antiparkinsonism drugs are also anticholinergic in nature. If a patient develops extrapyramidal side effects, and if he is not clinically improved to the point where the neuroleptic dosage may be lowered, then the use of antiparkinsonism drugs is indicated. Antiparkinsonism medication should be used for no longer than three months and should be withdrawn over a period of a few weeks. Should side effects emerge after antiparkinsonism medication has been discontinued, it may be reinstated.

In a Veterans Administration collaborative study (Klett and Caffey, 1972), 403 patients on antipsychotic drugs who had also been receiving antiparkinsonism agents for at least three months had the latter replaced by placebo for a six-week period. After this time, only 7% required resumption of antiparkinsonism medication. Similar results have been reported by other investigators. It would appear that only a minority of patients on antipsychotic medication require antiparkinsonism drugs for long periods (DiMascio, 1971).

LONG–ACTING NEUROLEPTICS

Fluphenazine enanthate and fluphenazine decanoate (Prolixin) are injected intramuscularly and remain active for approximately two weeks (Imlah and Murphy, 1973). These drugs are not recommended for treating the acute patient because of difficulties in titrating dosage and because of their slow onset of action (24 to 96 hours). These drugs should be started in inpatients who have been stabilized on oral medication and in outpatients who are unreliable about taking medication daily. Treatment is usually started with a dose of 25 mg, and this dose is repeated in one or two weeks. The usual dosage range is 6.25 to 50 mg: the more disturbed patient is given a higher dosage; the older or debilitated patient's dosage would fall at the lower end of the dosage range (Whitehead, 1973). It is estimated that approximately 80% of patients receiving long-acting medication will develop extrapyramidal side effects (Brauzer, 1975).* Because of this high incidence, patients should be warned of the symptoms and told to contact their physician or clinic if they occur. While the concurrent prophylactic use of antiparkinsonism medication with oral neuroleptics is discouraged, some clinicians feel that the high incidence of extrapyramidal side effects with the injectable, long-acting agents may make prophylactic administration of antiparkinsonism drugs clinically reasonable.

USE OF NEUROLEPTIC DRUGS IN OTHER CONDITIONS

For a patient suffering from an organic brain syndrome with psychosis, the neuroleptic drugs are effective in reducing psychotic symptoms, especially agitation, restlessness, hallucinations, delusions, and thought disorder. These drugs do not benefit the intellectual impairment, memory deficit, disorientation, or any of the symptoms resulting from the underlying etiology of the syn-

---

*B. Brauzer 1975: personal communication.

drome. Indeed, some patients with organic brain syndrome may show increased confusion or intellectual impairment when even small doses of antipsychotic medication are administered. These neurologic side effects of the neuroleptic drugs, plus orthostatic hypotension, are potentially serious side effects in the presence of cerebral damage because of the increased likelihood of dizziness which may result in falls and fractures.

In the elderly (Cole and Stotsky, 1976), changes in the central nervous system which accompany arteriosclerosis or senile brain disease may alter the sensitivity of cerebral tissues and result in highly variable and unpredictable effects (Salzman et al, 1970). The agitated or hyperactive elderly patient often may benefit from the use of neuroleptic drugs.

Evidence supporting the use of neuroleptic drugs in mixed anxious-depressed outpatients is controversial (Klein and Davis, 1969). In our own experience (Goldstein, 1974), neuroleptic drugs appear to be indicated in patients suffering from chronic mixed anxiety-depression who have not responded after reasonable periods of treatment (six to eight weeks) with anxiolytic drugs. The use of neuroleptic drugs in nonpsychotic patients should generally be discouraged.

Chronically anxious patients who have not had success with treatment with anxiolytic agents may be helped with the neuroleptic drugs. Use of neuroleptic drugs in treatment of anxiety should be reserved for chronic anxiety or for anxiety refractory to the benzodiazepines.

POLYPHARMACY

Combinations of psychotropic drugs should be avoided unless there is conclusive evidence that the combination is more effective than an appropriate single drug. Few controlled clinical trials document a greater efficacy of combinations of neuroleptics over single drugs; a possible exception is perphenazine/amitriptyline.

Surveys indicate that about 40% to 50% of hospitalized patients are receiving more than one psychotropic agent; it is not unusual to find patients receiving three, or even four, medications at the same time. These may include one or two antipsychotics, an antidepressant, and an antianxiety drug.

Drug interactions are a potential danger when multiple

drugs are used; this should make the clinician cautious about prescribing drug combinations. Furthermore, among outpatients, errors in taking medication increase with the number of drugs prescribed. Schizophrenics in particular are unreliable about following even a single-drug regimen; prescribing multiple drugs compounds the problem. Also, polypharmacy may make it difficult to determine which drug to adjust in the event of toxicity or a change in clinical state.

ADVERSE REACTIONS (SIDE EFFECTS)

Table 3 lists the major categories of adverse reactions and their treatment recommendations. Table 4 lists the nature and frequency of the side effects of the phenothiazines, thioxanthenes, and butyrophenones.

The two newest neuroleptic drugs, molindone (indole class) and loxapine (dibenzoxazepine), have been introduced too recently to fully evaluate their adverse reaction profiles. Molindone appears to be similar to the piperazine phenothiazines in regard to sedation, extrapyramidal symptoms, and autonomic nervous system effects. Weight gain and guanethidine reversal have not been observed with molindone to date (Davis, 1976). Loxapine appears to cause less sedation than do the aliphatic phenothiazines and fewer extrapyramidal symptoms than do the piperazine phenothiazines. If this observation is correct, the common practice of prescribing both a sedative phenothiazine and a stimulating phenothiazine would be obviated by use of loxapine, since its profile seems to lie midway between the two actions. Loxapine is similar to the phenothiazines in its autonomic nervous system effects.

Before we consider the individual side effects, it is important to recognize a distinction between those side effects which result from the pharmacologic activity of a drug and those which are due to allergic, hypersensitivity, or idiosyncratic factors in the patient. Some side effects are due to long-term use of a drug. At present, the bulk of our knowledge about the side effects encountered with neuroleptics comes from our experience with the phenothiazines. Thus, one will hear, for example, about lens opacities developing after long-term use of the phenothiazines, while this may not have been reported with similar use of another class of drugs. Yet one should not feel secure that such side effects not yet reported with a compound of a different chemical class will not occur. As our body of experience grows with the increased use of the drugs introduced after 1956, we will know if they will eventually exhibit the side effects already observed with the phenothiazines.

Allergic Reactions

Cholestatic jaundice is an allergic reaction seldom encountered today. In the late 1950s and early 1960s the incidence was about 5%. Recent reports cite an incidence of 0.1% to 2.0% (Shader et al, 1970). The etiology of this reaction may have involved manufacturing techniques.

Various types of skin eruptions and skin discolorations have been reported with use of the neuroleptics. Eruptions usually represent allergic reactions and appear early in treatment, while the discolorations are a photosensitivity reaction associated with long-term usage. The discolorations are generally purplish, thus the term "purple people" has been used to describe those who exhibit this photosensitivity reaction. Discoloration seems most marked about the face, arms, and hands. The condition can be treated by changing medications to a drug of another chemical class, or by the patient's wearing a hat and clothing which offer shade from the sun and by his using sunscreening creams (Baer and Harber, 1965).

Autonomic Nervous System Effects

The anticholinergic and the alpha-adrenergic blocking properties of the neuroleptics may give rise to side effects involving the autonomic nervous system. While most of these side effects are more uncomfortable than they are serious, the potential for development of serious problems exists, especially in elderly patients, who may experience glaucoma, paralytic ileus, or urinary retention. Complaints of constipation and difficulty in urinating should not be ignored.

Blurred vision due to impaired ciliary muscle accommodation may occur. Other symptoms include dry mouth and nasal stuffiness. In general, patients develop a tolerance to the drugs' anticholinergic properties and these effects soon disappear. This

Table 3
Adverse Effects of Neuroleptic Drugs and Their Treatment

Adverse Effects	Precautions and Treatment
Autonomic Nervous System	
Blurred vision, flushing, pallor	Reassurance, frequently subsides in 2–6 weeks
Dry mouth	Rinse mouth frequently; if severe, give neostigmine 7.5 to 15 mg PO or pilocarpine nitrate 2.5 mg qid PO
Hyperhidrosis, dysuria	Decrease dose if possible; if severe and cannot discontinue drug, give cholinergic drugs
Aggravation of glaucoma	Monitor with concurrent tonometry; local cholinergics; consultation
Fecal impaction	Mechanical aids
Paralytic ileus	Discontinue medication, hospitalize
Constipation	Mild laxative
Diarrhea	Atropine, belladonna
Nasal congestion	Neo-Synephrine nose drops
Inhibition of ejaculation	Change to a less potent antiadrenergic drug
Postural hypotension	Advise patient to get up slowly and to wear surgical elastic hose, if necessary.
Allergic	
Dermatitis	Discontinue medication or change to another neuroleptic; systemic antihistamine
Photosensitivity	Wear protective clothes; sunscreen (eg, Pabafilm)
Behavioral	
Impaired psychomotor function	Have patient avoid dangerous tasks (operating machinery, driving an automobile)
Drowsiness	Give single daily dose at bedtime
Fatigue, lethargy, weakness	Frequently decreases once patient gets up and gets moving
Oversedation	Give small initial doses to test tolerance
Anxiety, depersonalization	Reduce dosage or change to another phenothiazine
Insomnia	Use more sedating neuroleptic and give at bedtime
Depression, increased dreams, hallucinations, aggravation of schizophrenic symptoms in borderline patients	Reduce dose or substitute another neuroleptic
Cardiovascular	
Peripheral edema, thrombosis	Weigh benefits vs risk, consider discontinuing drug

Table 3 (*continued*)

Adverse Effects	Precautions and Treatment
Cardiovascular (*continued*)	
Tachycardia, bradycardia	Decrease dosage if possible
Hypotensive crisis	Levophed I.V. or ephedrine
Syncope	Give symptomatic treatment
Endocrine	
Abnormal lactation, menstruation; increased or decreased sex drive	Reassure patient; try another class of drugs
Weight gain	Monitor diet
Edema	Reassure patient; give diuretic if necessary; thiazines not necessary
Parkinsonian syndrome	Artane 4 to 15 mg or Cogentin 2 to 8 mg PO daily in divided doses
Dyskinesia, dystonia, oculogyric crisis	Cogentin 2 mg I.M. or Benadryl 25 mg I.V. or 50 mg I.M.
Tardive dyskinesia	Discontinue drug at earliest signs, or use drug most dissimilar chemically; try drug holidays with chronic patients; use low doses in elderly
Akathisia	Discontinue medication or change to another neuroleptic
Seizures from lowered convulsive threshold	Discontinue medication or decrease dosage, if possible; give anticonvulsant (eg, Dilantin 100 mg PO qid)
Respiratory depression	Reduce dosage or discontinue
Disturbed body temperature	Avoid extreme temperatures; treat hyperthermias as for heat stroke
Gastrointestinal	
Anorexia	Discontinue medication or institute frequent, small meals
Gastritis, nausea, vomiting	Discontinue medication or give symptomatic treatment; take medicine with milk after meals

is true of orthostatic hypotension, which may be minimized by instructing patients to sit up slowly when getting out of bed and, if necessary, to lie down after receiving medication. If treatment is needed for severe hypotension, epinephrine should not be used, since the neuroleptic drugs are alpha-adrenergic blockers. When the alpha-adrenergic system is blocked, the beta-adrenergic system is stimulated, and if epinephrine is then given, vasodilation of the arterioles and a further fall in blood pressure results. The term *epinephrine reversal* has been used to describe this phenomenon. In those rare situations where a vasopressor is required, noradrenaline should be used.

Electrocardiographic Changes

Electrocardiographic abnormalities consisting of broadened, flattened T waves and increased Q-R intervals have been observed in patients receiving neuroleptic drugs, especially thioridazine, in dosages as low as 300 mg per day. The clinical significance of these electrocardiographic changes is unknown. They are potentially dangerous in those patients with a preexisting cardiac disorder or electrolyte imbalance, as serious ventricular arrhythmia may develop. These abnormalities are reversible with the administration of potassium salts (Ayd, 1970).

Agranulocytosis

This blood dyscrasia is quite rare, but it is potentially toxic. It occurs within the first six to eight weeks of treatment and is heralded by fever, sore throat, and mucous membrane ulceration. Treatment consists of discontinuing the neuroleptic, giving medical treatment for the infection, and, if necessary, managing the psychosis with a drug from a different chemical class. Incidence is reported to be less than 1 in 500,000 (Cole and Davis, 1975), and it occurs most frequently in female patients over the age of 40.

Ophthalmologic Effects

Long-term high-dose administration of neuroleptic drugs has resulted in granular deposits in the cornea and in the posterior wall of the lens. To date, these changes have been reported most frequently with the phenothiazines; however, this has been the most extensively used group of neuroleptics in the United States. Retinal damage is not seen in these patients, and visual acuity is unaffected. The prevalence reported is between 1% and 30%. There appears to be a significantly higher incidence of pigmentation of the cornea and lens in those patients who have also had skin discoloration. The histochemical structure of the granules found in the lens, cornea, and skin resembles that of melanin.

Retinal pigmentation has been observed in patients receiving thioridazine in dosages exceeding 800 mg daily. Serious visual

Table 4
Nature and Frequency of Adverse Reactions
to Various Types of Neuroleptic Drugs

Adverse Reactions	Phenothiazines			Thio-xanthenes	Butyro-phenones
	Aliphatic derivatives	*Piperazine derivatives*	*Piperidine derivatives*		
Behavioral					
Oversedation	+++	−	+++	+++	−
Extrapyramidal					
Parkinsonian syndrome	++	+++	+	++	+++
Akathisia	++	+++	++	++	+++
Dystonic reactions	+	++	+	+	++
Autonomic					
Postural hypotension	+++	+	+++	++	++
Anticholinergic effects	+++	++	+++	++	+
Genitourinary					
Inhibition of ejaculation	++	++	+++	−	−
Cardiovascular					
EKG abnormalities	+	+	++	−	−
Hepatic					
Cholestatic jaundice	++	+	+	+	+
Hematologic					
Blood dyscrasias	++	+	+	+	++
Ophthalmologic					
Lenticular pigmentation	++	+	−	−	−
Pigmentary retinopathy	−	−	++	−	−
Dermatologic					
Allergic skin reaction	++	+	+	+	+
Photosensitivity reaction	++	+	++	+	+
Skin pigmentation	++	−	−	−	−

NOTE: +++ = common; ++ = uncommon; + = rare; − = not observed.

impairment, or even blindness, may result (Shader et al, 1970; Greiner and Berry, 1964).

Endocrine Effects

The effects of the neuroleptic drugs on the hypothalamus and pituitary seem to be responsible for the endocrine changes observed. Gynecomastia, galactorrhea, disturbances of glucose tolerance tests, false-positive pregnancy tests, and weight gain are among reactions which have been reported. Galactorrhea is generally the most troublesome. Sexual impotence which begins with delayed ejaculation and progresses to retrograde ejaculation and ultimately to loss of erection can probably occur with any of the neuroleptic agents, but it has not been reported with the newer drugs to date. It is most frequently observed with thioridazine and may be due to this drug's anticholinergic effects. Treatment consists of prescribing a neuroleptic with less anticholinergic activity.

Neurologic (Extrapyramidal) Effects

Drug-induced extrapyramidal reactions may be manifested in three ways: by a syndrome resembling naturally occurring Parkinson's disease; by a syndrome of uncontrollable restlessness known as akathisia; and by various dystonic syndromes, chiefly one resembling spastic torticollis. Age and individual susceptibility seem to be the most important determining factors.

The parkinsonian syndrome is managed by reduction of neuroleptic dosage or by administration of antiparkinsonism agents, or both. Daily dosages of some of the effective antiparkinsonism drugs are: procyclidine hydrochloride, 4 to 8 mg; benztropine mesylate, 1 to 4 mg; ethopropazine hydrochloride, 40 to 200 mg; biperiden, 2 to 6 mg. It is frequently possible, and always advisable, to reduce or discontinue the antiparkinsonism agent eventually. Sudden cessation of antiparkinsonism drugs should be avoided, since withdrawal effects may result. Prophylactic use of antiparkinsonism drugs is discouraged, as only a minority of patients develop extrapyramidal syndromes of any consequence, and the potential toxic effects of the antiparkinsonism drugs are considerable. Symptoms include mental confusion, dry mouth, blurred vision, and occasionally, paralysis of the bladder or bowel.

Akathisia may be alleviated by reducing the neuroleptic dosage or by concomitant administration of small doses of antiparkinsonism drugs or Benadryl. Akathisia (motor restlessness) presents a diagnostic problem and often is confused with an anxiety state. The patient feels he is unable to sit, and he has a need to pace. There is a generalized increase in motor activity. One schizophrenic patient used the neologism "too walkative" in describing his need to talk and walk excessively. The clinician should always consider the possibility of akathisia when called to see a patient who is receiving a neuroleptic drug and who is reported to be agitated, anxious, or restless. Careful questioning will establish the diagnosis.

Dystonic reactions are common in children and young adults. They usually appear soon after the drugs are started and are most frequently observed with the low-milligram phenothiazines, butyrophenones, and thioxanthenes. The dystonic syndrome is relieved by the parenteral administration of an antiparkinsonism drug, a barbiturate, or Benadryl, repeated, if necessary, an hour later. The neuroleptic drug causing the reaction should be temporarily discontinued, and an antiparkinsonism drug should be given when neuroleptic treatment is reinstated. It is preferable to resume therapy with a neuroleptic other than the one which caused the dystonic reaction.

Tardive Dyskinesia

Akathisia, parkinsonism, and dystonia usually appear within the first 70 days of neuroleptic treatment. These symptoms respond to antiparkinsonism drugs or disappear spontaneously a few days or weeks after the neuroleptic has been withdrawn or reduced in dosage. In contrast, tardive dyskinesia rarely occurs until after six months to one year of neuroleptic therapy. It does not respond to antiparkinsonism drugs and is not reversible when the drug is discontinued or the dosage reduced. In fact, the symptoms of tardive dyskinesia sometimes appear only after the neuroleptic medication has been discontinued.

Tardive dyskinesia is observed in about 20% to 40% of patients who have undergone long-term treatment with neuroleptics (Crane, 1973). Fann et al (1972) have reported an incidence of 36%. Involuntary movements of the oral region of the face—mostly of the lips and tongue (buccolingual syndrome)—are characteristic of the syndrome, but choreiform movements of the fingers and other muscle groups may also be observed. It is most likely to occur in elderly patients who have received large, cumulative doses of neuroleptics. Most patients who develop this complication are over 50 years old and are chronic, institutionalized patients who seem to be little distressed by their symptoms. The risk of tardive dyskinesia must always be considered when a patient is started on long-term neuroleptic treatment. Recent reports have indicated that children who have been treated for a long time with neuroleptic drugs may develop a similar condition.

The neurochemical mechanism of this disorder is believed to be linked to the development of dopaminergic hypersensitivity in the neostriatal pathways after long-term treatment (Klawans et al, 1974; Gerlach et al, 1974). This sensitivity might come about from an increase in the synthesis and release of dopamine by the presynaptic neuron due to feedback from the postsynaptic neuron, whose receptor for dopamine has been blocked. Another possibility is that some membrane damage occurs to the presynaptic neuron so that the postsynaptic neuron is essentially denervated, and characteristic "denervation hypersensitivity" to the neurotransmitter ensues. Either of these two mechanisms would explain the fact that more of the causative drug makes matters better and less makes matters momentarily worse. It would also explain the failure of anticholinergic drugs such as the antiparkinsonism agents to be effective in this disorder.

Tardive dyskinesia is a serious complication as no method has yet been found to reverse or cure it. The only relief that can be given for this condition is the discontinuation or increase of the neuroleptic medication that caused it. In a few exceptional cases, spontaneous recovery from the symptoms of tardive dyskinesia has been observed several months after the withdrawal of the neuroleptic. No certain way of preventing it is known, but there is reason to believe that periodic interruption of neuroleptic treatment for short periods of time may be helpful, since this reduces the level of accumulated neuroleptics. Such regular interruptions, or "drug holidays," are now recommended by many clinicians.

Sudden Death

This phenomenon has been reported in healthy young adults as well as in older patients (Moore and Book, 1970; Alexander, 1969). A number of mechanisms have been proposed, including microinfarcts in the myocardium; sudden, fatal ventricular arrhythmias; and laryngospasm with asphyxiation. At this time, there is no evidence that the mortality of patients receiving neuroleptic drugs is greater than a comparable sample of those not receiving medication (Peele and von Loetzen, 1972).

USE IN PREGNANCY

Since neuroleptic drugs have been administered to thousands of pregnant women with no well-documented reports that malformed children were born to these mothers, it seems safe to assume that neuroleptic drugs are not teratogenic. It is always best, however, to observe the usual precautions during the first trimester of any pregnancy; that is, to not administer any drug during this time unless there are important clinical indications for it. Two cases of extrapyramidal reactions in the neonate were reported by Tamer et al (1969) in mothers who were receiving the equivalent of 600 mg of chlorpromazine per day. The infants were born with dystonia, which was treated with Benadryl. The mothers had not shown extrapyramidal symptoms. The reader is referred to Shader and DiMascio (1970) for further and more detailed information on the medical complications of psychotropic drugs.

OVERDOSES

The high degree of safety inherent in the neuroleptic drugs has resulted in relatively few intentional or accidental deaths from these agents (Davis et al, 1968). Obviously, when neuroleptics are taken in combination with other drugs, the incidence of death greatly increases.

The clinical signs of neuroleptic overdose reflect the widespread pharmacologic activity of these agents and are a function of the amount of drug taken. The most frequently observed reactions to overdose are:

1. Impaired consciousness: initial sedation, eventual coma
2. Disorientation; symptoms of anticholinergic activity: blurred vision, dryness of mucous, nasal congestion, tachycardia, and hypotension
3. Extrapyramidal symptoms: dystonias, beginning with muscle spasms and tics and eventually developing into full-blown dystonic reactions (oculogyric crisis, spastic torticollis, etc); dyskinesias such as twitching
4. Convulsions: tonic, clonic, or startle seizures, which appear later
5. Temperature disturbances due to the effect of the neuroleptic on the temperature-regulating mechanism within the hypothalamus: chills, elevated and then lowered body temperature

Treatment

The first step in treating a neuroleptic overdose is to establish and maintain an open airway and to immediately follow this up with measures to facilitate elimination of the drug. If the patient is conscious, attempt to induce vomiting by the slow administration of 100 to 250 ml of a 25% solution of mannitol or a similar agent. (This may fail since the neuroleptics are anti-emetic.) Gastric lavage is helpful even hours after ingestion because the neuroleptics are water soluble. Peritoneal dialysis and hemodialysis do not appear to be very effective in treating this type of overdosage.

Convulsions should be treated with short-acting barbiturates. The sedative action of the barbiturate may potentiate that of the neuroleptic drug.

Stimulants are of little value; thus, amphetamines, methylphenidate, or caffeine should generally not be used.

Extrapyramidal symptoms should be treated with antiparkinsonism drugs, given parenterally or orally. Antiparkinsonism drugs are anticholinergic and must be used cautiously to prevent anticholinergic crisis.

Epinephrine should not be used to treat hypotension. If a vasopressor is required, use Levophed (0.2% solution) or Neo-Synephrine Hydrochloride. Maintain blood volume with I.V. fluids; elevate the feet; keep the patient warm with blankets, but do not apply external heat as it may worsen shock or produce local irritation.

Patients require close observation after initial treatment is given, as cardiac arrhythmia, respiratory failure, or shock may suddenly appear.

As stated at the beginning of the section, the neuroleptic agents are quite safe. The greatest danger lies with the patient who ingests multiple drugs and thus obscures the clinical picture (Kline et al, 1974).

SUMMARY

Laborit could hardly have been aware that his discovery of chlorpromazine in 1952 as a drug to reduce surgical shock would herald a new era in the treatment of the mentally ill. The neuroleptic drugs have made an impact on the treatment of all psychotic patients. The reduction of the resident population of mental hospitals by more than 64% in a 19-year period represents a better quality of life for many patients who would formerly have been destined to spend many years of their lives in mental institutions. The discovery and widespread use of the antipsychotic drugs also spearheaded the search for agents to treat depression and anxiety, and today the psychiatric armamentarium includes drugs to relieve the symptoms of these illnesses.

Perhaps the most important result of the discovery of the neuroleptic drugs is the impetus it has provided for the search for the biochemical basis of mental illness in the study of neurotransmitters, the chemicals within the brain that pass on stimuli and mediate emotion. Hopefully we will soon discover whether there may be an underlying biochemical lesion in psychotic patients.

While future historians will record the full impact of the discovery and use of the psychotropic drugs, their attendant problems—both medical and social—have already begun to surface. Medically, we are encountering some side effects such as tardive dyskinesia and lens and corneal opacities, which have been observed with long-term administration of these drugs. Only with time will we be able to knowledgeably assess the various benefit-to-risk ratios of the neuroleptics. In the social arena, community mental health programs which emphasize maintaining patients in the community and out of hospitals have been successful. Readmission rates of mental hospitals continue to rise. What the effect of this revolving door syndrome will be on patients, their families, and the economy is yet to be learned.

REFERENCES

Alexander, C.S.: Cardiac effects of psychotherapeutic drugs. *JAMA*. 208:366–368, 1969.

Ayd, F. A.: Cardiovascular effects of phenothiazines. *Int Drug Ther Newsletter* 5:1–8, 1970.

Ayd, F.A.: Rational pharmacotherapy: once-a-day drug dosage. *Dis Nerv System* 34:371–378, 1973.

Ayd, F.J., Jr.: A critique of chlorpromazine and reserpine therapy. In *Tranquilizing Drugs*, edited by H.E. Himwich, pp. 173–181. Washington, D.C: American Association for the Advancement of Science, 1957.

Baer, R.L. and Harber, L.C.: Photosensitivity induced by drugs. *JAMA*. 192:989–990, 1965.

Ban, T.A.: *Schizophrenia: A Psychopharmacological Approach.* Springfield, Ill: Charles C Thomas, Publisher, 1972.

Bein, H.J.: Discoveries in biological psychiatry. In *Biological Research with Reserpine in the Pharmaceutical Industry,* edited by F.J. Ayd and B. Blackwell, pp. 142–154. Philadelphia: J.B. Lippincott Co., 1970.

Blackwell, B.: Drug deviation in psychiatric patients. *Int Drug Ther Newsletter* 8:17–31, 1973a.

Blackwell, B.: Drug therapy: patient compliance. *N Engl J Med.* 289:249–252, 1973b.

Bobon, D.P.: Classifications and terminology of psychotropic drugs: a historical review. *Pharmakopsychiat.* 6:1–12, 1973.

Bradley, P.B.: (Rap) Research in psychopharmacology. *Wld Hlth Org Techn Ser.* 371, 1967.

Buckman, M.T. and Peake, G.T.: Prolactin in clinical practice. *JAMA.* 236:871–874, 1976.

Caffey, E.M., Jr., Diamond, L.S., Frank, T.V. et al: Discontinuation or reduction of chemotherapy in chronic schizophrenics. *J Chronic Dis.* 17:347–358, 1964.

Challas, G. and Brauer, W.: Tourette's disease: relief of symptoms with R1625. *Am J Psychiatr.* 120:283–284, 1963.

Cole, J.O. and Davis, J.M.: Antipsychotic agents. In *Comprehensive Textbook of Psychiatry,* edited by A.M. Freedman, H.I. Kaplan, and B.J. Sadock. Baltimore: The Williams & Wilkins Co., 1975.

Cole, J.O. and Stotsky, B.A.: Improving psychiatric drug therapy: a matter of dosage and choice. *Geriatrics* 83:74–78, 1974.

Crane, G.E.: Persistent dyskinesia. *Br J Psychiatr.* 122:395–405, 1973.

Curry, S.H., Marshall, J., Davis, J.M. et al: Chlorpromazine plasma levels and effects. *Arch Gen Psychiatr.* 22(4):289–296, 1970.

Curry, S.H., Samuel, G., and Mould, G.P.: Fluphenazine decanoate in patients absorbing oral chlorpromazine ineffectively. In *The Future of Pharmacotherapy: New Drug Delivery Systems,* edited by F.J. Ayd, Jr., pp. 53–60. Baltimore: International Drug Therapy Newsletter, 1973.

Davis, J.: Overview: maintenance therapy in psychiatry: I. Schizophrenia. *Am J Psychiatr.* 132:1237–1245, 1975.

Davis, J.: Recent developments in the drug treatment of schizophrenia. *Am J Psychiatr.* 133:208–213, 1976.

Davis, J.M., Bartlett, E., and Termini, B.A.: Overdosage of psychotropic drugs: a review. *Dis Nerv System* 29:157–246, 1968.

DiMascio, A.: Toward a more rational use of antiparkinsonism drugs in psychiatry. *Drug Therapy* 1:23–29, 1971.

Engelhardt, D.M. and Freedman, N.: Maintenance drug therapy: the schizophrenic patient in the community. In *International Psychiatry Clinics,* edited by N.S. Kline and H.E. Lehmann, pp. 933–960. Boston: Little, Brown & Co., 1965.

Engelhardt, D.M., Rosen, B., Freedman, N. et al.: Phenothiazines in prevention of psychiatric hospitalization. IV. Delay or prevention of hospitalization: a re-evaluation. *Arch Gen Psychiatr.* 16:98, 1967.

Fann, W.E., Davis, J.M., and Janowsky, D.S.: The prevalence of tardive dyskinesias in mental hospital patients. *Dis Nerv System* 33:182–186, 1972.

Gardos, G.E. and Cole, J.O.: Maintenance antipsychotic therapy: Is the cure worse than the disease? *Am J Psychiatr.* 133:32–36, 1976.

Gerlach, J., Reisby, N., and Randrup, A.: Dopaminergic hypersensitivity and cholinergic hypofunction in the pathophysiology of tardive dyskinesia. *Psychopharmacologia* 34:21–35, 1974.

Goldstein, B.J.: Clinical evaluation of thiothixene in chronic ambulatory patients. In *Modern Problems in Pharmacotherapy,* edited by H. Lehman and T. Ban. Basel: S Karger AG, 1969.

Goldstein, B.J., Brauzer, B. et al: The treatment of mixed anxiety and depression with loxapine: a controlled comparative study. *J Clin Pharmacol.* 14(8):455–463, 1974.

Green, D.E. and Forrest, I.S.: In vivo metabolism of chlorpromazine. *Can Psych Assoc J.* 11:299–302, 1966.

Greiner, A.C. and Berry, K.: Skin pigmentation and corneal and lens opacities with prolonged chlorpromazine therapy. *Can Med Assoc J.* 90:663–665, 1964.

Hasse, H.J. and Janssen, P.A.: *The Action of Neuroleptic Drugs.* Amsterdam: North Holland Publishing Co., 1965.

Hogarty, G.E., Goldberg, S.C., and the Collaborative Study Group: Drug and sociotherapy in the aftercare of schizophrenic patients: one year relapse rates. *Arch Gen Psychiatr.* 28:54–64, 1973.

Hollister, L.: *Clinical Use of Psychotherapeutic Drugs.* Springfield, Ill: Charles C Thomas, Publisher, 1973.

Hollister, L.: Adverse reactions to psychotherapeutic drugs. In *Drug Treatment of Mental Disorders,* edited by L. Simpson, pp. 267–288. New York: Raven Press, 1975.

Hollister, L., Overall, J. et al: Specific indications for different classes of phenothiazines. *Arch Gen Psychiatr.* 30:94–99, 1974.

Horn, A.S. and Snyder, S.H.: Chlorpromazine and dopamine: conformational similarities that correlate with antischizophrenic activity of phenothiazine drugs. *Proc Natl Acad Sci.* 68:2325–2328, 1971.

Hughes, J.S. and Little, J.C.: An appraisal of the continuing practice of prescribing tranquilizing drugs for long-stay psychiatric patients. *Br J Psychiatr.* 133:867–873, 1967.

Imlah, N.W. and Murphy, K.: The clinical use of long-acting psychotropic drugs. *Therapie* 28:587–594, 1973.

Itil, T., Keskiner, A., Heinemann, L. et al: Treatment of resistant schizophrenics with extremely high dosage fluphenazine hydrochloride. *Psychosomatics* 11:456, 1970.

Itil, T., Patterson, C.D., Keskiner, A. et al: Comparison of phenothiazine and nonphenothiazine neuroleptics according to psychopathology, side effects, and computerized EEG. In *Thiothixene and the Thioxanthenes,* edited by I.S. Forrest, C.J. Carr, and E. Usdin, pp. 35–45. New York: Raven Press, 1974.

Jacobsen, E.: The comparative pharmacology of some psychotropic drugs. *Bull WHO* 21:411, 1959a.

Jacobsen, E.: Classification of psychotropic drugs: discussion. In *Psychopharmacology Frontiers,* edited by N.S. Kline, p. 424. London: Churchill Livingstone, 1959b.

Jacobsen, E.: The classification of psychotropic drugs. *J Neuropsychiatr.* 4:241, 1963.

Janssen, P.A.J.: The butyrophenone story. In *Discoveries in Biological Psychiatry,* edited by F. Ayd and B. Blackwell. Philadelphia: J.B. Lippincott Co., 1970a.

Janssen, P.A.J.: Chemical and pharmacological classification of neuroleptics. In *Modern Problems in Pharmacopsychiatry: The Neuroleptics*, Vol. 5, edited by O.P. Bokon, P.A.J. Janssen, and J. Bokon, pp. 34–44. Basel: S Karger AG, 1970b.

Klawans, H.L., Bergen, D., Bruyn, G.W. et al: Neuroleptic-induced tardive dyskinesias in nonpsychotic patients. *Arch Neurol.* 30:338–339, 1974.

Klein, D.F. and Davis, J.M.: *Diagnosis and Drug Treatment of Psychiatric Disorders*. Baltimore: The Williams & Wilkins Co., 1969.

Klerman, G.: Pharmacotherapy of schizophrenia. *Ann Rev Med.* 25:199–217, 1974.

Klett, C.J. and Caffey, E.M., Jr.: Evaluating the long-term need for antiparkinsonism drugs by chronic schizophrenics. *Arch Gen Psychiatr.* 26:374–379, 1972.

Kline, N., Alexander, S. et al: *Psychotropic Drugs: Manual for Emergency Management of Overdosage*. Oradell, NJ: Medical Economics Publishers, 1974.

Labhardt, F.: Einteilung und Grundeffekte der Psychopharmaka. In *Psychiatrische Pharmakotherapie in Klinik und Praxis*, edited by P. Kielholz, pp. 15–29. Bern: Hans Huber Medical Publisher, 1965.

Lasky, J.J., Klett, C.J., Caffey, E.M., Jr. et al: Drug treatment of schizophrenic patients: a comparative evaluation of chlorpromazine, chlorprothixene, fluphenazine, reserpine, thioridazine, and triflupromazine. *Dis Nerv System* 23:698, 1962.

Leeds, A.A. and Levine, J.: *Psychotropic Drug Classification of the International Reference Center WHO-NIMH Network*. Chevy Chase, Md: National Institute of Mental Health, 1970.

Lehmann, H.E.: Pharmacotherapy of schizophrenia. In *Psychopathology of Schizophrenia*, edited by P. Hoch and J. Zubin, pp. 18–41. New York: Grune & Stratton, Inc., 1965.

Levitt, R.A.: *The Tranquilizers: Psychopharmacology, Biological Approach*. Washington, DC: Hemisphere Publishing Co., 1975.

Madsen, E. and Ravn, J.: Preliminary therapeutic experiments with a new psychotropic drug. *Truxal Nord Psykiatr Medlemski* 13:82, 1959.

Matthysse, S.: Antipsychotic drug actions: a clue to the neuropathology of schizophrenia. *Fed Proc.* 32:200–205, 1973.

Mental Health Statistical Notes, No. 9. Biometrics Division, National Institute of Mental Health, Public Health Service, 1969.

Mental Health Statistical Notes, No. 70. Biometrics Division, National Institute of Mental Health, Public Health Service, 1973.

Mental Health Statistical Notes, No. 97. Biometrics Division, National Institute of Mental Health, Public Health Service, 1974.

Mental Health Statistical Notes, No. 113. Biometrics Division, National Institute of Mental Health, Public Health Service, 1975a.

Mental Health Statistical Notes, No. 119. Biometrics Division, National Institute of Mental Health, Public Health Service, 1975b.

Mental Health Statistical Notes, No. 125. Biometrics Division, National Institute of Mental Health, Public Health Service, 1976a.

Mental Health Statistical Notes, No. 127. Biometrics Division, National Institute of Mental Health, Public Health Service, 1976b.

Mental Health Statistical Notes, No. 132. Biometrics Division, National Institute of Mental Health, Public Health Service, 1976c.

Michaux, M.H., Hanlon, T.E., Ota, K.Y. et al: Phenothiazines in the treatment of newly admitted state hospital patients: global comparison of eight compounds in terms of an outcome index. *Curr Ther Res*. 6:331, 1964.

Moore, M.T. and Book, M.H.: Sudden death in phenothiazine therapy. *Psychiatr Qtrly*. 44:389–395, 1970.

Møller Nielsen, I., Hougs, W., Lassen, N. et al: Central depressant activity of some thioxanthene derivatives. *Act Pharmacol Toxicol*. (Copenhagen) 19:87–100, 1962.

National Institute of Mental Health Psychopharmacology Service Center Collaborative Study Group: Phenothiazine treatment in acute schizophrenia: effectiveness. *Arch Gen Psychiatr*. 10:246–261, 1964.

Peele, R. and von Loetzen, I.S.: Phenothiazine deaths: a clinical review. Read before the Annual Meeting of the American Psychiatric Association, Dallas, Texas, May 1–5, 1972.

Petersen, P.V., Lassen, N., Holm, T. et al: Chemical structure and pharmacologic effects of thioxanthene analogues of chlorpromazine, promazine and mephazine. *Arzneim Forsch*. 8:395, 1958.

Prien, R.F. and Cole, J.: High-dose chlorpromazine therapy in chronic schizophrenia. *Arch Gen Psychiatr*. 18:482–495, 1968.

Prien, R.F., Gilles, R.D., and Caffey, E.M.: Intermittent pharmacotherapy in chronic schizophrenia. In *Veterans Administration Medical Bulletin*. Perry Point, Md: Central Neuropsychiatric Research Laboratory, 1973.

Prien, R.F. and Klett, C.J.: An appraisal of the long-term use of tranquilizing medication with hospitalized chronic schizophrenics. *Schizophrenia Bull*. 5:64–73, 1972.

Rifkin, A., Quitkin, R., Carrillo, C. et al: Very high dosage fluphenazine for nonchronic treatment-refractory patients. *Arch Gen Psychiatr*. 25:398, 1971.

Rivera-Calimlim, L., Astaneda, L., and Lasagna, L.: Effects of mode of management on plasma chlorpromazine in psychiatric patients. *Clin Pharmacol Ther*. 14(6):978–986, 1973.

Sachar, E.J., Gruen, P.H. et al: Thioridazine stimulates prolactin in man. *Arch Gen Psychiatr*. 32:834–836, 1975.

Salzman, C., Shader, R.I., and Pearlman, M.: Psychopharmacology and the elderly. In *Psychotropic Drug Side Effects*, edited by R.I. Shader and A. DiMascio, pp. 261–279. Baltimore: The Williams & Wilkins Co., 1970.

Shader, R.I., Appleton, W.S., and DiMascio, A.: Ophthalmological (pigmentary) changes. In *Psychotropic Drug Side Effects*, edited by R.I. Shader and A. DiMascio, pp. 107–116. Baltimore: The Williams & Wilkins Co., 1970.

Snyder, S., Greenberg, D., and Yamamura, H.I.: Antischizophrenic drugs and brain cholinergic receptors. *Arch Gen Psychiatr*. 31:58–61, 1974.

Stach, K. and Poldinger, W.: Strukturelle Betrachtungen der Psychopharmaka: Versuch einer Korrelation von chemischer

Konstitution und klinischer Wirkung. In *Progress in Drug Research*, edited by E. Jucker, pp. 129–290. Basel: Birkhäuser Verlag, 1966.

Stewart, R.B. and Cluff, L.E.: A review of medication errors and compliance in ambulant patients. *Clin Pharmacol Ther*. 13:463–468, 1972.

Swazey, J.: *Chlorpromazine: The History of the Psychiatric Discovery*. Cambridge, Mass: MIT Press, 1974.

Tamer, A., McKey, R., Arias, D. et al: Phenothiazine-induced extrapyramidal dysfunction in the neonate. *J Pediatr*. 75(3):279–280, 1969.

Whitehead, J.A.: Long-acting phenothiazines in the treatment of old people with mental illness. *Int Drug Ther Newsletter* 8:47–52, 1973.

10 Lithium

Allan B. Wells, M.D.
Myer Mendelson, M.D.

INTRODUCTION

Lithium salts were used medically in the nineteenth century for the treatment of gout, rheumatism, kidney disease, and a potpourri of other medical disorders. It has been sold in bottled waters for many years and is included, along with other salts, in such proprietary tonics as Perrier, Appolinaire, and Vichy water. Earlier in the century, some soda waters in this country contained lithium salts.

The first indication that lithium may have been used for manic attacks goes back to the second century AD, when alkali waters were prescribed for the treatment of excited states. Lithium reached a certain level of popularity in the late nineteenth century as a general curative and tonic, and it had become a part of medical mythology. By the turn of the century, it had been debunked by the medical community as an all-around nostrum.

273

In the 1940s lithium chloride was introduced as a salt substitute for cardiac and hypertensive patients. Since its taste was similar to that of table salt, it was thought to be an ideal seasoning for patients needing a salt-free diet. Its use in this way soon made it apparent, however, that an unrestricted dosage had toxic effects. Medical reports of severe illness and of several deaths related to the lithium salt-substitute began to appear. It was quickly withdrawn, and thereafter lithium carried a tainted reputation.

Also at this time, John Cade, a psychiatrist working in a small psychiatric hospital in Australia, began to develop a hypothesis regarding the etiology of manic-depressive illness. Although his basic idea later proved to be incorrect, it led him to the successful use of lithium salts in the treatment of manic and excited states. In 1949 he published a report of his work on nineteen patients which demonstrated not only the effectiveness of lithium in the manic state but also its safety when given in dosages that were not toxic.

It was approximately 20 years before lithium carbonate became generally available, and it has now become well established for the treatment and prevention of manic and hypomanic episodes. More recently, the benefits of its use in some depressive illnesses have also come to light.

RECOGNIZING MANIC STATES

Most textbook descriptions characterize manic states according to the classic triad of euphoric mood, pressure of speech, and hyperactivity. The descriptions of euphoria usually convey an image of zestful gaiety, an infectious, light-hearted good humor. The pressure of speech is described in terms of extreme talkativeness, flight of ideas, and rapid association of words by similarity of sounds and rhyme rather than by meaning. The psychomotor activity spans a spectrum ranging from purposeful but rapid action, to distractible restlessness, to frantic, ceaseless motion. This description represents the classic picture that clinicians have been taught. As in so many other conditions, the extremes are relatively easy to identify, but symptoms of intermediate stages may blend into those of other disorders. The characteristic features of mania are nearly always described as they might appear to the observer.

The assumption is generally made that the patient's euphoria or elation will be clearly apparent in his bubbling good humor, that his flight of ideas will be revealed in his pressured speech, and that his hyperactivity will manifest itself in restless, unceasing motion. These symptoms, however, may be concealed from the observer. If they are to be identified, as much emphasis must be placed on what the patient is experiencing subjectively as on what he is demonstrating objectively. Inquiries about racing or speeding thoughts may reveal their existence, independent of any pressure of talk and perhaps even coexistent with hesitant, slow, or drawling speech. High energy levels may be associated with a normal, even languid or lazy, appearance. Only careful questioning will reveal this. Elation may be present for months without being noted by spouses, parents, or siblings because of the absence of the behavior, speech, or facial expressions that ordinarily accompany this affect. It thus becomes important to inquire carefully about the patient's subjective experiences.

The elation that is usually described in textbooks may in fact be absent and be replaced by chronic complaining and irritable behavior that becomes a trial to the family. Or, the elation may be quickly transformed into hostility by the refusal of some trivial but inappropriate request.

Impulsivity has long been recognized as a major feature of manic states. It can be thought of as one manifestation of that pressure for activity which overwhelms the manic patient. He may change jobs, embark on distant trips, go on a buying binge, or manifest other signs of impaired judgment.

The term *flight of ideas* is almost universally used to refer to one of the most obvious symptoms of hypomanic and manic states. The implication is that one idea suggests another to the patient, and instead of his train of thought continuing to a predetermined goal, his ideas fly off in various directions. Though seemingly random, his ideas are interconnected. This is ordinarily contrasted with the *looseness of associations* manifested by schizophrenic patients, in which the listener cannot grasp the connections between the ideas expressed. However, the expressions flight of ideas and looseness of associations may often only betray the preconceptions of the clinician. If the patient is regarded as manic, then the flow of words is perceived as a flight of ideas; if the patient is seen as schizophrenic, the same flow of words is referred to as a loosening of associations. Even if one wishes to apply this differentiation properly, however, it is frequently not as easy to do as it may appear. For example, in some manic patients, perhaps only every second, third, or fourth thought will be reported, thereby making the connections between them incoherent and giving the appearance of loose associations.

A tendency that prevailed until very recently was that of classifying manic thought disturbances in an overly simplified stereotype of expansiveness and grandiosity. On the other hand, the presence of ideas of reference or persecutory ideas would incline one to diagnose schizophrenia. It is therefore worth noting that ideas of reference do occur in manic episodes; sometimes they are clearly grandiose. Moreover, persecutory delusions, misidentifications, and visual and auditory hallucinations have all also been reported. Mania may indeed have many faces, some of which very much resemble schizophrenia.

Treatment

In the treatment of acute mania and hypomanic states, lithium carbonate has proven unusually effective and safe. Nevertheless, it should be noted that success rates run at about 80% and that many patients will not respond to lithium alone. It should also be noted that, while many patients respond rapidly and dramatically within two weeks, our experience has been that for some patients treatment with adequate doses of lithium sometimes took several weeks to bring about a remission. In some patients it is necessary to add a phenothiazine or a butyrophenone (such as Haldol) to an adequate dosage of lithium carbonate before a response can be attained.

Prevention of Manic Episodes
with Lithium

Clinical and research evidence have established that lithium carbonate effectively prevents—or at least reduces the incidence of—recurrence of manic and hypomanic attacks. In a number of studies, the frequency of manic episodes before lithium treatment was significantly higher than during an equivalent period following inception of this treatment program. (Some researchers question the use of the term *prophylaxis* and prefer terminology such as *stabilization*, *normothymia*, or *mood compensation* to describe the patient's clinical status.) Some patients report a stability of mood which they had never before achieved. The prevention of relapses has given many people the ability to exercise much more control over their lives in terms of their family, social, and work adjustments. While many patients miss the elation of their manic episodes, the majority is grateful for the ability to operate in life free from the radical swings in mood which were previously so disruptive and destructive of normal functioning.

LITHIUM AND DEPRESSIVE ILLNESS

Manic-depressive disorder is a biphasic disease, with the depressive phases often outnumbering manic and hypomanic episodes. It is now often referred to as bipolar depression in psychiatric parlance to differentiate it from the condition of those patients experiencing only recurrent depressions (unipolar depression). It also frequently happens that an acute episode of mania has depressive features intermingled with the elation. A patient may be euphoric, talking rapidly and moving quickly, and he may suddenly stop, begin to cry, and experience intense depression. Just as quickly, the mood of elation can return. We have also noted that some depressive patients who have never had an overt manic attack experience racing thoughts during their depressions.

There is a growing body of evidence that lithium carbonate prevents recurrences not only of manic attacks but of the depressive episodes of bipolar depression as well. Additionally, some feel that lithium by itself can be an effective antidepressant for bipolar depressive patients. Some of these "lithium responders" have not responded to other types of antidepressants. Some researchers feel that lithium is also effective in unipolar depression.

In our experience, some patients with bipolar depression may initially present as having unipolar depression; that is, they have no previous history of overt manic or hypomanic episodes, only a history of recurrent depressive attacks. Careful inquiry into the history may reveal, however, that the patient recalls periods of racing thoughts and brief periods of exhilaration and accelerated activity. These periods may represent mood swings that are subtle and muted forms of the more florid "high" experienced in every manic episode. These depressed patients, and those who experience racing thoughts during a depression, probably deserve a trial of a month or more on lithium to determine if, in fact, they are "lithium responders."

OTHER INDICATIONS FOR LITHIUM

A number of studies have evaluated the use of lithium in schizo-affective schizophrenia. Some have demonstrated the effectiveness of lithium in controlling the mood component of this disorder, but not the schizophrenic symptoms. Other studies have suggested that lithium has some usefulness in treating emotional instability, character disorders, alcoholism, hyperactivity in children, some neurotic disorders, epilepsy, phobic reactions, and premenstrual tension. More investigation is required to establish its efficacy for these illnesses.

CLINICAL USE OF LITHIUM

During the acute manic or hypomanic stages, higher doses of lithium are generally necessary for therapeutic effectiveness. Maintenance therapy for the same patient often requires a lower dosage to achieve the same serum levels. During the acute period, serum lithium is determined after several days to help evaluate how much further the dosage should be increased. The usual, recommended therapeutic serum level is 0.9 to 1.6 mEq/liter. This represents a range of approximately 900 to 3000 mg daily, depending on the severity of the illness and on the patient's age, weight, and metabolism. Serum levels should not exceed 2 mEq/liter, as toxicity then becomes apparent. Sometimes a clinical remission can be obtained at lower serum levels, and it is our opinion that it is not necessary to push the dose to attain the usual desired serum level in these situations. Indeed, some patients may respond to exceptionally small dosages, occasionally to less than 300 mg daily.

Despite widespread publicity concerning the toxicity of lithium, it does not have to be administered in a hospital setting if it is prescribed by a physician familiar with its use. Hospitalization may be necessary because of the patient's disabling symptoms, but not purely for the administration of lithium. There is a certain amount of disagreement concerning the necessity of laboratory studies prior to treatment with lithium. Unless the patient presents with signs and symptoms of somatic disease, we do not consider such studies necessary; other clinicians feel that a physical and laboratory evaluation should be performed before lithium is used. Recommended laboratory studies include: complete blood count, renal function tests, thyroid tests, electrocardiogram, and urinalysis, or some combination of these.

Lithium carbonate is marketed in the United States as a 300-mg tablet or capsule. In the manic phase, dosages usually start at one or two pills per day (300 to 600 mg) and are increased by one or two pills daily until a therapeutic response is achieved or until serum levels fall in the range of 0.9 to 1.6 mEq/liter. Although the practice varies, serum lithium is measured once or twice weekly, depending on the dosage the patient is receiving and the degree to which the patient is experiencing side effects.

The importance of maintenance therapy after the initial manic episode has been controlled must be stressed to patient and family. During maintenance treatment, serum levels need not be taken frequently. When side effects are bothersome, when there are signs of toxicity, or when the patient experiences a febrile illness such as influenza, a serum level can be taken. Often this is not necessary, and the clinician familiar with lithium can adjust dosage without laboratory determinations of serum lithium.

In the treatment of depression, which more often takes place out of the hospital, increases in dosage can be added more leisurely. Relatively few serum levels need be taken, as the experienced clinician can modify dosage based on observations of the patient.

Rapid Cycles

There are some patients who go through extreme mood shifts within a relatively short period. They experience at least four such shifts per year and may experience them as often as every four to six weeks. Rarely, the cycles may last hours to days. Often there is no intervening period of mood stability, only swings from elation to depression, each having its own periodicity. These patients are particularly difficult to treat, as their condition is often resistant to lithium alone. They usually require antidepressants as well as major tranquilizers to control their mood shifts. Frequent changes and adjustments of medication are necessary.

Side Effects

When lithium therapy is first instituted, some patients report transient side effects which usually disappear as the dosage is stabilized. Occasionally a patient on a maintenance schedule who has previously been free of side effects will experience them for a brief period. It must be emphasized that there is an important distinction to be made between side effects and adverse effects, as the latter may require medical intervention. The most frequently reported side effects are nausea, gastrointestinal distress, diarrhea, fine tremor, fatigue, thirst, and urinary frequency. If the tremor persists, it can be controlled with low dosages (10 to 40 mg daily) of propranolol. When other symptoms persist, a temporary lowering of dosage—or even temporary cessation of treatment—is usually effective in controlling side effects.

Nausea can be a distressing side effect, and it is often treated by changing from the tablet to the capsule form. Antacids are also effective in relieving this symptom. Diarrhea is usually transient and can be managed by briefly lowering the dosage, or by using antidiarrheal agents if the condition persists. Other side effects which may occur include weight gain and muscle spasms (especially of the lower abdomen). A rare patient may experience severe, crampy pain which can mimic appendicitis. When the lithium is stopped, however, these pains rapidly disappear and therapy can usually resume without their recurrence.

Acne-like skin eruptions of the face, neck, and back are sometimes seen. While this may be distressing to someone who has been free of acne, it is not a sign of allergy and it disappears without treatment in most cases. It is not an indication that lithium must be discontinued. On the other hand, rashes are evidence of an allergic response and necessitate either a temporary discontinuation of the medication, or treatment with an antihistamine.

The list of potential side effects is longer, but these are usually rare. More common, but harmless, are the slightly blurred vision and the twitching (particularly as they fall asleep) which some patients report.

Toxicity

If lithium is taken in a controlled situation, under the guidance of those familiar with its use, toxicity is uncommon. Toxicity generally results when too much lithium is ingested relative to the body's ability to eliminate it. The phenomenon was first observed when lithium was used as a salt-substitute and taken in unrestricted amounts. Serum levels above 2 mEq/liter usually produce early toxic symptoms. A few patients may develop toxicity at much lower serum levels; they represent a small subgroup of persons who are intolerant of lithium. Elderly patients may also occasionally react adversely to lithium and tolerate only small doses and low serum levels, but they may still achieve a therapeutic effect.

Toxicity is usually a gradual process, beginning with several days of severe nausea, vomiting, diarrhea (an exaggeration of the early, transient side effects noted above), drowsiness, slurred speech, staggering walk, and muscle twitching.

Severe lithium toxicity has its greatest effects on the central nervous system, and the patient shows confusion and disorientation that may progress to coma and convulsions. Treatment consists of discontinuing lithium, taking the measures appropriate to hastening its clearance from the body, and preventing the complications of coma. Lithium is normally cleared quickly by the body, with the serum level dropping 50% within 24 to 48 hours after the last dose.

Again, it is important to note that, administered appropriately, lithium is not dangerous. Like most medications, if too much is taken it will have an adverse effect, but therapeutic dosages are not intrinsically a danger to the patient.

Conditions Which Dictate Caution

Since lithium is eliminated by the kidneys, impairment of kidney function can allow toxic levels of lithium to accumulate. Patients who have renal disease are at risk if placed on this medication. Cardiovascular disease also presents a situation where lithium should be used with caution, as heart patients are often on a therapeutic regimen which includes salt restriction and diuretics. The addition of lithium can lead to its retention and to the subsequent elevation of serum lithium to toxic levels, even though the dosage would normally be nontoxic. In fact, patients who do not have kidney or heart disease should be cautioned to keep their intake of fluids and salt normal in order to prevent lithium accumulation and toxicity.

Although many clinicians feel that lithium is contraindicated in patients with kidney or heart disease, others feel that its potential toxicity must be weighed against its ability to ameliorate symptoms and behavior which may contribute to the patient's physical disability. While lithium is not the treatment of first choice for such patients, it may be given if the patient is carefully monitored for toxicity by all who are taking part in the treatment.

Combining lithium with salt-depleting diuretics must also be undertaken cautiously. Some cases of toxicity have been reported after diuretics have been taken by patients on lithium. If, for example, a patient has concurrent hypertension and must use a diuretic, then use of lower dosages of lithium is advisable.

LITHIUM AND THE THYROID GLAND

Some patients on maintenance dosages of lithium manifest decreased thyroid function as measured in laboratory tests. Occasionally they may develop some enlargement of the thyroid gland. The patients can also experience some of the symptoms of hypothyroidism, such as fatigue. This is easily corrected by the addition of thyroid substitutes and generally does not mean that lithium must be discontinued.

LITHIUM AND PREGNANCY

The incidence of congenital abnormalities in children of mothers who took lithium during pregnancy is not higher than that in children of mothers who did not take lithium. However, some laboratory studies have shown that pregnant mice given lithium have borne offspring with a higher than normal incidence of cleft palate. This effect would occur during the first three months of pregnancy. The potential risk for humans who take lithium while pregnant appears to be slight, but again, risks must be weighed against benefits. When it is necessary to administer lithium to a pregnant woman, it is advisable to divide the dosage up as much as possible during the waking hours so that fluctuations in lithium blood levels will be small. For example: instead of one tablet four times per day, a pregnant woman could take one-half tablet eight times per day.

Because lithium appears in mothers' milk, infants of mothers taking lithium should not be breast-fed.

CONCLUSION

Lithium carbonate, a simple, inexpensive salt, seems to have found a firm place in modern psychiatric practice. Lithium's clinical effectiveness is now well established, and the indications for its use appear to be broadening. Psychiatrists, as well as other members of the health care system, are becoming more knowledgeable about its applications and its potential hazards. After a long sojourn on the fringe of accepted psychiatric therapy, lithium has come into its own.

REFERENCES

Bunney, W. and Hartman, E.: Study of a patient with 48-hour manic-depressive cycles. *Arch Gen Psychiatr.* 12:611, 1965.

Cade, J.: Lithium salts in the treatment of psychotic excitement. *Med J Austr.* 36:349, 1949.

Davis, J.: Overview: Maintenance therapy in psychiatry: affective disorders. *Am J Psychiatr.* 133:27, 1976.

Fieve, R., Kumbaraci, T., and Dunner, D.: The course of development of mania in patients with recurrent depression. *Am J Psychiatr.* 133:8, 1976.

Freedman, A. and Kaplan, H., eds.: *Comprehensive Textbook of Psychiatry.* Baltimore: The Williams & Wilkins Co., 1975.

Gershon, S. and Shopsin, B., eds.: *Lithium: Its Role in Psychiatric Research and Treatment.* New York: Plenum Press, 1973.

Karger, S.: *Lithium: The History of Its Use in Psychiatry.* New York: Brunner/Mazel, Inc., 1969.

Klein, D. and Davis, J.: *Diagnosis and Drug Treatment of Psychiatric Disorders.* Baltimore: The Johns Hopkins University Press, 1969.

Klein, D. and Gittelman-Klein, R.: *Progress in Psychiatric Drug Treatment.* New York: Brunner/Mazel, Inc., 1975.

Mendels, J. and Secunda, S., eds.: *Lithium.* New York: Gordon & Breach, Inc., 1972.

Mendels, J., Secunda, S., and Dyson, W.: A controlled study of the antidepressant effects of lithium carbonate. *Arch Gen Psychiatr.* 26:489, 1972.

Winokur, G., Clayton, P., and Reich, T.: *Manic-Depressive Illness.* St. Louis: C.V. Mosby Co., 1969.

Zall, H., Therman, P., and Myers, J.: Lithium carbonate: a clinical study. *Am J Psychiatr.* 125:549, 1968.

Zubin, J. and Freyhan, F., eds.: *Disorders of Mood.* Baltimore: The Johns Hopkins University Press, 1972.

11 Mind-Influencing Drugs in the Pediatric Patient

Dean T. Collins, M.D.
Harcharan S. Sehdev, M.D.

INTRODUCTION

All drugs, including the psychotropics, are potentially toxic substances. They can cause moderate, severe, or even fatal reactions (McAndrew et al, 1972). Fortunately, however, the ranges of safety of most psychotropic drugs are wide enough to permit a great deal of latitude in their use. Although the classes of drugs used in children are not different from those used in adults, their application is somewhat different. Neuroleptics (major tranquilizers) and stimulants are employed more frequently than are other classes of drugs. The decision to use medication in children, however, requires serious consideration (Blackwell and Ayd, 1975). Thorough assessment of presenting problems, a general review of the child's health, definition of target symptoms or behavior, careful choice of medication, and subsequent monitoring are all necessary. As with adults, other parameters—such as previous drug history, family history of drug responsiveness, and the use of concomitant medications, for either psychiatric or other disorders—need to be considered. In the light of now commonly known drug-drug interactions, these considerations are important.

Apart from the pharmacologic reasons for conscientious decisions on whether or not to employ medication, there are psychologic reasons which indicate that, everything else being equal, one should opt in favor of no drug use at all. In the course of growth and development, the child learns not only from his parents, peers, and others but also from his own experiences. Habit development is intricately related to and interwoven with experiential learning. The parents, or other care-givers, therefore impart significant messages if a drug in and of itself is viewed as a ready solution for ordinary problems, pains, and tensions. Early habits in confronting and solving problems serve as precursors to development of more permanent attitudes in life. It is therefore not surprising to learn that the child given drugs today becomes the adult who uses drugs to excess in the future. The principle that needs to be emphasized is that optimum tension is necessary for learning, and that successful struggle with and mastery of tasks gives gratification as well as incentive for further achievements. Easy remedies that obliterate optimum tensions and stresses in life are antithetical to growth and can create excessive dependence on the foreign substances used to relieve these tensions.

Certain symptoms in children are transitory and are related to developmental processes. In such situations, it may be best to leave them alone or to deal with them through means other than medication. For example, symptoms such as enuresis or episodes of anxiety in children which are related to family stresses or crises should not be construed as abnormal unless they persist for a long time or are of such severity as to be a significant impediment to growth. Dealing with these situations in a conservative way may constitute the best intervention (Sehdev, 1973).

When medication becomes necessary, one must be aware of the fact that idiosyncratic or paradoxical reactions can frequently occur in children. Sometimes the common reactions may be the reverse of what would be expected in an adult. Barbiturates, for example, are ordinarily sedating agents in adults, but they are frequently excitants in children. Why these paradoxical reactions occur in children is not clear. It is conjectured that perhaps the undefined characteristics of the developing brain, together with the processes of stratification of inhibition and control, make the site of action of these drugs less predictable and the behavioral manifestation of the drug effect therefore subject to impact on receptors at different foci than in the mature brain.

In regard to dosage, the pharmacologic axiom "The dose of any drug is that which is enough" holds true for psychotropic medications. The usual rule—that one should reduce medication for a child to one sixth the usual adult dosage—may be of value in initiating medication, but it may be best to calculate dosage on the basis of body weight by consulting the leaflet insert in the drug package. These guidelines, although helpful, may not always be clinically useful, and several pharmacotherapists now go far beyond the suggested dosages for some psychotropic drugs. As potent as they are, these drugs still have a wide dosage range within which therapeutic effects can be obtained. It would not be unusual to use a neuroleptic such as chlorpromazine (Thorazine) in a range of from 50 to 1500 mg per day. Particularly in children, it is desirable to reduce the dosage to the minimum effective level for maintenance purposes.

The side effects from the neuroleptics and other psychoactive drugs are at times irreversible—even lethal—and in initiating medication, the reaction that needs the most careful monitoring is hypotension. This is particularly true with the phenothiazines. Although extrapyramidal side effects can occur and are a nuisance, they are easily manageable. The anticholinergic syndrome has recently come to be recognized (DiGiacomo, 1975) as occurring with the use of both the tricyclic antidepressants and the phenothiazines. Lithium is only occasionally administered to children for various disorders and requires cautious and careful titration when used (Campbell et al, 1973; Warneke, 1975). The range of therapeutic blood levels of lithium is rather narrow, and its toxic effects can be very severe. Therefore, initiation of lithium therapy should not be undertaken outside of a hospital. After a maintenance dosage has been established, the blood level must be carefully monitored, at first every week and then once per month. The usual therapeutic blood level is 1.0 mEq/liter. The amphetamine-like substances have a unique use in children in the control of hyperactivity, usually considered to be associated with minimal brain dysfunction. Truly hyperkinetic children show a remarkable capacity for tolerating these drugs. It is suggested that the mechanism of action of the drugs is stimulation of cortical activity, which in turn serves to inhibit subcortical centers connected with motor functions.

With these general remarks as preamble, let us now present the classes of drugs and the conditions for which they are used in children. These indications should not be taken to mean that these drugs must be prescribed for these conditions. Rather, these indications are guidelines for the use of these drugs if it becomes necessary (see Table 1).

NEUROLEPTICS

These drugs are also referred to as major tranquilizers and antipsychotic drugs. The following four chemical groups of drugs are included in this class:

1. **Phenothiazines** are basically tricyclic compounds with various side chains which differentiate the compounds into three categories. *Aliphatic compounds*, such as chlorpromazine (Thorazine), typically have a sedating effect in addition to their antipsychotic action. The *piperidine group,* with thioridiazine

Table 1
Mind-Influencing Drugs with Pediatric Patients

Class of Drugs	Indication/Use

Neuroleptics
  Phenothiazines
  Butyrophenones
  Thioxanthenes
  Indolamines
	Psychosis, autism, severe anxiety, hyperactivity

Anxiolytics
  Benzodiazepines
  Meprobamate
	Restlessness, anxiety, insomnia

Hypnotics
  Chloral hydrate
  Flurazepam
	Insomnia, sleepwalking

Antidepressants
  Imipramine
  Desipramine
	Depression, enuresis

Stimulants
  Amphetamines
  Methylphenidate
	Hyperkinesis, narcolepsy

Anticonvulsants
  Diphenylhydantoin
  Mephenytoin
  Trimethadione
  Primidone
	Epilepsy (grand mal, petit mal, and psychomotor), aggressive behavior

Analgesics
  Aspirin
  Propoxyphene
	Pain

(Mellaril) as its prototype, has a minimal sedating effect. Among the *piperazine compounds* are trifluoperazine (Stelazine) and fluphenazine (Prolixin). Trifluoperazine is a stimulating compound, and fluphenazine, the prototype of the piperazine group, is known for its long duration of action and its availability for parenteral administration.

2. The **butyrophenones** include haloperidol (Haldol), a potent compound which produces therapeutic effects with very small doses. However, it also has a high potential for extrapyramidal side effects.

3. The **thioxanthenes** include thiothixene (Navane); this group of compounds has few side effects.

4. The **indolamines** are a newer group of neuroleptics. Molindone (Moban) has few side effects and therefore is of value as an alternative to other drugs. However, the indolamines are not as potent as are the other neuroleptics.

Basically, one must decide what specific symptom or behavior needs to be altered and then choose the agent accordingly. The choice of drug should also be based on consideration of potential side effects, some of which may be desirable and some of which may need to be avoided. For example, in an agitated psychotic patient, it may be best to use chlorpromazine (Thorazine), which would produce both sedative and antipsychotic effects. On the other hand, in a person with marked psychomotor retardation, the best choice of drug may well be trifluoperazine (Stelazine), a stimulant. Similarly, if hypotension occurs with administration of phenothiazines, use of a butyrophenone may be an appropriate alternative.

In general, it is desirable to become familiar with one agent from each of the categories—in regard to both the indications for its use and to anticipating and dealing with its side effects.

With the phenothiazines, atropine-like side effects such as dryness of the mouth, blurred vision, constipation, and tachycardia are common. Postural hypotension and extrapyramidal reactions (including dystonia) are also known to occur. Of particular significance is the infrequent occurrence of tardive dyskinesia and of skin and retinal pigmentation with the use of thioridazine (Mellaril), even in small doses.

If extrapyramidal reactions occur, they can be treated with

antiparkinsonism agents, which can usually be safely discontinued after several months. The routine use of antiparkinsonism agents in combination with neuroleptics is not justified. Interactions between antiparkinsonism agents and neuroleptics may in fact decrease the blood plasma levels of the neuroleptic and require that higher doses of the drug be given to obtain the same therapeutic effect. Whereas extrapyramidal reactions may be treated by antiparkinsonism agents such as benztropine mesylate (Cogentin) or diphenhydramine hydrochloride (Benadryl), the management of hypotensive states may be difficult. Atropine-like side effects such as dry mouth and constipation are usually only a nuisance, but they may sometimes be more serious. In view of this, "drug holidays" are frequently recommended—the patient is taken off the drug for a few days and resumes therapy on the minimum maintenance dosage.

ANXIOLYTIC (ANTIANXIETY) DRUGS

Many agents—bromides, paraldehyde, alcohol—have been used as anxiolytics in the past. More recently, barbiturates proved to be useful in the relief of anxiety, and they were used in the control of hypertension or to effect a general reduction in anxiety level. Other types of compounds, such as piperidinediones, including agents such as glutethimide (Doriden) and methyprylon (Noludar), were also developed. The most recent developments include benzodiazepine compounds such as chlordiazepoxide (Librium), diazepam (Valium), flurazepam (Dalmane), and oxazepam (Serax). The benzodiazepines are now very widely used (and misused).

Anxiolytic drugs are sedating when employed in higher dosages. Their mechanism of action seems to be based on their effects on the ascending reticular activating system; this accounts for their ability to induce unconsciousness. Their pharmacologic effects include relief of tension and anxiety, sedation, and, in higher doses, anesthesia. In contrast to the neuroleptics, they have anticonvulsant properties. Persistent use of these drugs may lead to habituation, and withdrawal symptoms may develop upon their discontinuance. Unlike the neuroleptics, these agents do not have striking autonomic or extrapyramidal side effects. If they are taken in toxic doses, however, cardiovascular or respiratory depression can occur.

The choice of agent is determined by the duration of action desired. The barbiturates' durations of action range from ultrashort, as in pentobarbital, to very long, as in phenobarbital. Chlordiazepoxide (Librium) is a long-acting agent; diazepam (Valium) is considered intermediate in its duration of action; flurazepam (Dalmane) is short-acting. Librium, therefore, is considered an agent of choice for relief of anxiety, whereas Valium, and particularly Dalmane, are used for nighttime sedation and sleep induction. When toxicity occurs, through either overdose or chronic use, the exaggeration of pharmacologic effects is noticeable and may include ataxia, nystagmus, and, eventually, respiratory depression, circulatory shock, and decreased tendon reflexes.

The clinical indications for these agents in children are limited to severe anxiety states which interfere with ordinary functioning and to emergency situations where an anticonvulsant is needed. The drug of choice for interrupting status epilepticus is diazepam (Valium), given intravenously.

HYPNOTICS

Hypnotics have limited use in children; they may be indicated for severe insomnia, especially when it occurs in reaction to extremely stressful events or crises. In younger children, diphenhydramine hydrochloride (Benadryl) can be used for its sedative side effects. This agent is primarily an antihistaminic, and, because of its safety, its sedative side effects can be employed as an adjunct for sleep induction. Benadryl is also considered extremely valuable in the treatment of extrapyramidal reactions resulting from the use of neuroleptics.

Chloral hydrate is another hypnotic of proven value. It may be given to young children in oral doses of 5 to 10 cc. As it is a safe hypnotic with minimal side effects, it is extremely useful and is often employed for minor procedures which require quietness, such as electroencephalogram recordings.

ANTIDEPRESSANTS

There are three types of chemical compounds in this class of drugs. *Tricyclic antidepressants* resemble the phenothiazines in their chemical structure. Commonly used tricyclics include amitriptyline (Elavil), doxepin (Sinequan), and imipramine (Tofranil). There is often a lag of about three weeks between the time treatment begins and the time therapeutic effects are obtained, and the patient or parents should be informed of this delay. The tricyclics also resemble the phenothiazines in that they may produce anticholinergic effects. Sedation is not uncommon with these drugs, especially with imipramine and related compounds. Other atropine-like side effects, such as dryness of the mouth, constipation, blurring of vision, tachycardia, and postural hypotension, also occur. In addition to causing confusion and disorientation, the drugs may exacerbate already existing psychotic-like behavior or symptoms, and it may be difficult to tell that this decline has been chemically induced by the drug and is not a primary manifestation of the illness. The specific antidote for this reaction is a 1-mg dose of physostigmine given parenterally and repeated after a brief interval if needed (DiGiacomo, 1975). Some of the tricyclics, such as imipramine, have been used in the treatment of enuresis in children (Poussain and Ditman, 1965).

Monoamine oxidase (MAO) inhibitors form another group of antidepressants. Tricyclics are preferred to MAO inhibitors because the latter's chemical interaction with tyramine-containing foods may lead to serious hypertensive crises. Also, special caution is required if MAO inhibitors are to be combined with tricyclic antidepressants. In view of these serious limitations, it is doubtful that any situation in children would require their use.

Amphetamines and amphetamine-like substances make up the third type of antidepressant. Their specific and sole use in children is the treatment of the hyperkinetic syndrome, rather than that of depression. Even in adults, the usefulness of these agents is limited because of their serious side effects: weight loss, agitation, hypertension, and the serious possibility of habituation.

In general, a diagnosis of depression in children is difficult to establish. Rather than presenting well-recognized symptoms as adults do, children may express depression through a variety of behaviors, including brooding, hyperactivity, delinquency, and self-destructive acts. This being the case, bipolar depressive illness (ie, manic-depressive illness) in children may go unrecognized, and treatment with lithium may therefore not be offered.

LITHIUM

Lithium is in a class by itself. Historically it was used in a variety of conditions, including rheumatoid arthritis. Its use in the treatment of manic-depressive illness is relatively recent. The use of lithium in the treatment of children has been erratic and empirical, and has yielded insignificant results (Campbell et al, 1973; Warneke, 1975; Feinstein and Wolpert, 1973; Brumback et al, 1975). When lithium is used, the maintenance dosage must be carefully established through blood level monitoring. Before lithium is given, it is necessary to ascertain that the renal and cardiovascular systems are both functioning well. Adverse side effects can include nausea, vomiting, tremor, anorexia, ataxia, stupor, convulsions, and coma.

ANTICONVULSANTS

These agents are not strictly mind-influencing drugs; their specific use is in raising the seizure threshold in convulsive disorders. The most commonly used anticonvulsants are diphenylhydantoin (Dilantin), methsuximide (Celontin), and mephobarbital (Mebaral). Claims of their efficacy in psychologic disorders are questionable; it may be that improvement in the seizure disorder brings concomitant change in the psychologic condition and in the behavior of the child.

ANALGESICS

These agents are traditionally used for relief of pain; their psychologic effects are minimal, except for those of the opiates. Since children rarely need analgesic agents stronger than acetylsalicylic acid, opiates are not to be employed except in conjunction with surgical procedures. The nonprescribed use of opiates will be discussed in the chapter devoted to drug abuse.

STIMULANTS

Originally, amphetamine-like compounds were used in the treatment of the hyperkinetic syndrome, construed to be secondary to minimal brain dysfunction. The hyperkinetic syndrome has been used at times as a wastebasket diagnosis, and overuse of stimulants to improve school performance in children has become notorious. In a recent study, a number of compounds—chlorpromazine, dextroamphetamines, hydroxyzine, and placebos—were used in the treatment of this syndrome in children

(Lipman, 1973). All active medication diminished hyperactivity; however, chlorpromazine and amphetamine were virtually equivalent to each other, and they produced significantly greater effects than did hydroxyzine. While amphetamines produced a significant reduction in hyperactivity, they also showed the greatest occurrence of side effects. Fish (1971) noted that only 10% of the children considered to be hyperactive responded to stimulants. This indicates that making a careful diagnostic evaluation and matching the medication to the individual (rather than applying a blanket policy of using only one group of drugs for the hyperkinetic syndrome) may be necessary.

ABUSE OF MIND-INFLUENCING DRUGS

From our own experience in an outreach facility, we know that many drugs are abused. Children 9 and 10 years of age are already using mind-influencing drugs, both prescribed and nonprescribed. Much of the drug use may not be known by the family doctor; this is obviously a hazard when any new drugs are added by prescription. Table 2 identifies drugs, prescribed and nonprescribed, frequently used by children. The table makes it

Table 2
Mind-Influencing Drugs Used by Children

Nature of Drug	Prescribed Drugs Used	Nonprescribed Drugs Used
Disinhibitor	Anxiolytics	Alcohol
Hypnotic	Antihistamines, chloral hydrate	Barbiturates, methaqualone
Stimulant	Amphetamines, methylphenidate	Amphetamines, cocaine
Neuroleptic	Phenothiazines, butyrophenones	Phencyclidine
Hallucinogen	None	LSD, hashish, marijuana, peyote, mescaline
Anticonvulsant	Diphenylhydantoin, barbiturates	None
Analgesic	Aspirin	Propoxyphene, heroin, codeine

readily apparent that the classes of nonprescribed, abused drugs are very similar to those of prescribed drugs.

Our knowledge of the use of mind-influencing drugs by youths comes mostly from listening to the children themselves. At our outreach facility, systematic efforts are made to help young people find other ways to deal with life's issues. A primary rule, however, is that a child who has taken drugs should not be helped with another drug if that is at all possible. For instance, bad trips from hallucinogens are, in most instances, best handled by psychologic measures—by talking the person down. This kind of help can be most effectively provided by someone who is not himself uncomfortable about illegal drugs, as he will not transmit anxiety to the child in distress.

Children today have available to them, without prescription, all the drugs we have discussed. They are available at schools and in friends' homes as well as on the streets. Even the child who is as young as nine is already making his own choices about mind-influencing drugs. One of our tasks as physicians is to develop in him not only an awareness of what he is choosing but also why he is choosing as he does. We need patience in listening to why he is taking drugs; tactics of coercion are not very successful. The most successful approach might be to help him find other ways to accomplish the purpose for which he is taking drugs.

REFERENCES

Blackwell, B. and Ayd, F.: Rational drug use in psychotherapy. *Audio Digest Fdn.* 4(20), Part II, October 27, 1975.

Brumback, R.A., Weinberg, W.A., and Herjanic, B.L.: Epileptiform activity in electroencephalogram induced by lithium carbonate. *Pediatrics* 56:831–834, 1975.

Campbell, M. et al: Drug studies. In *Annual Progress in Child Psychology and Child Development,* edited by Stella Chess and Alexander Thomas. New York: Brunner/Mazel, Inc., 1973.

DiGiacomo, J.N.: Treatment of psychoses. *Audio Digest Fdn.* 4(15), Side A, 23:40, and Side B, August 11, 1975.

Feinstein, S.C. and Wolpert, E.A.: Juvenile manic-depressive illness: clinical and therapeutic considerations. *J Am Acad Child Psych.* 12:123–136, 1973.

Fish, B.: One-child, one-drug myth of stimulants in hyperkinesis. *Arch Gen Psychiatr.* 25:193–203, 1971.

Lipman, R.M.: NIMH-PRB support of research in minimal brain dysfunction and other disorders of childhood. *Psychopharm Bull NIMH.* 1973, pp. 1–32.

McAndrew, J.B., Quentin, C., and Treffert, D.A.: Effects of prolonged phenothiazine intake on psychotic and other hospitalized children. *J Autism & Child Schizophrenia* 2:75–91, 1972.

Poussain, A.F. and Ditman, K.S.: A controlled study of imipramine (Tofranil) in the treatment of childhood enuresis. *J Pediatr.* 67:283–290, August, 1965.

Sehdev, H.: Do penguins really have turned-out feet, Daddy? (Treatment of a 4½-year-old boy via the parents). *Menninger Perspective* Winter, 1973.

Warneke, L.: A case of manic-depressive illness in childhood. *Can Psych Assoc J.* 20:195–200, 1975.

12 Mind-Influencing Drugs and Adolescents

Harvey A. Horowitz, M.D.

INTRODUCTION

The appropriate use of psychotropic medications in adult psychiatry is dependent on careful clinical diagnosis for which there are no laboratory tests nor radiologic studies. Differential diagnosis and chemotherapy in adolescent psychiatry is even more tenuous, due to the fact that adolescent psychopathology is rarely expressed in the typical adult syndromes and is more frequently expressed in the camouflage of behavior. These behaviors may be seen in recognizable symptom constellations which seem to be related to the major psychopathologic syndromes of adulthood, and which may be, in certain identifiable cases, amenable to specific chemotherapeutic interventions.

The goal of this chapter is not to exhaustively or completely review the vast literature in adolescent psychopharmacology, but rather to focus on several, common adolescent symptom constellations, and to then discuss the uses of a chemotherapeutic intervention as an integral part of the treatment plan. Where the uses of classes of mind-altering drugs in adolescent patients do not differ from those in adults, we refer the reader to the appropriate sections of this book.

THE MASKS OF ADOLESCENT PSYCHOPATHOLOGY

The myth of normative adolescent turmoil—that adolescence is a period of predictable and expectable developmental chaos which will be survived without sequelae—has been challenged and refuted by several authors in recent years (Weiner and Del Gaudio, 1976; King and Pittman, 1970; Masterson, 1967, 1968; Offer and Offer, 1971). "The stage they're going through" has often concealed extremes of maladaptive, self-destructive behavior. Diagnoses such as *adolescent adjustment reaction* and *situational stress disorder* are inaccurately and excessively used and mask the confusion around and the significance of adolescent psychopathology. Disturbed adolescents themselves find some security and comfort in the camouflage of various socially acceptable teenage roles, roles which hide their struggle and their pain. Several of these typical adolescent "costumes" are described below, that they might be recognized and, perhaps, treated.

Acting–Out and Rebelliousness

The acting-out, rebellious boy is an early- to mid-adolescent (aged 13 to 17) who expresses himself and his feelings of anger, tension, and depression through his behavior. Although he was always an active, energetic, and restless child, puberty brought drastic, catastrophic changes. Groping to master these changes in his body, his emotions, and his environment, and fearing overdependence on his family, he becomes tense, unable to concentrate, and charged with energy he is unable to control. Difficulties at school, where he fails and gets into disciplinary trouble, and at home, where he is irritable, aggressive, and negative, all lead to increased tension, a sense of failure, loss of self-esteem, and feelings of hopelessness. The tension mounts; vague feelings are inexpressible and leave only a sense of confusion, isolation, and unrest which must be acted on. Fighting, running away, truancy, stealing, and using drugs are all acts of rebellion and self-definition, and provide relief of tension through what seems to be the only available outlets.

The acting-out adolescent girl, once a friendly, energetic, and happy child, is now a frightened, anxious, and lonely teenager looking for another person, a gang, or an experience to ease her fears, her loneliness, and her emptiness. Unable to be alone with herself and unable to communicate her needs to her parents, from whom she drifts in an effort to be independent, she is left alone with unmanageable panic and despair. To combat her distress, she moves out into her world, becomes promiscuous, and enters into a series of sexual experiences which relieve her of tension and give her a sense of self-worth and attachment. She gets into drugs; she fails in school; she attacks her family; and ultimately, she hates herself. Self-loathing brings more despair, and the cycle continues.

Boredom and Withdrawal

The bored, withdrawn teenager is tired, dissatisfied with everything (particularly himself), negative, angry, and unhappy. He is passive—he can't find anything that interests him, and he can't find anything to do. He spends most of his time watching television, and then he slips away, isolated, to his room. Once a good student, he now is an "underachiever" and is uncooperative and irritable. He wants only relief from the painful, agitating boredom. Relief comes from detachment and withdrawal—either physically, into his room; emotionally, into his headphones; or chemically, into drugs.

Pseudomaturity and Pseudosophistication

The pseudomature, socially precocious teenager is in flight: she wants to escape adolescence as quickly as her womanly body or her bright mind will carry her. Frightened by the struggle for acceptance, a place in her peer world, and mastery over her feelings of inadequacy, she flees, emotionally unprepared, into what she perceives to be the adult world. Lonely, isolated, lost, and bewildered, she imitates those around her whom she idealizes.

She throws herself into the arts, music, fashion, and personal relationships, not solely out of genuine curiosity but more out of desperation and despair. She functions well superficially with adults but can't seem to connect with those her own age, finding them uninteresting, boring, and childish. In fact, she doesn't know how to enter into or enjoy what is appropriate to her age, nor can she face her sense of defectiveness and failure. Her imitation of the adult world does not work well for her and leaves her only with vague feelings of unrest and dissatisfaction. In her search for warmth, affection, and a sense of belonging, she may get into drugs, become promiscuous, or run away.

RECOGNITION OF DISTURBANCES OF AFFECT IN ADOLESCENTS

Although clinically diverse, the four "typical" adolescent patients described above share a single psychopathologic entity: a severe disturbance of mood. The behavioral expression of mood, and hence the clinical presentation of dysphoric affect in adolescence, is determined by the stage of psychosocial and personality development of the adolescent. The diversity of clinical manifestations of adolescent disturbances of mood results from the varying relationships of mood to the available age-specific repertoire of cognitive and affective behaviors. These behaviors are an effort, albeit maladaptive, to modulate and control the intense mood swings which are frequently the adolescent's inner experience. Thus, adolescent patients, like children, do not present with typical, adult depressive syndromes or with chief complaints of sadness, inexplicable feelings of pessimism, or feeling "blue." Rather, they exhibit disturbances of behavior, the behavioral equivalents of mood. The clinician must, therefore, recognize and demonstrate the relationship between the psychopathologic substrate of depression—that is, low self-esteem—and the behavioral expression of that mood—that is, "acting-out" behaviors such as drug abuse and delinquency.

Disturbed behavior in adolescence as an expression of disturbed affect (ie, affective equivalents) is clinically recognizable as distinct symptom clusters or syndromes. Descriptions of three such syndromes follow (Feinstein and Wolpert, 1973; Conners, 1974; Toolan, 1974; Glaser, 1967; Chwast, 1974; Klein and Davis, 1969).

The Hyperactive Dysphoric Behavior Syndrome

This syndrome represents the behavioral expression of manic disorders and is characterized by behaviors which reflect intense underlying mood swings and social, sexual, and motor impulsivity and hyperactivity. Symptomatic behaviors which appear in this syndrome include: rebelliousness, hyperaggressiveness, violence; inability to concentrate; superficial confidence and optimism; drug abuse; promiscuity; delinquency; and truancy and running away.

The Hypoactive, Withdrawn Behavior Syndrome

This syndrome represents the behavioral expression of depressive disorders and is characterized by behavior which reflects underlying depression and anxiety, and psychomotor retardation. Symptomatic behaviors include: depressed mood; apathy; negativism; passivity; dependency; irritability and restlessness; social, scholastic, and sexual withdrawal and failure; avoidance and anxiety; wanderlust, philosophizing, and religiosity; sleep and eating disturbances; and drug abuse.

The Hysteroid Dysphoric Behavior Syndrome

The hysteroid dysphoric syndrome has both manic and depressive equivalents and is characterized by behavior which both reflects and defends against underlying mood swings, particularly, intense depression resulting from a heightened sensitivity to disapproval, rejection, and loss. It is more commonly seen in females. Symptomatic behaviors of this syndrome include: emotional lability; anger and aggressiveness; egocentricity, histrionics, manipulativeness; inability to be alone; possessiveness, dependency; low frustration tolerance; overeating, oversleeping; an activity and achievement orientation; drug abuse; promiscuity; and somatization and hypochrondriasis.

CHEMOTHERAPY OF THE DISTURBED ADOLESCENT

In discussing the chemotherapy of the disturbed adolescent, one must consider the psychologic and developmental consequences of massive emotional insult to the immature, incompletely formed adolescent personality. Obviously, chemotherapy alone does not consititute adequate treatment for the adolescent patients we have described. The therapeutic plan for the disturbed adolescent must take into consideration the conflicts and developmental tasks of the individual, his relationships with his peers, and his place in his family. Thus, comprehensive treatment of the adolescent patient must include individual, group, and, particularly, family psychotherapy in addition to the chemotherapy to be described.

The use of chemotherapy with adolescent patients is a difficult enterprise with significant risks and should be initiated only by the clinician experienced with this patient group. General practitioners and general psychiatrists should seek consultation prior to undertaking such treatment.

Treatment of the Hyperactive Dysphoric Behavior Syndrome

Clinical experience with hyperactive dysphoric adolescents indicates that lithium is of considerable value in controlling the lability and explosiveness of affect and the social, sexual, and motor hyperactivity of the behavior of these patients. As a result of the effectiveness of lithium in stabilizing mood and reducing affective excitability, there is a consistent and predictable reduction in chronic self-destructive behaviors. Promiscuity, drug abuse, delinquency, running away—behaviors which previously were impulsive and the result of an inner pressure to act without reflection—diminish significantly. Patients describe the subjective changes as a reduced pressure to act, as a sense of having more time to reflect, or as a sense of operating at a slower internal speed. Issues and concerns which formerly brought inappropriate, excessively hostile reactions tend to be more available to discussion. Limits, authority, and frustration tend to be better tolerated. Control of feelings and behavior, the lack of which formerly brought shame which was frequently hidden behind anger, now becomes an attainable skill. Perhaps the most significant therapeutic effect of lithium in these cases is the patient's increased ability to reflect upon his thoughts and feelings, which allows him to participate and become more involved in his psychotherapy.

Our clinical experience with lithium in hyperactive, impulsive, dysphoric adolescents is supported by the reports of several investigators who describe, in controlled studies, the effectiveness of lithium in reducing aggressive affect in adult prisoners (Sheard, 1971, 1975; Tupin et al, 1973); in diminishing aggressive, explosive affects and hyperactivity in severely disturbed children (Campbell et al, 1972) and adolescents (Annell, 1969); and in stabilizing the mood swings and impulsivity seen in character disorders in adolescents (Rifkin et al, 1972).

The efficacy of lithium treatment is dependent upon adequate blood levels, which fall in the range of 1.0 to 1.5 mEq/1liter, and which can be achieved with dosages of 1200 to 1500 mg per day. Our method of lithium treatment is to prescribe dosages which increase by 300 mg (one tablet) per day and to make serum determinations weekly until dosage and serum concentration are stabilized. Therapeutic blood levels of lithium can be reached in 5 to 10 days, and a therapeutic response to treatment should be seen in 10 to 14 days. Because lithium is a potentially toxic drug, serum determinations must be made at regular intervals, scheduled according to the patient's reliability in taking the medication and the nature of the psychotherapeutic relationship. However, we have found adolescents to be as tolerant of lithium as adults are and to show no greater frequency or severity of side effects.

Duration of treatment for lithium-responsive hyperactive dysphoric adolescents should be anologous, in our view, to lithium prophylaxis in manic-depressive disease in adults. At this writing, lithium-responsive adolescent patients are kept on their medication and followed up weekly with clinical evaluations and serum concentration determinations.

The tricyclic antidepressants are effective in treating hyperactive dysphoric adolescents who are unresponsive to lithium. Imipramine, which has been shown to be useful in the treatment of hyperactive and aggressive behavior in children (Rappaport, 1965), is also efficacious in stabilizing mood and in reducing hyperactivity and impulsivity in hyperactive dysphoric adolescents. The use of tricyclics in adolescents parallels that in adults, and one must ensure an adequate therapeutic trial with adequate dosages (200 to 300 mg per day) over a sufficient amount of time (three to four weeks).

Treatment of the Hypoactive, Withdrawn Behavior Syndrome

Clinical experience with hypoactive dysphoric adolescents indicates that the drug treatment of first choice is the tricyclic antidepressant group of drugs, particularly imipramine or amitriptyline. Imipramine is useful in controlling depression and in reversing the behavioral depressive equivalents: apathy, withdrawal, low energy, and low activity. Withdrawn adolescents treated with imipramine are less negative, more optimistic and assertive, more interested and active in school and in their social world, and less likely to use other chemical mood stabilizers, such as alcohol or marijuana. As are adults, responsive adolescents are more receptive to psychotherapy as negativism and depression diminish. Our experience with imipramine in the treatment of the withdrawn, apathetic adolescent coincides with that reported by Frommer (1968) in England, who has successfully treated a group of depressed, withdrawn, enuretic children with amitriptyline.

In those patients in whom the phobic anxiety component of the syndrome predominates and in whom marked avoidance of social and scholastic situations is noted, monoamine oxidase (MAO) inhibitors, such as phenelzine, are also quite useful. Frommer has reported success with the MAO inhibitors in treating this disorder, which she calls a depressive phobic anxiety state.

Treatment of the Hysteroid Dysphoric Behavior Syndrome

Our own clinical experience and the experience of others (Klein and Davis, 1969) with mood-dominated, dramatic, demanding, and manipulative hysteroid dysphoric adolescents has indicated that the MAO inhibitors are the drug treatment of choice. Adequate treatment provides these patients with a stability of affect which enables them to tolerate frustration and limits and to deal more effectively with the anger and depression which results from loss and rejection. The use of MAO inhibitors in adolescents presents special problems because of dietary precautions and the nature of the adolescent psychopathology. For this reason, treatment should be initiated either during hospitalization or within a substantial, durable, and trusting therapeutic relationship. The use of MAO inhibitors in adolescent patients is not otherwise different from that in adults.

CHEMOTHERAPY OF THE PSYCHOTIC ADOLESCENT

Drug treatment of the psychotic adolescent does not substantially differ from that of the psychotic adult, and treatment decisions for both age groups depend on differential diagnosis. The clinician faced with a psychotic adolescent who can benefit from chemotherapy needs to be aware of the increased likelihood of a bizarre, regressive presentation in this age group—again, the consequence of the effects of overwhelming psychosocial stress on an immature and vulnerable ego. Because a bizarre, psychotic clinical picture in an adolescent patient is frequently misdiagnosed as schizophrenia (Carpenter et al, 1973), it must be emphasized that primary affective disorders (manic-depressive disease) do occur in adolescence, often with "atypical," bizarre, psychotic presentations (Horowitz, 1976). A clinical indication helpful in the differential diagnosis, and therefore in determining specific drug treatment, is the affective quality of the patient. The presence of a prominent disturbance of affect, with lability, elation, hostility and depression, is strong presumptive evidence of manic-depressive disease, and mood-stabilizing drugs are indicated. Those psychotic adolescents presenting with blunted affect and a formal thought disorder (as opposed to an affective disorder) are presumptively diagnosed as schizophrenic, and neuroleptics are indicated. (The specifics of the usage of mood-stabilizing and antipsychotic drugs are presented in the chapters on these drugs.)

Chemotherapy of Drug-Induced Psychotic Reactions

Drug-induced psychotic reactions, in which adverse effects persist beyond the 48-hour pharmacologic life of the drug itself, are not uncommon among adolescents and are precipitated by illicit mind-altering substances such as lysergic acid diethylamide (LSD), amphetamines, and marijuana. The drug is thought to release an underlying predisposition or vulnerability to psychosis. The clinical picture of the drug-induced psychotic reaction may resemble either manic-depressive disease or schizophrenia, and drug treatment is based on the psychiatric evaluation (Horowitz, 1975).

Use of Sedatives and Minor Tranquilizers in Adolescence

Because of their enormous potential for abuse and for inducing dependence and addiction, minor tranquilizers such as diazepam, and sedatives such as the barbiturates, should rarely, if ever, be used with adolescents. Sleep disturbances and anxiety in adolescent patients respond equally well to tricyclic antidepressants (amitriptyline) and related drugs given in therapeutic dosages at bedtime. When anxiety in the teenager is chronic, overwhelming, and diffuse, anxiolytic drugs may be indicated while intensive psychotherapy is undertaken.

REFERENCES

Annell, A.: Lithium in the treatment of children and adolescents. *Acta Psychiatr Scand.* 207(Suppl):19–30, 1969.

Campbell, M. et al: Lithium and chlorpromazine: a controlled crossover study of hyperactive, severely disturbed young children. *J Autism & Child Schizophrenia* 2:234–263, 1972.

Carpenter, W.T., Strauss, J.S., and Muleh, S.: Are there pathognomonic symptoms in schizophrenia? *Arch Gen Psychiatr.* 28:747–752, 1973.

Chwast, J.: Delinquency and criminal behavior as depressive equivalents in adolescents. In *Masked Depression,* edited by S. Lesse, pp. 219–235. New York: Jason Aronson, Inc., 1974.

Conners, C.K.: Classification and Treatment of Childhood Depression and Depressive Equivalents. Paper presented at International Symposium on Depression, New Orleans, November 13–15, 1974.

Feinstein, S.G. and Wolpert, E.A.: Juvenile manic-depressive illness. *J Am Acad Child Psychiatr.* 12:123–136, 1973.

Frommer, E.A.: Depressive illness in childhood. *Br J Psychiatr.* 2:117–136, 1968.

Glaser, K.: Masked depression in children and adolescents. *Am J Psychother.* 21:565–574, 1967.

Horowitz, H.A.: The use of lithium in the treatment of the drug-induced psychotic reaction. *Dis Nerv System* 36:159–163, 1975.

Horowitz, H.A.: Lithium and the treatment of adolescent manic-depressive illness. *Dis Nerv System,* in press.

King, L.F. and Pittman, G.D.: A six-year follow-up study of 65 adolescent patients: natural history of affective disorders in adolescence. *Arch Gen Psychiatr.* 22:230–236, 1970.

Klein, D.F. and Davis, J.W.: *Diagnosis and Drug Treatment in Psychiatric Disorders.* Baltimore: The Williams & Wilkins Co., 1969.

Masterson, J.F.: The symptomatic adolescent five years later. He didn't grow out of it. *Am J Psychiatr.* 123:1338–1345, 1967.

Masterson, J.F.: The psychiatric significance of adolescent turmoil. *Am J Psychiatr.* 124:1549–1554, 1968.

Offer, D. and Offer, J.L.: Four issues in the developmental psychology of adolescents. In *Modern Perspectives in Adolescent Psychiatry,* edited by J.G. Howells. New York: Brunner/Mazel, Inc., 1971.

Rappaport, J.: Childhood behavior and learning problems treated with imipramine. *Int J Neuropsychiatr.* 1:635–642, 1965.

Rifkin, A. et al: Lithium carbonate in emotionally unstable character disorder. *Arch Gen Psychiatr.* 27:519–523, 1972.

Sheard, M.H.: Effect of lithium on human aggression. *Nature* 230:113–114, 1971.

Sheard, M.H.: Lithium in the treatment of aggression. *J Nerv & Ment Dis.* 16:108–118, 1975.

Toolan, J.M.: Masked depression in children and adolescents. In *Masked Depression,* edited by S. Lesse, pp. 141–164. New York: Jason Aronson, Inc., 1974.

Tupin, J.P., Smith, D.B., Classon, T.L. et al: Long-term use of lithium in aggressive prisoners. *Compr Psychiatr.* 14:311–317, 1973.

Weiner, I.B. and Del Gaudio, A.C.: Psychopathology in adolescence. An epidemiological study. *Arch Gen Psychiatr.* 33:187–193, 1976.

13 Interaction of Mind-Influencing Drugs with Other Prescribed and Nonprescribed Agents

Henry H. Swain, M.D.

INTRODUCTION

A single drug, administered to a large group of individuals, will produce a wide spectrum of responses which will differ both quantitatively and qualitatively from person to person. If these individuals are also receiving a second drug simultaneously, the variety of responses is increased and the pharmacologic complexity compounded. Of course, most patients are receiving more than one drug at a given time, so the potential for drug-drug interactions is usually present. Furthermore, it has become apparent that substances other than prescribed medications (eg, alcohol, over-the-counter drugs, and even certain foods) can modify pharmacologic effects of drugs.

The subject of drug interactions has attracted a marked increase in interest recently, but it is still difficult to maintain a sense of perspective in dealing with this topic. There is a bewildering array of data available, but much of it is anecdotal and fragmentary. The likelihood of a particular reaction and the seriousness of that reaction if it should occur should each be defined. Some drugs (eg, oral anticoagulants, digitalis, morphine) are dosage-sensitive, while other drugs (eg, penicillin, aspirin, diazepam) are not. An interaction which alters the effectiveness of one of the former drugs would be expected to have clinically significant consequences, while alterations in the effectiveness of one of the latter would be much less likely to have serious results.

The pharmacologic basis for drug interactions is apparent in some cases and quite unknown in others. A knowledge of the underlying mechanism is useful not only as a device for remembering that the interaction occurs but also for predicting what related drugs can be expected to act similarly.

In the presentation which follows, each of several classes of mind-influencing drugs will be considered from the points of view of (1) pharmacologic mechanisms which lead to drug interactions, (2) the types of interactions which are known to occur, and (3) the seriousness of the interactions.

INTERACTIONS WITH MAO INHIBITORS

Monoamine oxidase (MAO) inhibitors interact with a variety of other drugs, sometimes with disastrous consequences. Some of the interactions can be explained directly on the basis of MAO inhibition, while others suggest that other types of drug-metabolizing enzymes are inhibited as well. The consequences of inhibiting MAO can be seen by comparing the effects of an MAO inhibitor such as phenelzine (Nardil) on the responses to four different sympathomimetic agents: norepinephrine, phenylephrine, amphetamine, and tyramine.

All of the clinically available MAO inhibitors act to irreversibly depress the activity of this mitochondrial enzyme. The cells in which this action is important are: (1) those of the liver and gastrointestinal tract, in which orally ingested phenylephrine or tyramine are normally deaminated; and (2) the nerve endings of the sympathetic nervous system, in which the enzyme normally (a) inactivates norepinephrine (unless it is protected in storage granules) and (b) destroys any tyramine which reaches the nerve ending.

With exogenously administered norepinephrine (or epinephrine, or isoproterenol), there is little change in the magnitude of the blood pressure response as a consequence of pretreatment with an MAO inhibitor. By the oral route, these catecholamines are not absorbed to any significant extent; therefore, it makes no real difference whether MAO in the intestine and liver is active or not—no drug reaches these sites to be destroyed. Parenterally administered norepinephrine and other catecholamines are carried by the bloodstream directly to the adrenergic receptors of tissues and act without the intervention of sympathetic nerve endings. Therefore, inhibition of intraneuronal MAO has no effect upon the response to these agents. It is possible that chronic administration of an MAO inhibitor, which decreases norepinephrine release from adrenergic nerve endings, could lead to a "denervation supersensitivity" of the receptors, with a slight increase in the response to intravenous norepinephrine, but the magnitude of this effect would never be great and the consequences would be trivial. Thus, the responses of the body to orally or parenterally administered norepinephrine, epinephrine, and isoproterenol are not modified by the inhibition of MAO.

Phenylephrine (Neo-Synephrine) given by the oral route is potentiated by MAO inhibition, but parenteral phenylephrine is not. Phenylephrine is a direct-acting sympathomimetic, which means that it acts upon the adrenergic receptors rather than through the adrenergic nerve endings. When the drug is given parenterally, the bloodstream carries it to the receptors, where it exerts its characteristic effects, whether or not intraneuronal MAO is inhibited. Unlike the catecholamines, however, phenylephrine is absorbed from the gastrointestinal tract following oral administration; like the catecholamines, it is deaminated by MAO. Under normal circumstances, a significant portion of an oral dose of the drug is destroyed by intestinal and hepatic MAO before it reaches the main circulation. After enzyme inhibition, more of the oral dose reaches the tissue receptors, and the pressor effect of the drug is increased significantly. Since many nonprescription cold remedies contain phenylephrine, they represent a hazard to patients taking MAO inhibitors. It is not clear whether there is danger in topical applications of phenylephrine as a nasal decongestant in a patient taking an MAO inhibitor.

Amphetamine's pressor effect is potentiated by MAO inhibition not because of action upon amphetamine, but because of action upon intraneuronal norepinephrine. Amphetamine is not a substrate for MAO. The drug is well absorbed when given by mouth, and it passes through the liver without being destroyed, whether MAO is active or inhibited. Amphetamine is an indirect-acting sympathomimetic agent: it does not act directly upon the adrenergic receptors but instead causes the release of norepinephrine from adrenergic nerve endings; the released norepinephrine activates the receptors. The enzyme MAO exerts two related effects upon the nerve endings: (1) it destroys any norepinephrine which is free in the neuronal cytoplasm and not bound to storage granules; and (2) it destroys part of the norepinephrine which is released from storage granules (by indirect-acting agents like amphetamine) before it can leave the neuron and pass to the receptors. Therefore, inhibition of MAO permits accumulation of norepinephrine in the neuronal cytoplasm (some have referred to this as "supercharging" the neuron with norepinephrine) and also permits the escape from the neuron of a greater proportion of the norepinephrine released from the storage granules. By either or both of these mechanisms, MAO inhibition causes an enhanced blood pressure response to amphetamine and related drugs (including ephedrine). The sudden rise in blood pressure can lead to a cerebrovascular accident and death.

Tyramine, like amphetamine, is an indirect-acting sympathomimetic amine which releases norepinephrine from adrenergic nerve endings. Tyramine differs from amphetamine in that it is a substrate which is deaminated readily by MAO. Tyramine is not used as a drug but is a component of a number of foods, including sauerkraut, wines, beers, and particularly cheeses. Thus, the oral route is the natural one by which tyramine enters the body. The enzyme MAO normally provides a double barrier against the norepinephrine-releasing effects of ingested tyramine. In the gastrointestinal tract and in the liver, the enzyme deaminates the substance as rapidly as it is absorbed, and no significant amount appears in the general circulation. Even if tyramine reaches the adrenergic neurons, its releasing effects are minimized by its rapid inactivation by intraneuronal MAO. When the enzyme is inhibited by drugs, however, there is a different chain of events: (1) tyramine in the diet is absorbed into the general circulation; (2) it is free to act intraneuronally to release norepinephrine; (3) the neurons are "supercharged" with cytoplasmic as well as granular-bound norepinephrine; and (4) norepinephrine released by tyramine's action is free to leave the neurons and reach the adrenergic receptors. Thus, with MAO inhibition there is an enormous enhancement of the response to dietary tyramine, and this often has disastrous consequences.

In summary, MAO inhibition enhances the blood pressure raising effects of these substances as follows: with norepinephrine, any slight enhancement is the result of receptor supersensitivity; with phenylephrine given orally, enhancement is the result of increased absorption of the drug into the general circulation; with amphetamine, the action of the inhibitor on intraneuronal MAO considerably increases the pressor response; with tyramine-containing foods, which normally cause no pressor response at all, the combined inhibition of hepatic and neuronal enzymes leads to hypertensive episodes (which have proven fatal in at least 15 cases). These interactions are illustrated in Figure 1.

The inhibitors of MAO affect other enzyme functions as well, including those responsible for the metabolism of other drugs. In this manner, MAO inhibitors increase and prolong the responses to barbiturates, alcohol, potent analgesics, and antiparkinsonism agents. Meperidine is a drug which normally is metabolized rapidly in the body and which shows quite clearly the consequences of delayed inactivation. Two different clinical pictures have been noted in patients who have received meperidine after inhibition of MAO: narcotic-type respiratory depression is the prominent sign in one group of patients; the other group manifests the atropine-like effects of excitation, delirium, hyperpyrexia, and convulsions. It is interesting to note that these effects have not been reported when morphine has been given to patients on MAO inhibitors. Perhaps the fact that morphine is normally metabolized more slowly than meperidine could explain this difference.

INTERACTIONS WITH TRICYCLIC ANTIDEPRESSANTS

Most of the interactions between the tricyclic antidepressants and other drugs are related to the ability of the former to produce sedation, cholinergic blockade, and interference with the uptake mechanism of the adrenergic neuron. The sedative effects appear to be additive to those of a number of central nervous system depressants. The tricyclic antidepressants also show summation with other drugs (certain antihistamines,

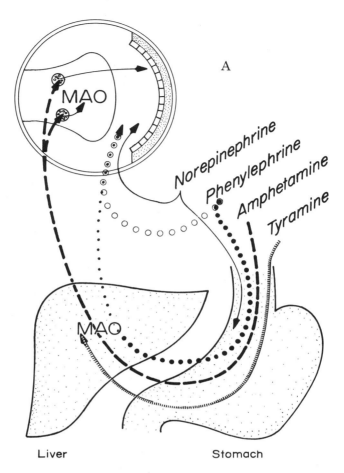

A

NORMAL

Figure 1. Diagrammatic representation of the effects of MAO inhibition on sympathomimetic agents. **A.** The effects in a normal individual (no inhibition of MAO). Norepinephrine (slender line) is not absorbed from the stomach or intestine when given parenterally (upper slender line), but passes via the bloodstream to the **adrenergic receptors** (represented symbolically at the right side of the round microscopic field). Phenylephrine can be given either orally (solid circles) or parenterally (open circles). A portion of an orally administered dose of phenylephrine is destroyed by MAO in the liver (shown by smaller solid circles beyond the liver). Like norepiniphrine, phenylephrine acts directly on the adrenergic receptors. Amphetamine (heavy, dashed line) is not destroyed by MAO. When given by mouth, it is carried by the blood to the adrenergic nerve endings (shown at the left of the microscopic field), where it releases norepinephrine from storage granules. A portion of the amphetamine-released norepinephrine is destroyed intraneuronally by MAO, and a portion passes out of the neuron to activate adrenergic receptors. Tyramine (shaded line), when given by mouth, is totally destroyed by mucosal and hepatic MAO before it reaches the general circulation, and therefore it exerts no systemic effects.

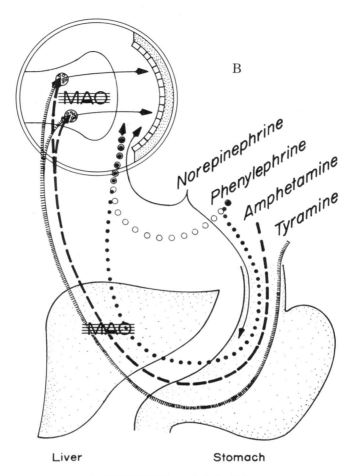

B

Norepinephrine

Phenylephrine

Amphetamine

Tyramine

Liver   Stomach

AFTER MAOI

B. The corresponding effects after inhibition of MAO. Extracellular norepinephrine is not attached by MAO; therefore, parenterally administered norepinephrine is not poteniated by MAO inhibition. Parenteral phenylephrine is unchanged in its actions by the inhibition of MAO, but oral phenylephrine is somewhat potentiated because the drug is no longer partially destroyed in its passage
through the liver. While amphetamine is not a substrate for MAO, the norepineph-
hrine which it releases intraneuronally is susceptible to enzymatic destruction;
thus, after MAO inhibition, a greater portion of the amphetamine-released
norepinephrine is free to leave the neuron and activate adrenergic receptors.
Tyramine's actions are potentiated markedly by MAO inhibition through
several different mechanisms: (1) ingested tyramine is no longer destroyed in
the gut and liver and therefore reaches the general circulation; (2) it releases
norepinephrine from adrenergic nerve endings; (3) the released norepinephrine is
free of MAO destruction and therefore can pass from the nerve ending to the
adrenergic receptors; and (4) it is possible that the inhibition of neuronal MAO
permits the cytoplasmic accumulation of extra amounts of norepinephrine in the
nerve ending.

313

antiparkinsonism drugs, meperidine, and a variety of over-the-counter preparations) which have atropine-like side effects.

The uptake mechanism in the adrenergic neuron is the most important factor in terminating the action of norepinephrine which has been released by sympathetic nerve stimulation. This energy-dependent pump returns norepinephrine molecules into the neuron, where they are once again stored in granules. The pump is also necessary for amphetamine to release norepinephrine and for the initiation of the action of guanethidine (Ismelin) as an antihypertensive agent. The pump is blocked by cocaine and by the tricyclic antidepressants. The consequences of this blockade include potentiation of the pressor effects of epinephrine and norepinephrine, blockade of the pressor effects of amphetamine, and interference with the antihypertensive effects of guanethidine.

The combination of a tricyclic antidepressant with an MAO inhibitor can lead to an interaction characterized by atropine-like signs, including hyperpyrexia, convulsions, and coma. There is some disagreement as to whether this interaction occurs only when one or both drugs have been given in excessive doses, or whether it may also be encountered with "therapeutic" doses of each. Since the effects of MAO inhibition persist for a number of days after the drug has been discontinued, most clinicians would agree that a period of two weeks should elapse between the discontinuation of an MAO inhibitor and the initiation of a tricyclic.

INTERACTIONS WITH PHENOTHIAZINES

Substituted phenothiazines potentiate the actions of a variety of central nervous system depressant drugs. They share with the tricyclic antidepressants the ability to interfere with the amine uptake pump in the adrenergic neurons; they lower the threshold to seizures, both drug-induced and epileptic; and they have quinidine-like properties.

Their potentiating effect on central nervous system depressant drugs was first noticed in the ability of promethazine (an antihistaminic which lacks antipsychotic properties) to prolong the sleeping time of barbiturate-treated mice. Meperidine's respiratory depressant effects are both intensified and prolonged by the simultaneous injection of a phenothiazine, and this interaction has been induced in attempts to increase the efficacy of meperidine as an analgesic agent. The potentiation of morphine by phenothiazines is much less marked than that of meperidine.

Blockade of the amine pump alters the body's response to amphetamine. Phenothiazines have been used in treating amphetamine overdosage, and they interfere with the weight-reducing effects of amphetamines. It would be expected that phenothiazines would block the antihypertensive action of guanethidine by the same mechanism.

The administration of a phenothiazine in epileptic patients who are receiving either no treatment or only marginally effective doses of their antiseizure medication may precipitate convulsions. Similarly, persons who are withdrawing from either barbiturates or alcohol, and are therefore prone to seizures, are even more likely to have them if given a phenothiazine.

The piperidine group of substituted phenothiazines (thioridazine, mesoridazine), and to a lesser extent the aliphatic group (chlorpromazine, triflupromazine, promazine), exert quinidine-like effects upon the heart, with prolongation of the refractory period and depression of intracardiac conduction. In the rare instances in which these quinidine-like actions of the phenothiazines lead to cardiac arrhythmias, the administration of quinidine is absolutely contraindicated, since it would intensify rather than relieve the problem.

Tricyclic antidepressants and the substituted phenothiazines appear to inhibit each other's metabolism, so that administration of either causes an elevation of the blood level of the other. This is not surprising, as there is great similarity in the chemical structures of the two families of drugs. However, the interaction is probably of no clinical significance.

INTERACTIONS WITH BENZODIAZEPINES

There are few, if any, troublesome interactions between the benzodiazepines and other drugs. Because they are sedative agents, they naturally show summation of action with other drugs with this type of action. A few brief reports suggest that diazepam may interfere with the antiparkinsonism effects of levodopa, but the effects of this latter drug are sufficiently variable as to raise some question as to the reproducibility of the observed drug interaction.

INTERACTIONS WITH BARBITURATES

The sedative effects of the barbiturates are additive with the sedative effects of many other drugs. Phenobarbital provides the classic example of a drug which can induce drug-metabolizing enzymes. Associated with the endoplasmic reticulum of liver cells is a mixed-function oxidase system which is responsible for the biotransformation of a large number of drugs and other chemical substances. Under the influence of repeated doses of phenobarbital, the amount of enzyme protein increases and the rate of drug metabolism increases also, a process referred to as "enzyme induction." Many drugs are now known to cause this induction of drug-metabolizing enzymes, but phenobarbital is the best known case. Other barbiturates exhibit this property to varying degrees.

As a consequence of the increased rate of drug metabolism, the blood levels of affected drugs fall. Thus, giving phenobarbital can cause a lowering of the blood level of the oral anticoagulant warfarin and of the anticonvulsant phenytoin. When the administration of phenobarbital is stopped, the metabolic rate falls, and the blood levels of affected drugs rise again. In the case of a dosage-sensitive drug such as an oral anticoagulant, these changes in blood level can be clinically significant.

INTERACTIONS WITH ETHYL ALCOHOL

Beverage alcohol can interact with a variety of drugs, and it is the nonprescribed agent most likely to be involved in this way. With barbiturates and with meprobamate (Miltown), which is pharmacologically similar, the interactions with alcohol involve three different factors: induction of drug-metabolizing enzymes, competition for drug-metabolizing enzymes, and additive central nervous system depression. Alcohol resembles the barbiturates in that it induces the synthesis of hepatic drug-metabolizing enzymes; therefore, persons who regularly ingest large quantities of alcohol metabolize barbiturates more rapidly and are somewhat resistant to their action. On the other hand, if an individual ingests alcohol and a barbiturate at approximately the same time, each substance delays the metabolism of the other. Therefore, when an alcoholic is sober, he is more resistant to the actions of a barbiturate; when he has been drinking, he is more sensitive to them. Finally, there is nonspecific summation of the sedative effects of alcohol with those of the barbiturates.

Benzodiazapines, such as diazepam (Valium), and phenothiazines, such as chlorpromazine (Thorazine), also show nonspecific summation of sedative effects with alcohol.

Tricyclic antidepressants such as imipramine (Tofranil), particularly during the first day or two of therapy, add to the effects of alcohol and cause marked central nervous system depression. Apparently, tolerance develops after a few days of therapy with a tricyclic agent, and the effect of alcohol is less deleterious. Nevertheless, some clinicians would caution patients on tricyclic antidepressants to limit their intake of alcohol.

Finally, there is the phenomenon of paradoxical reaction to these drugs: substances which normally cause sedation and drowsiness produce central nervous system stimulation and excitation instead. Patients are said to "climb the walls" instead of going quietly on the nod. The phenomenon is often seen in children and is not uncommon in the elderly. It is encountered with alcohol, barbiturates, the benzodiazepines, and probably with all sedative agents.

Disinhibition is the clue to this paradoxical response. In the process of maturation, we all learn to inhibit certain forms of behavior. These inhibitions seem to be particularly susceptible to the actions of sedative drugs, which produce *dis*-inhibition at doses which do not also cause incapacitating ataxia or paralyzing stupor. The various responses to alcoholic drunkenness—belligerence, amorousness, lacrimation, somnolence—are so well known as to require no documentation. It is much simpler to explain these varying responses as the removal of different inhibitions in different people. It seems reasonable to suggest that the more tenuous the inhibition, the more likely is a breakthrough in response to a disinhibiting drug. In many elderly patients, the veneer of civilization has worn a little thin; with little children, the inhibitions are still incompletely formed. It is therefore not surprising that these are the age groups most likely to show the disinhibitory response to the various sedative drugs. Under the duress of sickness and hospitalization, even the mature adult may be susceptible to this paradoxical response, which manifests an interaction not with another drug, but with the patient's life situation.

14 The Use of Mind-Influencing Drugs in the Preoperative Period

Alan Jay Ominsky, M.D.

This chapter is addressed to the physician whose patient will be undergoing surgery within a few hours to a few days. It will have two sections. The first will discuss care of the emotionally well-adjusted patient facing surgery, for whom no psychiatric intervention is sought or necessary. The second section will discuss some of those less common situations, where preoperative psychiatric consultation can be of considerable help to both the patient and the physician.

THE EMOTIONALLY WELL-ADJUSTED PATIENT

Preoperative Anxiety

Today the care described below is often initiated by the family doctor and then continued in the preoperative period by the anesthesiologist and the surgeon. While sharing of responsibility can theoretically result in superior management of the patient's emotional needs, as well as of his physical problems, a real risk exists that each person treating the patient will assume that someone else has ministered to the patient's questions and emotional needs. Since the anesthesiologist is often the last physician to see the patient on the night before surgery, it behooves him to verify that the emotional aspects of the patient's care have been tended to. Indeed, this is occasionally the opportunity to provide part or all of a patient's emotional support during the preoperative period, and it can constitute one of the major gratifications of anesthesiology as a medical specialty.

Most human beings faced with a situation that carries a potential risk to their survival or to their continued normal ways of functioning experience at least some degree of fear. Surgery is an obvious example of a situation that induces such anxiety. Any patient facing surgery necessarily faces, to varying degrees, the possibilities of pain, disability, or death, either from disease itself, or as a consequence of things the surgeon or anesthesiologist will do. Other sources of preoperative anxiety include having to face the unknown and having to give up, at least temporarily, control of one's daily activities and place oneself in a highly dependent position. Relinquishing control and becoming dependent on others can be the hardest part for certain patients to face. Finally, some patients fear they may act in an unacceptable or hysterical manner or say embarrassing things during the anesthetic induction or in the postoperative period.

Unfortunately, many physicians respond to preoperative anxiety as something which is all bad, which will obviously respond to sedatives, and which should routinely be treated with such drugs. All three of these assumptions are erroneous. All standard textbooks on anesthesiology carry recommendations for multiple possible preoperative medication regimens; however, most patients facing elective surgery do not need sedative premedication of any kind and, indeed, are probably better off without it.

For one thing, the average lay patient facing surgery (or even death) is usually less anxious than is the average physician placed in the same position. In addition to the other motivations they may have, many physicians (consciously or unconsciously) choose their profession out of a greater than average concern about death and out of a stronger than average desire to be in control of most situations. For these physicians, a personal surgical experience may be truly terrifying. Also, many physicians are more reluctant than are laymen to recognize their fears, to accept them as appropriate, and to talk about them openly with other, trusted human beings. For a physician to admit to a colleague (or in some cases even to himself) that he is "scared" before an exploratory laparotomy might be regarded by some physician-patients as an intolerable show of weakness. Such a physician may not discuss his anxiety (or even recognize it as such) and may therefore never come to learn that fear is often made more manageable simply by sharing it with another caring and empathic human being. Too many physicians prefer to avoid discussing feelings with their patients, and if indeed they do detect the existence of anxiety, they invariably handle it by prescribing a sedative. Some physicians go even further and routinely prescribe preoperative sedation for virtually every patient, on the assumption that this is somehow helpful.

Let us look at these assumptions more critically. First, is preoperative anxiety harmful? Anxiety does carry certain harmful physiologic sequelae: for example, increased release of catecholamines with resultant tachycardia, and increased cardiac work and cardiac output. In a patient with heart disease, increased cardiac work can result in angina, arrhythmias, or even in myocardial infarction. Moreover, in any patient, significant increases in cardiac output will increase both the total quantity of anesthetic agent required and the time it takes to achieve a satisfactory level of surgical anesthesia. However, this prolongation of anesthetic induction by anxiety was more important 20 or 30 years ago, when anesthesia usually started with a gas induction using unpleasant, slow-acting agents such as ether. In those days, the time to achieve surgical levels of anesthesia was often as long as 20 to 30 minutes, and 10 or 15 of those minutes were spent in the hazardous "second stage" of anesthesia, where the chance of injury from laryngospasm, vomiting, or uncontrollable agitation was much increased. With the modern intravenous induction agents (eg, thiopental), the more rapidly acting, nonirritant inhalation agents (halothane, enflurane), and the rapidly acting intravenous neuromuscular blockers (such as succinylcholine), anesthetic induction is swift and comfortable. The "second stage" of anesthesia, when identifiable, is very brief, and the risks of second stage injury to a healthy patient with an empty stomach are minimal.

While it is true that most patients facing surgery will experience some anxiety, the amount of that anxiety will be determined largely by the patient himself—that is, by what stage of life he is in and by the emotional significance to him of what he has to face. Some patients are stoic and placid in the face of most stress, while other patients tend to be more excitable and histrionic. An elderly patient may well be more accepting of a major illness than will a teenager. Some patients regularly handle their daily anxiety by reaching for a sedative (most commonly alcohol), while others find anything that dulls their intellectual functioning to be more of a burden than a blessing. Perhaps preoperative sedation is most clearly indicated in the case of the patient who normally consumes several ounces of alcohol or several doses of Valium daily even when not in the hospital. For such patients, preoperative sedation represents primarily a continuation of their normal sedative usage. For the remainder of the population, however, the routine administration of preoperative sedation is more difficult to justify.

It was demonstrated a number of years ago that the level of identifiable preoperative anxiety in the average patient is reduced significantly by a routine preoperative visit from the anesthesiologist, but no such demonstration has ever been provided by a sedative. For the great majority of patients, a preoperative visit by the physician is all that is required to reduce the patient's anxiety to satisfactory levels as judged by the following criteria:

1. The patient appears reasonably comfortable, cooperative, and at ease when he comes to the operating room.
2. The patient states when asked that he feels reasonably comfortable and at ease.
3. The patient's pulse, blood pressure, and respiration are within their previously established acceptable range.
4. The patient states when asked postoperatively that the experience was satisfactory.

There is no clear evidence that adding sedatives (in doses short of those which produce sleep) to the preoperative preparation of most patients will demonstrably reduce the patient's anxiety level more than will the preoperative visit. What sedatives will do (since virtually all have effects which last at least several hours) is to prolong the fuzziness and confusion that follows general anesthesia. Especially after short procedures (such as dilatation and curettage), this fuzziness or confusion can be more of an annoyance and a danger to the patient than anything the sedative was supposed to prevent.

Nonpharmacologic Anxiety-Reducing Measures

There are a number of nonpharmacologic measures the physician can take to decrease the patient's preoperative anxiety and to make the patient's postoperative experience safer and more comfortable.

First, the preoperative visit itself can serve to rapidly establish a comfortable personal relationship. Medical history taking and the act of physical examination have "fall-out" value far beyond the information obtained thereby. In our society, people come to know and trust others primarily as a consequence of encounters which usually have some other, formal purpose. As an example, close friends almost always turn out to have originally met because of physical proximity or as a result of a shared task or mutual hobby. The first requirement for any meaningful relationship is simple human contact. So, the first step a physician can take to help his patients with their anxiety is to personally establish contact with them well before surgery.

The next most important anxiety-reducing function of the preoperative visit is to make sure that the patient knows what to expect in sufficient detail that he does not have to worry about possibly unpleasant surprises. This includes such details as the fact that he will have to wear a (rather unattractive) hospital gown, that transportation to the operating room will be on a litter, and that the experience of being transported in this manner (where passersby can look down at him) may itself be somewhat unpleasant. The patient is told that he will be quite aware of his surroundings when he arrives in the operating room. Some people will express a desire to be asleep during all of this, but virtually all patients quickly accept the fact that to anesthetize them in their room (which is what being asleep would amount to) would be unacceptably hazardous. I discuss in detail such items as the application of a blood pressure cuff, the starting of an intravenous infusion, and how anesthesia will be initiated.

Whenever possible, the physician may wish to compare the experience a patient is about to have with something he has already experienced and found tolerable. For instance, before most elective surgery in healthy patients, he can tell them that the risk of death or injury from anesthesia is actually less than that of being killed or injured in an automobile accident. He can tell them that starting an intravenous infusion is usually no more uncomfortable than receiving an intramuscular injection. If he believes that spinal or local anesthesia is indicated (as he often may for certain procedures) he can usually put it in terms similar to these: "If I were having this done for myself or were taking care of a close personal friend, I would want to have a spinal (or local) anesthetic." He can then state why he feels this way and can discuss the hazards and discomforts involved without exaggerating or denying them.

It is certainly true that one physician may see and premedicate a patient in his room and a different physician may provide anesthetic care in the operating room. But consider how helpful it would be to you (were you the patient) to have established a trusting relationship with the actual person in whose hands you were placing your life and capabilities. Also, consider how helpful it would be to you to learn exactly what was expected of you and what you were going to experience directly from the person responsible for your care, rather than from a representative.

Once a trusting relationship has been established with the patient, the next most useful way to reduce problems created by preoperative anxiety is to bring the existence of such anxiety into the open as something which is expected, appropriate, and, indeed, useful. For many patients, especially those who will have chest or abdominal surgery, the postoperative period will be uncomfortable and will carry some real risks, especially those of pneumonia and thromboembolism. I have found it useful to tell the patient that I, and indeed most others, would certainly be somewhat anxious if I were facing what he or she has to face. This simple act of confidentiality usually helps the patient open up if he wishes to talk about feeling anxious. I have certainly found it more effective to state that I myself would have some anxiety than to ask the patient if he is afraid.

I next tell the patient that I believe that having a reasonable amount of anxiety before surgery is usually a good sign—it shows he is approaching things realistically and makes him more likely to take such steps as he personally can to minimize any danger and discomfort. For instance, it is extremely important that the patient know that he will be asked, in his own interests, to bear a reasonable degree of postoperative pain or discomfort. Postoperative coughing, deep breathing, and getting out of bed soon after surgery are all measures of major importance in minimizing the chances of pneumonia or thromboembolism. These latter complications pose the greatest risks to most patients, yet they are risks which the patient himself can do as much, or more, to minimize than can his physician. A patient who has no anxiety before major surgery really scares me, because such a patient is ignoring the real risks and discomforts involved, and he is much less likely to be cooperative later when he is faced with the need to do things that produce unanticipated discomfort.

On the other hand, I also want the patient to know that, while we will ask him to bear some discomfort in his own interests, we will not allow that discomfort to become overwhelming. Patients who know that they will get enough medication to keep pain bearable will accept a greater degree of discomfort before asking for medication than will those who are afraid that they may be forced to endure overwhelming discomfort if they delay their requests for medication.

THE ANXIOUS OR DEPRESSED PATIENT

I would now like to discuss the management of patients who differ considerably from routine preoperative management problems. Some of these patients may be greatly benefitted by the involvement of a psychiatrist as early as possible prior to any planned surgical procedure.

Fears of Death

The first category consists of those patients who tell the surgeon (or some other member of the medical team) that they expect to die during the procedure. Such patients usually have no history of any psychiatric disorder and often have had uneventful anesthesias and operations in the past. Most seasoned clinicians have learned through experience not to ignore any patient who tells them that he is "going to die." It has certainly been my own experience that this type of communication can be ignored only at both the patient's and the surgeon's peril. The patient is certainly communicating something important; it behooves the physician to try to identify the exact nature of that communication. If not responded to, the belief that one is going to die during a procedure could produce massive sympathetic nervous system stimulation.

It seems plausible that such sympathetic hyperactivity might predispose to serious cardiac arrythmias and even to ventricular fibrillation. The pathophysiology of such extreme anxiety may resemble that of "voodoo death," in which a member of a primitive tribe believes that a curse is upon him and becomes so anxious about it that he does in fact die unless the spell is relieved (at least in the victim's mind) by the intervention of an acceptable authority figure.

The statement "I am going to die during this procedure" can mean a number of quite different things. Each of these different meanings carries with it a different prognostic significance and requires a somewhat different response from the physician. For instance, such a statement might be the patient's way of indicating his continuing extreme anxiety—which may arise from misunderstandings or misgivings about the procedure itself. This can be the case even though the surgeon has taken time to explain the procedure and respond to questions. In some cases it is not so much the answers to the questions as the emotional support represented in the act of answering them which is what the patient really needs and wants. In such a situation, the patient may benefit greatly from having another physician, particularly one who possesses specific training and skills in interpersonal process, sit down with and listen to him or her, and spend the extra time that the patient seems to desire. If an interested, interpersonally skillful psychiatrist is available, having him talk with the patient may be of great help. However, such a patient must be told in advance that the consultant has been called in because of special skills and interest in communicating with anxious preoperative patients and not because anyone thinks that the patient is "crazy." If the psychiatric consultant is not interpersonally skillful, or if his visit lacks the patient's consent, the result is likely to be worse than useless. In such an event, it is wiser to seek help from an interpersonally skillful and interested nurse, social worker, or clergyman.

Extreme anxiety often stems from either a newly developed or a long-standing phobia about surgery or anesthesia. If so, it is important to establish that the problem is indeed a phobia and not simple anxiety. Of still greater importance is the investigation of whether that phobia still serves an important function in the patient's overall life adjustment, as would be the case if the phobia served to maintain a state of invalidism on which the patient had beome unconsciously dependent. Most laymen (and most nonpsychiatric physicians) try to reason phobias away, even though severe phobias are usually quite refractory to simple reason. However, many phobias, provided they do not play an important role in the patient's present adjustment (see below) do respond rapidly to a combination of supportive psychotherapy, antianxiety drugs, behavioral modification techniques, and/or hypnosis.

Another possible meaning of the communication "I am going to die" is that the patient is depressed and wants to die; a desire for death accompanies many severe depressions. As with extreme anxiety, the very existence of untreated severe depression in a patient facing major surgery may serve to decrease the patient's chances for survival. One possible detrimental consequence of an untreated depression is that the patient will not exert the necessary effort to get better. For example, a depressed patient with a diminished desire to live is far less likely to cooperate with necessary but painful postoperative activities (such as deep breathing and early mobilization) than is a patient who is determined to survive. Also, if a depression is endogenous and severe, at least one of its causes (or perhaps one of its results) may be a decreased level of sympathetic activity in the central nervous system.

Whether such decreased sympathetic activity might contribute to circulatory problems remains conjectural, but it is certainly within the realm of possibility. In any event, acute depression, even when severe, is one of the most rapidly treatable of psychiatric disorders. Depending on the cause, supportive psychotherapy, antidepressant drugs, electroconvulsive therapy, or some combination of these is almost always effective.

Still another possible meaning of the statement "I am going to die during this procedure" is that the patient regards the procedure as producing symbolic death. For instance, a woman who feels that her sexual appeal and her self-worth are dependent on having attractive breasts might consider mastectomy the equivalent of death. This type of symbolic identification can occur without its meaning being obvious, even to the patient. A less disturbed patient might, in fact, be able to say, "Living without a breast, for me, would be the same as being dead." However, other patients convert simile (it is *like* being dead) to metaphor (it *is* being dead) and hence to "I will die during this procedure."

Anxiety over Loss of Symptoms

Perhaps the most difficult of all patients to treat are those who have unconsciously become dependent on invalidism to maintain a life-style or to control a spouse relationship. Two examples of such patients are discussed below.

A 35-year-old man was referred to me on an emergency basis because he had refused surgery despite almost complete intestinal obstruction caused by scarring from severe colitis. Surgery had been scheduled and the patient heavily premedicated, but he had become panic-stricken on his way to the operating room and had refused to proceed.

Careful history taking (from both the patient and his spouse) revealed that the patient had never made a very successful occupational or marital adjustment, even prior to the onset of his disease. He had little education and poor interpersonal skills and had been unable to hold any job for more than a few months. This situation had existed for some years prior to the onset of his colitis and had been the cause of much conflict between him and his wife, a practical nurse whose job was the main source of family income. With the onset of severe colitis, the patient acquired a medical justification for his life of invalidism at home. Because of his illness, his wife made fewer demands on him and complained less about having to support him. Additionally, because of the painful nature of the patient's condition, his family physician provided him with narcotics, the effects of which the patient found quite to his liking.

When the patient's disease progressed to the point of intestinal obstruction, he was admitted to a university hospital many miles from his home. His surgeon, with little real knowledge of the patient as a person, tried to cheer him up by suggesting that the progression of his disease actually was a blessing in disguise since the now necessary operation would likely not only correct the immediate obstruction but would also effect great improvement in the disease and allow the patient to return to a normal life. Unfortunately, the surgeon had no way of knowing that a requirement to return to "normal life" seemed to this particular patient a fate worse than death.

We were only able to get the patient to agree to life-saving surgery by having his family doctor impress upon the patient that the surgeon's initial optimism was unrealistic. The patient was told that, in fact, a procedure extensive enough to cure him would probably be more than he could physically tolerate, and that the surgical intervention would relieve the obstruction but would be very unlikely to completely cure his disease or to completely remove his symptoms. Only when the patient was told this did he accept the surgery needed to preserve his life. Naturally, we made no attempt to interpret to the patient the relationship between his family doctor's statements and his own, superficially paradoxical acceptance of surgery. To have confronted this patient directly with the connection could only have had undesirable results.

With most patients who unconsciously use somatic symptoms (whether they are of an organic etiology or not) as a major way of dealing with life's problems, insight is useful primarily as a means of devising a successful way to deal with the patient. Insight is vital to me as a psychiatrist because it affords me an understanding of the ways the patient may (unconsciously) use symptoms (physical or emotional) as solutions to present-day life problems. It has been my experience, though, that such patients rarely benefit from such insight themselves. They recognize and gain from these insights only if and when they have already begun using other, more workable solutions for their problems. Only then can they afford to realize the extent to which they used their original symptoms as solutions. Unfortunately, the more severe somaticizers never develop more workable solutions, and hence insight never comes.

Another example of a patient whose symptoms were inextricably bound up in her life-style is a 40-year-old woman with a long history of back pain. She has already undergone two laminectomies, as well as a spine fusion. I was asked for my opinion about whether further organic intervention made sense from a psychologic viewpoint. Under such circumstances, I always ask several key questions. First, what are the most important things that the patient says he or she wants to accomplish which the symptoms are interfering with? Second, how successful has the patient been in actually doing those things before he or she became symptomatic? Third, did anything else (other than the symptoms) also occur that might have made it difficult or impossible to continue to do the things the patient says his or her symptoms are preventing? Fourth, what objective evidence exists that, despite the existence of his or her symptoms, the patient has at least continued to try to do some of the things he or she says she wants to do? Finally, for any patient who is married (or living with someone else), does the other person independently provide the same answers as the patient does to the above questions?

When I asked this woman, "What is the most important thing that your back pain is interfering with?" she replied (to my astonishment), "Entertaining my husband's friends." It quickly became apparent that this woman despised her husband's friends, and that prior to her illness his demands on her to play hostess to his business associates (in order to further his career) was a serious cause of strife. Most of their other conflicts (eg, his desire for frequent sexual intercourse) were also "solved" by her symptoms, because they made it impossible for her to meet his demands. I must emphasize that her illness was in no way feigned—it was real. However, once she had learned (without conscious awareness) that she could control and punish her husband through her symptoms, she was not about to relinquish those symptoms, even if it meant submitting to (but failing to improve after) repeated surgery.

Under the circumstances, the surgeon and I agreed that surgery was contraindicated. Understanding the situation helped to provide a useful, if unorthodox, strategy. I offered to treat the woman with hypnosis, provided that hypnotherapy was limited to helping her to relax despite pain rather than aimed at "curing" her pain. My justification to her was that to remove her pain, in view of the pathology in her back, might be dangerous. I further insisted that if I was to treat her at all, her husband had to attend each session, since even the increased ability to relax might cause her to try to resume a schedule that had already proven "back-breaking," and such a schedule, under the present circumstances, might produce irreparable injury. My therapeutic strategy could be summarized as follows: first, I felt I had to reassure this particular patient that nothing that I or anyone else could do would suddenly or completely cure her back problem. Only when she felt secure in this belief (although she could never admit this even to herself) did I have any chance of making a therapeutic impact on the problem. Then, by making the husband's presence at hypnosis sessions mandatory, I introduced a situation where, with myself as catalyst, the husband and wife might begin to learn to communicate in a less pathologic way. (A hypnosis session in their case consisted of 10 minutes of hypnosis and 40 minutes of what was essentially couples' therapy—never, of course, described to them in those terms.)

While the results were not perfect, both the woman and her husband obtained considerable benefit. I knew from my experience with other such situations that, had either husband or wife been told initially that what was really needed was a change in their communications system, they would have met such a suggestion with a combination of massive denial and hostility.

This is another example of where insight was important for the therapist (provided the therapist acted wisely) but was initially both unimportant to and inadmissible by the patient.

In discussing this couple, I do not wish to oversell what can usually be accomplished. Psychiatrists and nonpsychiatrists alike need to realize that patients who have long used somatization as a primary way of dealing with interpersonal or emotional problems rarely, if ever, modify this pattern for very long. Often the only insight gained into the situation is that of the therapist, who comes to realize that attempts to cure such a patient (via surgical or pharmacologic or psychotherapeutic means) may end up with both iatrogenic complications and the therapist having the headache (produced by his banging his head repeatedly against a stone wall).

There are case reports, but no controlled studies, that suggest that some fraction of these patients respond to a neuroleptic and an antidepressant used in combination. The daily dosages usually recommended have been on the order of 150 mg of amitriptyline and 2 mg of Prolixin for a 70-kg, otherwise healthy adult. When I use this combination, I usually start with 75 mg of amitriptyline for two or three nights, then double it for the next two or three nights, and then add the Prolixin (also at night). If such a regimen is to work, the patient often has to tolerate an initially incapacitating level of drowsiness for several days, but that particular side effect usually subsides within a week. One must also warn the patient about dry mouth and the other less common but more serious anticholinergic, cutaneous, neurologic, and vasomotor side effects. Whether or not such a drug regimen will ultimately prove demonstrably better than placebo remains to be seen. It certainly will not work for many of those patients who are dependent on their symptoms for secondary gain.

Finally, in regard to the use of electrical stimulators, biofeedback, hypnosis, and acupuncture: with each of these therapies it remains to be demonstrated that beneficial results, when they do occur, occur with greater frequency than they would after use of a placebo. Certainly if the patient's symptoms are really interpersonal "solutions," it would be difficult to see how these therapeutic interventions could provide more than transient benefits. However, since the intensity of situationally induced stress does vary (even if problem-solving mechanisms by which people respond to stress tend to be constant), it may be that any one of the above therapies will provide a supportive relationship with the therapist and will thereby sustain a patient through a particularly stressful period and result in an apparent "cure" when (and if) the external stress lessens.

REFERENCES

Coping with surgery and other painful medical procedures. Hoffman-LaRoche Inc. Series on Coping #13. *Med Trib.* October, 1976.

Egbert, L.D., Battit, G.E., Turndorf, H. et al: The value of the preoperative visit by an anesthetist. *JAMA.* 185:553–555, 1963.

Egbert, L.D., Battit, G.E., Welch, E.E. et al: Reduction of postoperative pain by encouragement and instruction of patients. A study of doctor-patient rapport. *N Engl J Med.* 270:825–827, 1964.

Kennedy, J.A. and Bakst, H.: The influence of emotions on the outcome of cardiac surgery. A predictive study. *Bull NY Acad Med.* 42:811–849, 1966.

15 Illegal or "Street" Drugs

Dana L. Farnsworth, M.D.

INTRODUCTION

"Assessing the full extent of drug abuse in the United States is comparable to describing the color of a chameleon on the basis of an instantaneous view of the animal," explained Dr. Vernon Patch, a very experienced and astute observer and researcher of the drug scene (National Commission on Marihuana and Drug Abuse, 1973, Appendix, Vol. 1, p. 997).

In this chapter a wide variety of substances will be discussed primarily in terms of their method of distribution but with the understanding that many of them can be considered in various other classifications as well. For our purposes, a "street" drug will be defined as any substance which is passed from person to person, with or without monetary consideration, and which will influence the mind when ingested in sufficient quantity. Some of these drugs, such as heroin and cocaine, are totally illegal. Others, such as tobacco, alcohol, and solvents of various kinds, are not even regarded as drugs by many people. Still others, such as amphetamines, barbiturates, and tranquilizers, are legal when prescribed by a physician, but illegal under other circumstances.

It may not seem to those who want exact or literal definitions that alcohol, coffee, and tobacco qualify for inclusion in this list. However, since alcohol is illegal in every state for those under a certain age and is the most abused of all drugs, we are including it. Tobacco is not illegal, but we choose to include it because of its danger to health and because of the blatant disregard smokers exhibit to all warnings by health officials. Coffee is practically a universal beverage, but for those who use so much of it that its stimulant drug, caffeine, causes disturbing symptoms, there is a drug problem. Because several of these substances are treated at length in other chapters, the emphasis in this discussion will center on the informal—particularly, the illegal—aspects of their distribution and use.

When an individual is believed to have a drug problem, several aspects must be considered. For example, no one could be said to have a drug problem who used alcohol in moderation, but he certainly would have one if he used it excessively. A person might be considered to have a drug problem, however, if he used any LSD or other psychedelic drugs, including marijuana. Anyone who is addicted to a drug or is otherwise drug-dependent does indeed have a drug problem.

Another problem, and one which has social implications, occurs when the use of drugs, either moderately or excessively, puts a person into conflict with other people. This may be due to violation of existing laws or to a clash between the values and moral standards of drug users and nonusers. Alcohol is probably the most common cause of drug problems: it can lead to arrest for driving while under its influence; it may lead to absence from work because of using too much of it; or it may cause the individual not to take care of members of his family who are dependent upon him. The alcoholic may contract a variety of physical and emotional difficulties which range from delirium tremens to cirrhosis of the liver.

In one sense, coffee, tea, and tobacco may be classified as drugs, yet the harm from using them varies a great deal: from none at all to the severe forms of injury—carcinoma of the lung and emphysema—seen in the case of heavy cigarette smoking. Overuse of cigarettes harms the individual smoker but not usually other people, although it may annoy them. With most of these substances, the physical and psychologic dependence they engender are intricately interwoven and often cause the subtle pressure for their use to take precedence over any consideration of danger to health.

If one were to judge the nature and extent of the use of street drugs from the publicity given them in the news media, it would be reasonable to surmise that such drugs were no longer used extensively. Conversations with those physicians who see large numbers of young people, however, give quite the opposite impression—such drugs continue to be used, but the complications they engender are no longer the prime source of interest to most news reporters that they were in the late sixties and early seventies.

The National Commission on Marihuana and Drug Abuse (1973, pp. 93–94) delineated five usage patterns of drugs to aid in the understanding of the vastly complicated experience of drug users. These are:

1. *Experimental drug use.* This is the short-term, non-patterned trial of one or more drugs (not more than ten times per drug) motivated by curiosity about new feelings or mood states.
2. *Social or recreational drug use.* This occurs among friends or acquaintances desiring to share an acceptable and pleasurable experience.
3. *Circumstantial or situational drug use.* This stems from a perceived need or desire to achieve a known and anticipated effect, such as alertness during examinations or relief of fatigue.
4. *Intensified drug use.* This refers to long-term, patterned use of drugs to achieve relief from a persistent problem or stressful situation.
5. *Compulsive drug use.* This includes frequent use of high dosages of a drug over a long period which produces dependence such that the individual cannot discontinue such use without experiencing physical or psychologic disruption. This type of use poses the highest risk to the health, welfare, and safety of any community.

MARIJUANA

One of the most extensively used products in the illegal drug category is cannabis. *Cannabis sativa,* the hemp plant, grows in almost all parts of the world but flourishes best in hot, dry climates such as those of Mexico, Jamaica, Morocco, and various portions of India. Marijuana consists of the chopped leaves and stems of the cannabis plant. Hashish is formed of resin scraped from the flowering top of the cannabis plant. It also can be smoked or eaten and is much more potent than marijuana. The chief psychoactive ingredient of cannabis is tetrahydrocannabinol (THC). There is no accepted medical use for cannabis, although a few conditions, such as glaucoma, may be relieved by its use.

The main effect of cannabis is a subtle mood change in which the individual has a sense of increased well-being. However, this is quite dependent on the setting and expectations of the user. Perception of colors, sounds, patterns, textures, and taste is greatly enhanced. Space and time are often distorted in ways that can be either pleasing or disconcerting. Time seems to pass slowly. Inhibitions may be relaxed in a manner similar to that experienced with low doses of alcohol. True hallucinations do not occur.

When strong forms of cannabis, such as hashish, are used, the individual may experience a simple depression, a panic state, a toxic psychosis, or a psychotic break. The risk of a psychotic break is greater in those persons who already have a history of mental disorder. Physical dependence does not develop, nor are withdrawal symptoms noticeable when its use is discontinued.

It has often been stated that the use of marijuana leads to the use of "hard" drugs such as heroin or cocaine. Strictly speaking, this is not true. Rather, the entrance of young, inexperienced, or troubled persons into a group that has a high incidence of use of any drug increases the likelihood that these new members will try other drugs. In short, one particular drug does not lead to another, but the pressures or other influences prevalent in a given group increase the likelihood that a new addition to the group will try the drugs prevalent in it. An examination of the patterns of other drug usage by the regular user of marijuana is likely to reveal increased use of alcohol and tobacco.

The weight of evidence indicates that marijuana does not cause violent or aggressive behavior and in fact serves to inhibit such behavior. Neither does it promote criminal behavior. Strong opinions about its presumed harmful effects continue in many quarters, but these are based more on feelings than on facts.

After a year's study of marijuana and its derivatives, the National Commission on Marihuana and Drug Abuse (1972, p. 152) came to the conclusion that this substance, though harmful in various ways, was far less harmful than nearly all other drugs, including alcohol and tobacco, which are both not only legal but also widely advertised. There was no evidence that marijuana per se leads to the use of stronger drugs, but such use is encouraged by peer group pressures of various kinds. Although it is a harmful drug, it is far less dangerous than most other street drugs.

For these reasons, the Commission strongly recommended that marijuana not be legalized, since this would result in its being advertised extensively and in its being used by many people. On the other hand, the Commission recommended that it be decriminalized: that small amounts (1 oz or less) be subject to seizure and possibly small fines to the owner. Since 1972, when this recommendation was made, eight states—Alaska, California, Colorado, Maine, Ohio, Oregon, Minnesota, and South Dakota—have passed such legislation.

HEROIN

When the term drug addiction is introduced into almost any conversation, most people think almost automatically of addiction to heroin. Yet when individuals are taking heroin from a readily available supply, the social effects are rather limited. In brief, heroin does not by itself lead to crime; rather, its absence after a person's body has become accustomed to the drug does lead to acquisitive crimes (notably burglary or shoplifting), committed for the purpose of securing money to buy more of the drug. In contrast, assaultive offenses are more frequently committed by users of alcohol, amphetamines, or barbiturates. Also, some of the nonbarbiturate sedatives, notably methaqualone, do occasionally lead to violent behavior.

One recent survey in the United States revealed that heroin had been tried by 1.3% of the adults and 0.6% of the youth, and an additional 1% of the adults and 3% of the youth indicated that they might like to try it at some time to see what it was like (National Commission on Marihuana and Drug Abuse, 1973, p. 69). No accurate data are available regarding how many persons in the United States are dependent upon heroin, but the respected estimates (most in favor) suggest that there are more than 500,000 at any particular time, most of them in the larger cities. It is quite probable that heroin use is gradually increasing. The incidence is greatest among young people in urban centers where living conditions are unfavorable. About 25% to 50% of those who experiment with heroin may become dependent on it.

More opiate-dependent persons are in methadone maintenance programs than are in any other modality. Other forms of treatment, including group therapy, family counseling, vocational training, and social services, should accompany such therapy. The ultimate effectiveness of such treatment remains under debate. Heroin maintenance programs have had considerable support in the past but have not been generally accepted.

COCAINE

Cocaine is less widely available and is more expensive than heroin. In a recent national survey, 3% of the adults and 1.5% of the youth in the sample reported that they had tried cocaine at least once, and an additional 3% of the adults and 1.5% of the youth indicated that they would like to try it in the future, particularly if it were legal (National Commission on Marihuana and Drug Abuse, 1973, p. 69).

The actual relationship between cocaine use and criminal behavior is not clearly demonstrated, but the pharmacologic effects of the drug would seem to suggest a potential for drug-induced violent behavior similar to that shown by amphetamine and barbiturate users (National Commission on Marihuana and Drug Abuse, 1973, p. 165). Like the opiate user, the user of cocaine is more prone to commit crimes against property than against people.

The supply of illegal drugs of all kinds varies greatly from time to time and from place to place. Therefore, when the supply of addicting drugs becomes limited, drug pushers will try to sell other varieties. In such situations, cocaine enters the black market in increased amounts. In the last few years, cocaine has been illegally imported from South America, especially when the supply of opium from the usual sources in Southeast Asia or Mexico has been intercepted. Cocaine, like marijuana and LSD, is used for its positive effects rather than for the relief of immediate distress that motivates heroin intake.

A recent monograph on cocaine, its history and all other aspects of its use and effects, has just been published and is by far the most informative and reliable of any publications up to this time (Grinspoon and Balakar, 1976).

HALLUCINOGENS

One of the most intriguing of the drugs which produce hallucinations in the user is *peyotl,* or *mescal,* a substance found in significant quantity for use or study in the dried extract of a cactus plant in the form of button-shaped discs one to two inches in diameter and from an eighth to a quarter of an inch thick. The plant grows along both the Mexican and the United States sides of the Rio Grande. Mescaline is an alkaloid of the peyote cactus and was first isolated in 1896. It is much less potent than LSD in producing an altered state of consciousness. It has been used by American Indians for centuries in elaborate religious ceremonies. Typically, three to seven of the mescal buttons are ingested. The active principle causes "visions," or vibrant hallucinations, characterized by brilliantly colored, shimmering mosaics of great variety. Dr. S. Weir Mitchell and William James both tried the drug but concluded that "one time was enough" (Kluver, 1966). The volume referred to has extensive descriptions of varieties of vivid hallucinations. Mescal has not been as prominently featured in drug use in the last two decades as have LSD and psilocybin, possibly because its effects are usually by no means pleasant.

There are few, if any, recognized medical uses for the hallucinogens, even though serious searches have been conducted to find such uses for a long time. For a considerable period in the early stages of interest in these drugs, there was hope that mental illness might be minimized in some instances or that the drugs could be used in psychotherapy. The reason for such interest is that certain effects of these drugs tend to imitate the symptoms of schizophrenia. This raised the hope that studying drug-induced, model psychoses might contribute to the understanding of those which occur apparently spontaneously.

Various attempts to use the hallucinogens in the treatment of terminal cancer patients or for the treatment of alcoholism and other drug addictions have also not been particularly noteworthy.

The hallucinogens do not produce hallucinations in the classic sense; rather, they alter perception somewhat. After-images may be prolonged and overlap with present perceptions. Objects seem to move in a wave-like fashion or to melt. Sensory impressions become overwhelming. Sometimes it may appear that colors are heard and that sound is seen. Time seems to pass very slowly. Self boundaries appear to disintegrate, and the user may come to feel a sense of oneness with the universe. Moods may change radically from gaiety to depression, from elation to fear, or vice versa (Delong, 1972).

Adverse effects with LSD ingestion are not very common—possibly not more than 10% of those who try it will experience any—but they may occur more frequently among the young (15 to 25 years old), who have not yet established a satisfying pattern of life. Psychoses are relatively rare and mostly occur in persons already vulnerable to them. A more common reaction is the so-called bad trip, which often occurs among young people who are not firmly settled in a life-style that gives them guidelines to follow. Visual images may be distorted and may contribute to panic reactions by arousing immense anxiety and fear. Some individuals may experience psychotic episodes with paranoid behavior. There can even be feelings of omnipotence, such as that exhibited by a young man who stepped in front of a speeding automobile under the assumption that he was invincible. (Needless to say, the automobile won, though the experimenter survived after spending several weeks in a hospital.)

After taking LSD several times, an occasional individual will experience a flashback—a recurrence of some aspect of the drug experience when the individual is not directly under the influence of the drug. The mechanism of such flashbacks is not known.

An occasional older person who experiments with LSD several times gradually loses his former capacities, retreats from his usual style of life, and ceases to carry out any productive activity. The prevailing behavior is usually one of innocuous uselessness (Freedman, 1970). These cases are seldom reported in the medical literature because of the complexity and subtlety of the changes, and out of concern that privacy might be violated.

As this is written, there is no reliable evidence that LSD causes birth defects; nor does it produce chromosome damage detectable by available methods. But, we must not allow ourselves a false sense of security, for this is not the final word on LSD. Additional investigation into this compound may very well change the value of today's data. One must also keep in mind that the LSD in the possession of a drug user or experimenter is of necessity a street drug, illegally prepared and illegally distributed. The effects of such drugs are unpredictable, and their use is dangerous.

One very serious apparent result from extensive use of LSD is a rather drastic personality change. Some individuals may believe that they have been immensely improved by the whole experience, and yet they may be unable to carry on in a regular job or to demonstrate in any way to their friends that they have benefitted by the experience.

In spite of many statements to the effect that LSD is mind-expanding, there is no evidence that the hallucinogenic drugs have freed anyone's mind for any activity which it could not have done as well, or better, without having been influenced by the drug.

LSD is effective when taken by mouth, which is the usual method of administration. It produces effects such as pupillary dilation, increased blood pressure, tremor, nausea, muscular weakness, and increased body temperature; but these effects are usually minor. Human deaths as a result of the pharmacologic action of LSD are very few in number, and when they do occur, they are usually the result of faulty judgment on the part of the individual who is having the hallucinogenic experience.

AMPHETAMINES

The amphetamines have had a highly varied use in this and in many other countries during the last few decades. They have been quite helpful in controlling narcolepsy and in reducing appetite in the treatment of obesity. They have been effective in reducing nasal obstruction, fatigue, or mild depression. Unfortunately, they lend themselves to abuse, and in sufficient quantities they can cause hallucinations, delusions, and suspiciousness to the point of paranoia. Their use in athletic contests has been known to have produced fatalities. Few ethical uses of the amphetamines now remain, and what use is made of them must be supervised closely.

The epidemic of amphetamine abuse of the late 1960s was described by one authority as a white, middle- and upper-class phenomenon affecting persons who were bored and frustrated, and who had no particular need to work to support themselves (Cohen, 1970).

ALCOHOL

Alcohol continues to be the drug most used to excess. Discussion of its misuse raises numerous, complex issues. Children may ask their parents how an adult's use of alcohol differs from their own actual or potential use of marijuana or other drugs taken for nonmedical purposes. Attempts to be logical by stressing the fact that such drugs are dangerous and may seriously threaten one's life and future career will be countered by well-informed youngsters with the fact that alcohol use is far and away the most dangerous of our drug problems (National Commission on Marihuana and Drug Abuse, 1973, p. 43). More than $24 billion were spent in the United States during 1971 on alcoholic beverages, a sum amounting to at least 10 times the amount spent on all other types of psychoactive drugs, both prescribed and illicit. Estimates for more recent years run to over $30 billion per year. Of the nearly 100 million people who use alcohol, 9 to 10 million become chronic alcoholics. From these ranks come a terrifying array of serious, and often fatal, automobile and other accidents; crime; suicide; emotional and physical illness; family disintegration; and unemployment. The final irony is that more than half the people in this country do not even identify alcohol as a drug.

A recent survey (Straus, 1973) points out that alcohol is a substance which permeates, pleases, and yet plagues most of the world. In social situations it relieves tension, promotes a sense of well-being, and enhances relaxation and conviviality. Its use to excess produces disaster. The question then arises: what constitutes discreet or indiscreet use of alcoholic beverages?

For drinking to become a threatening problem, a person must usually use alcohol to excess over a period of several years and must also have a serious family or personal problem which he cannot resolve. Under these circumstances, alcohol's temporary relaxing effects may be sought both by drinking it more often and by drinking it in greater amounts. When a person has become dependent upon alcohol, most methods of dealing with the problem are notably unreliable; prevention is easier, less expensive, and, in the long run, far more rewarding.

No society or country has ever solved the alcohol problem, though some do better than others. Some societies treat those who use it very severely, even with capital punishment, but this does not stop its use. Prohibition of alcohol has never been entirely successful in any society. The most notable extensive attempt to prohibit the use of alcohol was made by the United States from 1920 to 1933, but it was a dismal failure. Numerous programs are underway throughout the United States today to aid the chronic alcoholic in limiting or stopping his or her use of alcohol.

Practically no group advocates a return to prohibition. But the problem persists, and much sentiment is being developed to help people learn to stop using alcohol self-destructively.

The following practices, if followed on a wide scale, might reduce significantly the human tragedy that is now so obvious:

Never drink alone.

At home or at parties, the usual rule should be one or two drinks (1½ ounces of 86 to 90 proof liquor) over a period of at least an hour. The more concentrated the drink, the more quickly complications arise, especially when the drinks are consumed rapidly. The liquor should therefore be diluted, and the individual should always have some food when drinking.

All parents, especially if they themselves drink, should teach their children within the home setting about alcoholic beverages—their nature, effects, and risks—and how to use them. Those parents who do not drink should feel free to uphold their ideas in discussions with their children but not to impose them with such fervor as to invite rebellion.

Never drive after more than one drink unless two to three hours have intervened. This is the time required for sufficient metabolization of alcohol in the body; coffee or a sandwich will not speed up this process.

Never drink to solve a problem.

Keep danger signs in mind. Many listings of these have been compiled; the ones we would stress are: drinking twice a day, having three or more drinks daily, binge drinking, and a tendency to need more alcohol in order to achieve a desired effect.

It is especially important not to drink when taking other drugs unless one's physician has specifically stated that it is safe to do so. Drugs often enhance each other's effects. Most people know that combining sleeping pills and alcohol is dangerous, but this danger also accompanies the combination of alcohol and many other medications, including some over-the-counter preparations. A physician's warning in such situations may be life-saving.

No specific rules such as these are applicable to all persons or situations. The important thing is to maintain a cautious and thoughtful attitude, so that one can enjoy the perceived advantages of alcohol without suffering the distressing consequences of its abuse.

TOBACCO

As they do with alcohol and coffee, relatively few persons look upon tobacco (or the nicotine it contains) as a drug. Since the vested interests of the tobacco industry are so strong, and since many thousands of persons are dependent on it for their livelihood, it is not likely that the rate or manner of its consumption will change greatly in the foreseeable future.

Changes are occurring in cigarette-smoking habits in that adults are smoking less and teenagers, particularly girls, are smoking more. Peer-group pressures appear to be at work in each instance. For adults, pressures against smoking in public places, such as airplanes, are mounting. Among teenagers, the campaign against smoking has had little effect, and for girls, the idea that they have the same "right" to smoke as boys is gaining credence. For them the prospect of developing cancer of the lung or emphysema seems too far in the future to be taken seriously—and besides, these usually occur in "someone else."

SOLVENTS AND INHALANTS

Inhalation of solvent vapors is not particularly new; a century or more ago people went on ether jags, and in more recent times gasoline sniffers have become known. Sometimes workers in industry will expose themselves to solvents to see whether or not jags will occur. In recent years, however, sniffing epidemics have occurred and have been reported by various authors (National Commission on Marihuana and Drug Abuse, 1973, Appendix, Vol. 1, p. 107).

This type of substance abuse has become a more or less permanent form of deviant behavior among a proportion of adolescents. The incidence of solvent sniffing varies considerably and depends upon the changing attitudes of young people, which are usually stimulated by publicity of various kinds. The age range of participants is usually from 13 to 17 years. Boys are involved much more often than girls. Sniffing usually begins as a fad and often accompanies a variety of antisocial acts, which are frequently caused by the inhalants. Children of minority groups, but not blacks, are frequently involved. Most families are in low socioeconomic circumstances. There is usually a high degree of family disorganization.

Among the substances that are misused are model airplane glue, plastic cements, fingernail polish remover, lacquer thinners, cleaning fluids, gasoline, deodorants, hair sprays, antiseptics, antitussives, shampoo, and cocktail glass chillers. A chronic sniffer will try various products and then select those which give him the kind of reaction he wants to experience. Many of these sniffers may test numerous materials randomly without knowing their composition. This type of experimentation has resulted in fatalities. Toluene is relatively safe, but the chlorinated hydrocarbons of cleaning fluid are much more toxic. The popularity of many of these drugs derives from the fact that they are easily available and inexpensive. Abused inhalants are usually taken by placing a rag or piece of gauze which has been soaked in the substance over the mouth and nose. Alternatively, cements that have solvents in them will be rolled into the form of a tube and placed in the mouth. Some individuals put the material in a paper or plastic bag or balloon and use it as an inhalation chamber by placing it over the nose or mouth.

The effects of these various substances range from mild inebriation, resembling that of alcohol intoxication, to a chemical psychosis with hallucinations, delusions, and gross behavioral disturbances. Feelings of drunkenness, dizziness, and euphoria are frequent, but these are also accompanied by a sense of reckless abandon, grandiosity, invincibility, and omnipotence. This combination is thus likely to cause impulsive, destructive, and accident-prone behavior, just as it would with alcohol, but judgment and reality testing are even more affected. Serious crimes, including homicides, have been committed by persons so affected. Accidental suicide may occur, because some persons develop the feeling that they are capable of any feat, including jumping from a rooftop or stepping in front of an oncoming train. Distortions of space and visual perception are common and may lead to sensations that the walls are closing in or that the sky is falling. Visible objects may change shape, identity, or color. Hallucinations are common. The psychosis produced by the inhalants is temporarily more dangerous than that produced by LSD and other hallucinogens. The action of the inhalants more closely resembles that of the amphetamines or cocaine than some of the other frequently abused drugs. Death may occur, particularly

when plastic bags are used and when the method of administration of the inhalant is not well planned (Press and Done,
1967). Occasionally, "sudden sniffing death" occurs when tri-
chloroethylene and fluoridated refrigerants or propellants are
used. Sometimes toluene, benzine, and gasoline are involved in
such cases. Aside from those already mentioned, there are few
acute adverse physical effects of inhalant abuse upon the individual. The more unstable the individual before he starts such
experimentation, the more likely he is to experience adverse
reactions.

SOCIAL MILIEU OF UNSUPERVISED
DRUG USE

The numerous studies of the nature and causes of unsuper-
vised drug use have brought forth so many different conclusions
that a combination of factors, rather than single specific causes, is
indicated. A variety of findings is contained in the papers published in the appendices of the Second Report of the National
Commission on Marihuana and Drug Abuse (1973), from which
the following generalizations are derived.

In many groups of drug-using youngsters, particularly during the late 1960s and early 1970s, the use of marijuana, speed, or
LSD was an excuse to make a contact: buying some of the drug
would get a conversation started that would eventually find them
a place to stay. There was also a good deal of sexual posturing
which paralleled somewhat the hair-combing rituals of the
black-jacketed, motorcycle group of an earlier era.

Many of the youngsters were trapped in an aimless and
endless cycle and were looking for something to share with
others. Survival was an accomplishment. Sex was as much a
commodity for survival as spare change might be. These young
people were not, as a rule, mentally ill in the traditional sense.
Instead, they were unable to deal appropriately with authority;
nor could they get along at home. Since their home environments
were unsatisfactory, they tried to move in any direction that
would give them more satisfaction. Often their odd manners, bad
judgment, and great emotional demands on others shaped a way
of living which they could not carry on in their home environments, which demanded more conformity and obedience.

The families or former homes of many of the street
youngsters using illicit drugs were characterized by high

incidences of alcoholism, desertions, incest, and violence. Drug use was found to be greater among those youngsters who considered their mother of little importance and among those whose fathers had frequently appeared in court to answer charges for their behavior. Some were members of minority groups who were discriminated against; some had previous police records for vandalism, gang fighting, and so on. It is well known that violence, delinquency, and drug use are outgrowths of other, possibly psychosocial, situational, or economic factors that are not causally related to one another. Consequently, delinquency does not necessarily lead to drug use.

An obvious psychologic corollary of drug use is that it becomes woven into the fabric of the user's life to replace something that is missing. Certain very basic needs and desires are common to all, but they are especially important to the young. These include the need to be wanted and loved and to participate fully in the social system of which they are a part. Drug use itself is not the cause of the alienation of youth, of the decay of values and the search for new and often radical values, of the spiritual malaise, or of the decline of economic incentive. Rather, it derives from these phenomena, and it is most often observed when young people feel neither needed nor wanted by key persons in their lives. Thus, the young person who already has problems compounds them when he becomes involved with psychedelic or other drugs.

Pope (1971) has reported that homosexuality is much more prevalent among drug users than among those who abstain. He believes that it satisfies many of the feelings that also lead to drug use; that it serves as a way to deal with loneliness, as a response to the drug subculture's approval of acting out, and, in some instances, as a reaction to a family constellation of a distant father and a dominant, intimate mother.

Popular music is often blamed for encouraging the use of illicit drugs, but proof for this is very difficult to obtain. In a survey of the possible effects of popular music and lyrics about drugs, it was determined that references to drugs are almost as frequently discouraging of their use as encouraging of it (National Commission on Marihuana and Drug Abuse, 1973, Appendix, Vol. 2, p. 723). It seems probable that developing policy through public opinion would be much more effective than making rules or laws on what could or could not be expressed in lyrics. It seems quite reasonable that drug use is encouraged more by person-to-person recommendation within groups of young people than by anything that comes through in lyrics to music.

Because of lessened publicity about illicit drugs in recent years, many people believe that their use is decreasing. However, most people who work closely with young people, especially with those in trouble, find that there is still widespread use of these drugs, and that there is an abundance of reasons for continuing effective drug education programs.

DRUG EDUCATION

The goal of an efficient drug education program should theoretically be that of aiding its students or recipients to deal with the drugs they encounter—whether these are totally illegal (heroin, cocaine, psychedelics), prescribed by physicians, or widely used but not under supervision (alcohol and tobacco)—in such a way as to do no harm to themselves or others. Obviously there is no single correct way to do this, at least at present. The variables in such programs are practically infinite. Almost no one can avoid using all drugs, nor should they. Few people are kept away from drugs by fear tactics, particularly if truth is replaced by exaggeration. The individual's decision to use drugs in non-medicinal ways is far more dependent upon the attitudes and opinions of his friends and associates (set and setting) than on the biochemical or pharmacologic factors involved.

Children learn about drugs from one another, from the attitudes and comments of their parents and their schoolteachers, and from advertisements on television, as well as by formal instruction in the classroom through lectures, discussions, or films. Practically the only certainty in this field is that no single effective system has yet been devised for imparting information and developing attitudes among the young which will enable them to act sensibly with respect to drugs. Yet even in this field, knowledge is preferable to ignorance, and low-keyed attempts to teach young people how to deal with drug problems on their own are highly desirable. Support of efforts toward making drug education programs effective must come from parents, physicians, schools, churches, service clubs, and, one hopes, the mass media. Nearly all forms of drug abuse make money for someone, and this places a difficult obstacle in the path of preventive programs.

Drug education which emphasizes pharmacology and which

is taught in special classes created for this sole purpose is giving way to a tendency to teach about the effects of misused drugs in any course in school or college when it becomes appropriate and natural. Rather than taking a solely negative approach in drug education programs, we can portray the use of drugs in terms of human need and thus make it possible for issues to be discussed positively. In this way, the impact upon students or patients is likely to be more favorable than in a system in which drugs always seem to be culprits of some kind.

One of my middle-aged friends, a college physician, became aware of how often it seemed that the attitudes of students toward drugs had developed, in part at least, from attitudes exhibited by their parents. He spoke of this to his wife, and, as an experiment, they searched their house and collected their own supply of drugs. To their surprise and dismay, they gathered more than 40 kinds of drugs which they had used at some time in the past. Fortunately, their own children had been brought up in such a way that they did not feel the need to experiment with drugs.

A significant service that all physicians and health educators could render society is to encourage everyone to dispose of drugs they no longer need and to put those that may be useful in the future out of the reach of those who might harm themselves by their irresponsible use.

The attitude of the physician is a crucial factor in dealing with patients who are involved with illegal or street drugs. If he "lays down the law" and tells his patients what they already know about the harmfulness of such drugs, his time is wasted. The focus should be on the attitudes of, and the patients' relationships with, family and friends rather than on the particular drug with which they are involved at the moment. Helping young patients to understand the nature and extent of their motivations encourages them to make decisions in their own best interest, whereas telling them what they should do may invite rebellion.

REFERENCES

Cohen, S.: Speed: The risk you run. In *What Everyone Needs to Know about Drugs*, edited by Joseph Newman, pp. 148–159. Washington, D.C: U.S. News and World Report, 1970.

Delong, James V.: *Dealing with Drug Abuse*. New York: Praeger Publishers, 1972, pp. 90–98.

Freedman, D.X.: A psychiatrist looks at LSD. In *What Everyone Needs* to Know about Drugs, edited by Joseph Newman, pp. 160–177. Washington, D.C: U.S. News and World Report, 1970.

Grinspoon, L. and Balakar, J.B.: *Cocaine: A Drug and Its Social Evolution.* New York: Basic Books, Inc., 1976.

Kluver, H.: *Mescal and Mechanisms of Hallucinations.* Chicago: University of Chicago Press, 1966, pp. 13–32.

National Commission on Marihuana and Drug Abuse: Marihuana: a signal of misunderstanding. *First Report of the National Commission on Marihuana and Drug Abuse.* Washington, D.C: U.S. Government Printing Office, 1972. Appendices: 2 Vols.

National Commission on Marihuana and Drug Abuse: Drug use in America: problem in perspective. *Second Report of the National Commission on Marihuana and Drug Abuse.* Washington, D.C: U.S. Government Printing Office, 1973. Appendices: 4 Vols.

Pope, H.J.: *Voices from the Drug Culture.* Cambridge, Mass: The Sanctuary, 1971, pp. 56–57.

Press, E. and Done, A.K.: Solvent sniffing. *Pediatrics* 39:451–461, 611–622, 1967.

Straus, R.: Alcohol and society. *Psychiatr Ann.* 3:9–108, 1973.

SUGGESTED READING

American Medical Association: *Drug Dependence, A Guide for Physicians.* Chicago: American Medical Association, 1969.

Bonnie, R.J. and Whitebread, C.H.: *The Marihuana Conviction, A History of Marihuana Prohibition in the United States.* Charlottesville, Va: University of Virginia Press, 1974.

Canadian Commission of Inquiry into the Non-Medical Use of Drugs: *Cannabis.* Ottawa: Information Canada, 1972. Interim Report, 1973. Final Report, 1973.

Farnsworth, D.L.: Substitute for competence: drug dependence and its amelioration. In *Further Explorations in Social Psychiatry,* edited by B.H. Kaplan, R.N. Wilson, and A.H. Leighton. New York: Basic Books, Inc., 1976.

Glasscote, R.M., Sussex, J.U., Jaffee, J.H. et al: *The Treatment of Drug Abuse.* Washington, D.C: Joint Information Service of the American Psychiatric Association and the National Association for Mental Health, 1972.

Grinspoon, L.: *Marihuana Reconsidered.* Cambridge, Mass: Harvard University Press, 1971.

Group for the Advancement of Psychiatry: *Drug Misuse, A Psychiatric View of a Modern Dilemma.* New York: Charles Scribner & Sons, 1973.

Levin, Peter A., ed.: *Contemporary Problems of Drug Abuse.* Acton, Mass: Publishing Sciences Group, Inc., 1974.

Lindesmith, A.R.: *Addiction and Opiates.* Chicago: Aldine Publishing Company, 1968.

Marin, P. and Cohen, A.Y.: *Understanding Drug Use.* New York: Harper and Row, 1971.

Mayor LaGuardia Committee on Marihuana: *The Marihuana Problem in the City of New York*. 1944. Reprint. Metuchen, N.J.: Scarecrow Reprint Corporation, 1973.

Mikuriya, T.H., ed.: *Marijuana Medical Papers, 1839–1972*. Oakland, Calif: Medicomp Press, 1973.

Musto, D.F.: *The American Disease*. New Haven, Conn: Yale University Press, 1973.

Ray, O.S.: *Drugs, Society, and Human Behavior*. St. Louis: C.V. Mosby Co., 1972.

Rosenthal, M.S.: *Drugs, Parents, and Children*. Boston: Houghton Mifflin Co., 1972.

Rubin, V. and Comitas, L.: *Ganja in Jamaica*. Paris: Mouton & Co., 1975.

Snyder, S.H.: *Uses of Marijuana*. New York: Oxford University Press, 1971.

Winick, C.: *Sociological Aspects of Drug Dependence*. Cleveland: CRC Press, Inc., 1974.

Wittenborn, J.R., Smith, J.P., Brill, H. et al: *Drugs and Youth*. Springfield, Ill: Charles C Thomas, 1969.

Wittenborn, J.R., Smith, J.P., and Wittenborn, S.A.: *Communication and Drug Abuse*. Springfield, Ill: Charles C Thomas, 1970.

16 The Positive Power of the Placebo and the Art of Prescribing

Martin Goldberg, M.D.

INTRODUCTION

Prescribing medication for a patient today is a very different process than it was in years gone by. Physicians in the past had relatively few drugs to work with, and most of them, we now know, were ineffective in terms of physiology and pharmacology. The prescription was written in a strange language, Latin, to ensure that the patient knew nothing of what he was receiving, and perhaps to add a certain dignity to the whole process. "Mistura Rhei et Sodae plus Tinctura Opii Camphorata" was not only unintelligible to most patients, but it also sounded a good deal more impressive than the mundane English "Mixture of Rhubarb and Soda plus Paregoric." A respectable prescription in those days almost always called for the mixing and compounding of three or more different ingredients. This compounding was carried out by the pharmacist, who had to be truly skilled in making up powders, capsules, and suppositories as well as in preparing

351

tinctures, elixirs, and the like. When a patient took his prescription to the pharmacy, he expected that it would take some time for it to be compounded. If the pharmacist looked at the prescription, whistled softly to himself, and said, "This will take at least an hour to make up," the patient glowed with quiet satisfaction, knowing that any medicine that difficult to prepare must indeed be strong and effective. And patients would have been shocked and dismayed if any druggist had informed them that they could have their prescription right away because it only had to be poured from one bottle into another. In short, prescriptions were surrounded by the aura of ritual and were mysterious medications known only to the doctor and druggist and were far beyond the patient's ken. There was much that was bad about such a system, yet surely there was also much that was good. How else can we explain the fact that those few, simple, largely "ineffective" medications which the doctor in times past had at his command so often proved to be most effective and remedial indeed in calming apprehension and in relieving suffering?

Today, the writing and filling of a prescription is a far different matter. Courses in prescription writing have long since disappeared from medical school curricula, and Latin is a language for bright high school students, rather than for doctors and pharmacists. If our prescriptions are unintelligible to patients, it is not due to the language they are written in but rather to the barely readable scrawls we cultivate. Nonetheless, many of our patients know a good deal about the drugs they are receiving, and at times some of them (thanks to *Time* magazine, *The New Yorker*, *The New York Times*, etc) seem to have a knowledge about medications and therapeutics that rivals our own. We have a plethora of drugs available to us now, with any number of medications available for a specific purpose or complaint. (Should anyone doubt this, let him simply glance at the glossary in the back of this book, which lists the abundance of remedies for psychic ills.)

The pharmacist's task is still a most important one, but no longer does it consist of mixing, pulverizing, or compounding in any way. Virtually all prescriptions, even those involving combinations of drugs, are ready-made by the manufacturers. And if the patient waits for his prescription in the drug store today it is not because the pharmacist is compounding it, but simply because there are many other orders to fill first. Whatever the patient does not know about the drug he is receiving, the pharmacist should and generally does know, and quite often this knowledge is shared. In summary, the mystery is gone, and the ritual, if any remains, is of a far different nature.

Much of this is for the better. Surely it is better that we have so many more drugs: many of them highly effective, some slightly or questionably effective, some ineffective. Surely it is better that the patient knows something, and perhaps a good deal, about the medications he receives. Surely it is better that the doctor can write a prescription in a matter of seconds and that the pharmacist can fill it almost as quickly. Yet there is a strong likelihood that the mysterious processes of prescribing and preparing medication have become much too simple and have lost some effectiveness even as the drugs available have become more effective. How else can we explain the many cases in which a patient is given a prescription for a drug that is undoubtedly effective for his complaint, yet he subsequently achieves no calming of his anxiety or relief of his suffering? In order to explore this question a bit further let us consider two case examples.

PATIENT COMPLIANCE WITH THE THERAPEUTIC REGIMEN

Comparison of Two Cases

First, there is the case of a gentleman we will call Mr. Wright. He is a 45-year-old salesman who comes into his physician's office complaining of lack of energy, loss of appetite, insomnia with early morning awakening, and a tendency to develop sudden and unexplained spells of sadness and crying. His physician takes a thorough history and does a complete physical examination. That examination and some routine laboratory tests are all quite normal, and the physician astutely makes a diagnosis of depressive disorder. He prescribes amitriptyline (Elavil), 100 mg daily, for Mr. Wright and asks him to return in two weeks. Mr. Wright does just that, and on his return appointment his doctor is delighted to find that his patient is much improved. Mr. Wright reports that he is now sleeping well, his appetite has improved, and although his sadness and lethargy persist, these symptoms are also beginning to lessen.

Now, let us look for a moment at another case, that of a man we will call Mr. Rong. Mr. Rong is also a 45-year-old salesman, and he presents himself to his doctor with complaints identical to

Mr. Wright's: some melancholy with crying spells, loss of appetite, lack of energy, and insomnia with early morning awakening. Here, also, the physician takes a complete history and performs a thorough physical examination plus routine laboratory studies. Once again, since the physical and laboratory studies reveal no pertinent findings, the doctor makes a diagnosis of depressive disorder, prescribes 100 mg of amitriptyline daily for his patient, and asks him to return in two weeks. When Mr. Rong appears for his second visit, however, the results are not so pleasing. Mr. Rong looks worse than ever; he is now obviously very slow and lethargic, seems to have lost more weight, and appears almost despondent. He reports that his symptoms are uniformly worse and that the medicine has not helped at all.

Here we have, apparently, two very similar patients receiving the same treatment and responding to it in opposite ways. There are several possible explanations for this phenomenon. Perhaps Mr. Wright and Mr. Rong, although both are depressed, have very different types of depressive disorder: one of which is responsive to amitriptyline and one of which is not. Or perhaps Mr. Wright has coincidentally received some psychologic boost in the two-week therapy period that would account for the improvement in his condition while Mr. Rong has had no such luck. It may even be possible that Mr. Wright has simply gone into a spontaneous remission quite independent of the medication he received. In the case of these two particular men, however, there is a totally different explanation for the varying results. To understand it, we will have to go back and examine how each of their physicians prescribed the medicine and how each of these patients used it.

Mr. Rong's physician used the short, sweet, and simple approach. He said to Mr. Rong, "I think you may be suffering from a depression; this medicine should straighten you out," whereupon he wrote out the prescription for amitriptyline, 25 mg four times per day, handed it to his patient, and told him to return in two weeks' time. Total time elapsed in prescribing: one minute. Mr. Rong took the prescription to his friendly pharmacist, and since his doctor had told him nothing about the medication, when the pharmacist handed him his pills, Mr. Rong asked, "What is this stuff, anyhow?" Somewhat at a loss, the pharmacist answered, "It's pretty strong medicine and it ought to calm you down." By now, Mr. Rong was frankly puzzled. He did not much like the idea of being given "strong" medicine, and he did not think he needed to be calmed down at all! On the contrary, he wanted something to pep him up. But his doctor had prescribed this medication for him, and he decided to try it and see what help it might give him.

That day he took a 25-mg tablet on four different occasions, as directed. By the time he took his third pill, he felt groggy and sleepy, and after taking the fourth pill he went to bed early, taking a half-grain phenobarbital tablet that another physician had previously prescribed for his insomnia. He slept *very* soundly. Perhaps he slept too soundly, for in the morning he slept right through his alarm clock's call and was barely able to drag himself out of bed and get to work an hour late. All day long, he felt awful. It seemed to him that he was in a daze or stupor and was just going through the motions of what he had to do in robot-like fashion. There was a strange, metallic taste in his mouth and his mouth was oddly dry. In an effort to counteract this, he doubled his usual quota of luncheon martinis from two to four. At dinner, he took his third dose of 25 mg of amitriptyline for the day. He felt so sleepy afterwards that he barely made it to his bed. The next thing he knew, it was morning and his wife was shaking him to wake up. Mr. Rong never did make it into the office that day. He felt almost stuporous and slept off and on throughout the morning, afternoon, and evening. His wife asked him if he was remembering to take his new medicine, but he refused to answer her. By the next day, Mr. Rong got himself back to work, but the new medication was a thing of the past. He had decided that the amitriptyline made him feel a "helluva lot worse," not better, and he was not about to take any more of it. When he arrived back to see his physician after the two-week interval, he had been off the medicine for 12 days, having used it faithfully for just 48 hours.

Now let us examine how Mr. Wright's physician went about the process of prescribing. He also began by giving Mr. Wright his opinion that the latter was suffering from a depression and by telling him that he was prescribing some appropriate medication. He then said, "I want to explain a few things about this medicine to you. It's generally very helpful in clearing up depressions, once we get the right dosage. Some people aren't helped by it. If that should prove to be the case with you, there are other good medications we can try. Now, this medicine takes a little time to build up in your system to a level where it will be helpful, and you'll have to take it steadily and faithfully. It's not like taking aspirin for a headache; it's not the kind of drug where you take one or two pills and feel better. You have to stay with it, taking regular doses, and then it can help you.

"There are a couple of effects of the medicine I want to

explain to you. First off, it will probably help your sleep problem a great deal. For that reason, take the entire dose at night, an hour or so before bedtime. Most people, when they first start using it, get almost too much help with their sleep. In other words, it just might make you feel really groggy and dopey for a few days. Don't worry about that—it's a normal reaction. Start the medicine on a weekend if you think it might interfere with your work, but by all means stick with it, and you'll find that as you get used to it, the grogginess will wear off, but your sleep pattern will be much better. The other thing is that this medicine almost always dries up your mouth and may give you a slightly strange taste in your mouth. When that happens, you'll know the medication is working in your system. Unfortunately, it can't be avoided, so just use some hard candy or some glycerine cough drops to counteract it."

The physician then went on to ask Mr. Wright several questions. Was he using any sleeping pills? It turned out that Mr. Wright had been using phenobarbital each night in an attempt to sleep. The doctor, realizing that barbiturates can speed the breakdown and metabolism of amitriptyline in the liver and thus interfere with development of a therapeutic level, advised Mr. Wright to discontinue the sedation. The physician also asked Mr. Wright whether he used any alcoholic beverages. When the latter confirmed that he did indulge a bit (a martini or two at lunch each day), he was told that alcohol and the prescribed medicine tend to interact with each other in such a way that "one drink is going to feel like two to you." Consequently, Mr. Wright was advised to either eliminate or minimize his drinking while using the amitriptyline.

Finally, the doctor explained to Mr. Wright that it was good to build up a level of his medicine gradually and thus give the body a chance to get used to it. Consequently, he was advised to use only one pill the first day, and then increase the dose by a pill each day until he was up to four pills. Since all doses were taken before bedtime, Mr. Wright took one 25-mg pill the first night, two the second night, three on the third, and four pills each night thereafter, until the day of his return visit with the doctor.

Although all this advice may sound a bit complex, the total time elapsed in prescribing for Mr. Wright was just under five minutes. Mr. Wright followed his physician's very clear instructions quite faithfully. He did indeed find that the medication helped with his insomnia immediately, and he was pleased to discover that the initial grogginess his doctor had predicted was moderate and did wear off in a few days. His mouth was dry and there was a metallic taste in it. But Mr. Wright had been warned of this and kept taking the medicine, finding, to his delight, that by the second week he definitely felt better and his symptoms were abating. He arrived back at his physician's office for his second visit having taken the medicine faithfully throughout the intervening two weeks. Even more important, he arrived back at the office with additional confidence and trust in his doctor, who had clearly and accurately predicted for him the course of his therapy.

Maximizing Patient Compliance

What are we to make of these two clinical cases? Our research scientists would analyze the data scrupulously and come up with the following profound conclusion: Mr. Wright is doing well in recovering from his illness because he is a *compliant patient.* Mr. Rong, on the other hand, is doing poorly because he is that unfortunate and bothersome creature, a *noncompliant patient.* As an experienced clinician, I have a different explanation, which is just this: there is probably no significant difference between these patients, but there is a difference in the way they were treated. Mr. Wright's doctor practiced the *art of prescribing,* and although that is taught but little these days, it is still quite often the difference between successful and unsuccessful treatment.

Obviously, the noncompliant patient who receives a prescription but never takes the medicine, or who uses it only sporadically or briefly, cannot benefit from his prescribed therapy. The physician's art is to prescribe in such a manner as to maximize compliance (Kabat, 1976). To accomplish this, we want to make it fairly easy for the patient to take his medication, and we want to prevent him from encountering any surprises. ("The best surprise is no surprise" is the advertising slogan of a national motel chain, and this is quite true in therapeutics, also.) We also want to maximize the patient's faith and confidence in his physician by prescribing in such a manner that the patient comes to believe we know what we are doing. To achieve these goals, I would suggest the following general rules:

1. Whenever possible, prescribe medication in a simple, once-a-day dosage form. The more doses a patient has to take per

day, the more likely he is to be noncompliant and to forget or skip doses. If once-a-day dosage is not feasible, prescribe the minimum number of doses per day.

2. Always be certain to prescribe enough medication to last the patient unitl his next visit with you. "Running out of medicine" increases noncompliance, even when the patient can renew the prescription, because it adds another step to the process of remaining faithful to a treatment regimen.

3. Prescribe that medication be taken at definite, set times. Rather than prescribing "one pill four times per day," prescribe "one pill before (or after) each meal and one pill at bedtime." Rather than prescribing "one pill at night," prescribe "one pill an hour before bedtime." Rather than "one pill every eight hours," prescribe "one pill at 8 AM, one at 4 PM, and one at 12 midnight." The more definite the times, the more likely the patient is to establish a good pattern of taking the medication regularly.

4. Ascertain what other medications the patient is currently taking. This allows you to avoid incompatibilities and disturbing interactions. Also, find out what medication of a similar nature to the one you are about to prescribe the patient has used in the past and with what results. If you are going to prescribe amitriptyline and the patient says something like, "Another doctor gave me Elavil once, and it didn't help me at all," this should give you pause. Under the circumstances, this is not the drug to prescribe (even though the patient's previous trial on it may well have been unsuccessful because the dosage was inadequate or the therapy was not sustained for a sufficient period of time), because the patient has lost confidence in this particular medication. So if you wish to prescribe a tricyclic antidepressant, you will do better to prescribe a different one, such as imipramine, protriptyline, nortriptyline, or doxepin.

5. Despite the fact that most experts and virtually all textbooks warn against prescribing combination drugs, give them careful consideration. There are many clinical situations where you may want to prescribe two different medications for two different purposes. A common example of this involves the patient who is depressed but who also has a great deal of agitation or tension stemming from anxiety. In this situation, you may well decide to prescribe both a tricyclic antidepressant and a strong antianxiety drug. If you prescribe dosages of two different pills for your patient, that complicates his therapy and reduces the likelihood of his compliance in taking the medication. If you prescribe a

combination medicine such as Triavil or Etrafon, which combines amitriptyline with perphenazine, your patient has only one pill to take and the chances of precise compliance are far better.

It has been pointed out that combination drugs employ a fixed ratio of the two ingredients and hence lack flexibility. This is a valid objection, but one that can be minimized when various ratios are available in the combination. On reflection, one is startled to find that so much criticism is directed at combination drugs for lacking dosage flexibility. It would seem more appropriate to criticize the lack of flexibility of most single-drug dosage forms, since these single drugs are often marketed as the sort of tablet or capsule that cannot be compounded with another ingredient by a pharmacist. Moreover, the average patient today may be hard put to find a pharmacist who will accept a prescription that calls for actually compounding several ingredients. Pharmacists will often decline such rare prescriptions with the alibi that they don't have the ingredients in stock.

6. Consider the possibility that your patient may be using nonprescribed substances which may interact or interfere with the therapeutic effects of the drug you are prescribing. Alcohol is one of the very common substances in this category and it interacts with many medications; it potentiates the central nervous system sedative effects of barbiturates, benzodiazepines, phenothiazines, tricyclic antidepressants, and the like. Stimulant drugs such as caffeine and nicotine are used even more widely than alcohol. The amount of diazepam (Valium) that you prescribe to calm an anxious patient may prove to be inadequate if that patient is regularly consuming large amounts of caffeine in his daily coffee ration or is stimulating himself with the nicotine from 20 to 40 cigarettes each day. Therefore, ascertain just what nonprescription drugs your patient is using and either adjust the dosage of your prescription accordingly or warn the patient of the possible pitfalls of drug interaction.

7. Tell your patient something about the medication you are ordering for him. If you do not do so, many patients will develop misconceptions. They may get erroneous, partial, or misleading information about the drug from a friend or neighbor, or from a pharmacist, as Mr. Rong did. It is generally neither necessary nor desirable to give the patient a long, complex chemical name to identify the medication you are ordering, but it is helpful to let him know about the sort of drug it is and what can be expected from it.

8. The more precisely you can predict for your patient what his prescription is going to do or not do for him, the more compliant he will be in using the drug. (Remember, the best surprise is no surprise.) This is where Mr. Wright's physician did such a beautiful job. He predicted for Mr. Wright the sedative effects of the amitriptyline, the dryness of the mouth that was apt to develop, and other effects he was likely to notice. Of course, we often cannot predict the exact effects that a drug is going to have in the human organism, but even that fact can be explained to the patient honestly in advance. For example, in prescribing an antidepressant, the physician may well say something like, "This medicine helps many people who are depressed, but it doesn't work for everybody. You take it faithfully for several weeks, and when we get to the right dosage, it should help you. If it doesn't, we will have learned something and we can put you on another type of antidepressant drug that may do a much better job for you."

Tell the patient what he can and cannot expect from the medicine. Can he expect immediate relief if the drug is to be effective, or should he anticipate that he must take the drug for a period of time? Is he supposed to use the medicine for only a brief period—only until relief of his complaints is achieved—or should he stay on the drug for a long time, indefinitely, or until he checks with you?

9. Where side effects from a drug are so common as to be almost universal, inform the patient of those, also. With other side effects that occur quite often but not in a majority of cases, simply mention them to your patient. As for the myriad possible side effects that may be produced by any drug, from aspirin on up, it is generally neither necessary nor therapeutically wise to frighten the patient by mentioning or listing all these.

10. If for any reason you suspect that a patient might intentionally overdose on the medication you are prescribing, do the following: (a) Prescribe that drug which has the widest margin of safety if taken in excessive dosage. For example, if you are prescribing a sedative/anxiolytic, give diazepam (Valium), which is far safer than meprobamate, the barbiturates, or any of the major tranquilizers. Similarly, if you must prescribe a hypnotic, prescribe flurazepam (Dalmane), a much safer drug than chloral hydrate, the barbiturates, or the bromides. (b) Prescribe only a small amount of medication, and insist that the patient have a return visit with you (not a telephone call!) before any further

amounts of drug are ordered. (For further suggestions relative to preventing a patient from overdosing on medication, see the section on detecting the suicidal patient, in the chapter "Recognizing the Depressed Patient.")

Rules for the Patient

There is another, briefer set of rules that our patients might observe which will help greatly in maximizing the effectiveness of prescribed medications. We need to instruct our patients to do the following as their part of the therapeutic process:

1. Take the prescription exactly as it is ordered: in the precise amount, in the precise manner, and at the specified time or times.
2. If some unanticipated effect develops from the medicine, call the doctor and tell him about it immediately. Similarly, if symptoms seem to worsen, or if new symptoms develop after taking the prescription, call at once and convey this information to the doctor.
3. It is generally not desirable to take *less* of a medication than was ordered without checking with the physician.
4. *Never* take *more* of a medication than was ordered. If one pill makes you feel good, that does not indicate that two pills will make you feel excellent. More likely, two pills will make you feel quite ill.
5. If you have to stop taking your medicine for some reason, call your physician and tell him about it.
6. Don't discuss your prescription with family, friends, or acquaintances, and if you must discuss it, don't take their comments about the medication too seriously. Your 21-year-old nephew may be a sophomore in nursing school or in pharmacy college, but that does not make him an expert. Rely on the advice of the physician you have consulted.
7. Your prescription is a specific medication ordered for you by your physician. Never offer it to another person for some complaint with which they are suffering. Similarly, never take a medication that has been prescribed for someone else.

THE MIGHTY AND MYSTERIOUS
PLACEBO

Let us now turn to another aspect of the art of prescribing and consider the placebo. Some people would describe it as the "lowly" placebo, but I choose to speak of the "mighty and mysterious" placebo.

According to *Dorland's Illustrated Medical Dictionary* (1974), the term placebo comes from the Latin verb meaning "I will please" and indicates "an active substance or preparation given to satisfy the patient's symbolic need for drug therapy, and used in controlled studies to determine the efficacy of medical substances. Also, a procedure with no intrinsic therapeutic value, performed for such purposes." This rather lengthy definition does not tell us much about the placebo. In reality, no patient has a "symbolic need for drug therapy." Rather, he has a need for the alleviation of his complaints: for his pain to diminish, for his headache to go away, for his nervousness to subside. Since placebos can produce such results at times, they are still used quite often in clinical practice, sometimes with the premeditation of the physician and sometimes without it. That is, at times we prescribe inert or relatively inert substances knowing that they are inactive but may be helpful, and at other times we prescribe such substances because we truly believe that they possess some medicinal qualities.

The term placebo has fallen into disfavor, however, except when employed in the second sense of our dictionary definition: "an inactive substance . . . used in controlled studies to determine the efficacy of medicinal substances." We have been made to be somewhat ashamed of the "sugar pill" and to regard it as a bit of quackery, deception, or at the very best, highly unscientific medicine. Yet Evans (1974a) has shown that "the ingestion of placebo medication can significantly reduce pain and suffering in approximately one patient in three." Perhaps even more relevant is Evans' deduction from his research that "under appropriate conditions a placebo is about half as effective as morphine in relieving pain." One would have to suppose that if a new pain-killer were introduced on the market, and if it could be truthfully advertised that it reduces pain and suffering for one patient in three—is proven half as effective as morphine—and has absolutely no side effects, no incompatibilities, no toxicity, and no potential for physiological addiction, then that painkiller would soon be a very successful product indeed.

THE PLACEBO EFFECT

To understand more about the placebo, let us look a bit further at Evans' work. He reports (1974a) that the placebo effect recorded in double-blind studies equals about half the effectiveness of the assumed capacity of the analgesic being administered, which indicates that the context in which the medicine is given is highly influential on therapeutic outcome. This is an extremely important and thought-provoking statement for any clinician to contemplate and understand. If the context in which the medicine is given is highly influential on therapeutic outcome, then we, as practitioners of medicine, certainly want to utilize the potent forces involved to help our patients. Moreover, if the "placebo effect" derives from the context in which medication is administered, then it must be present in a patient's response to an active therapeutic substance, just as it is present with the giving of an inactive agent.

McGlashen et al (1969) have discussed how the placebo effect is achieved, particularly in analgesia. Noting that there is a relationship between anxiety reduction and the alleviation of pain, they feel that "placebos apparently act upon the secondary component of pain, particularly by reducing anxiety." If this is true, then we might hypothesize: if an analgesic agent such as aspirin relieves pain to a certain extent, and if an inactive placebo also appears to relieve pain by acting on the secondary component (anxiety), then if and when a physician prescribes aspirin for a patient in a manner such as to evoke the placebo effect, the patient will have the benefit of both the pain relief from the aspirin and the anxiety reduction from the placebo effect, with the net result that the relief of symptoms will be definitely greater and more effective.

What I am suggesting is that the placebo effect may well result with any prescription that is given to a patient, regardless of whether the prescription is for an inactive or an active substance. Also, the placebo effect may well be additive in many instances to the physiologic effects of active agents in the process of symptom relief.

In another of his papers, Evans (1974b) recognizes this when he states: "The placebo responder has a marked advantage when he does have to take other pain-killing drugs. He will be much more responsive to them. For example, in one study a standard dose of morphine was only 54% effective for patients who were insensitive to placebos but 95% effective for placebo responders."

McGlashan et al (1969) note that "when associated with ingesting active drugs, the placebo effect, broadly conceived, occurs in a situation surrounded by an aura of expectancy and implied change. Because of the patient's belief that the medication should work, changes in behavior or experience are anticipated. In this sense the placebo response is a nonspecific effect of the drug treatment."

When we discuss the positive power of the placebo, then, we are dealing with the patient's anticipation of changes in his behavior or experience based on his belief that the medication should work. More than this is involved, however. We have considered the medication and we have considered the patient, but we have thus far not considered the third important factor in the therapeutic situation: the doctor. Not surprisingly, it has been found that the placebo effect depends not only on the patient's belief that the medication should work but also on the physician's conviction that the medication will be effective. This is precisely why the prescribing of sugar pills is no longer practiced and, indeed, simply cannot be practiced by most of us. Since we know that such sugar pills are inactive, we have no belief or conviction in them as medication; but our medical predecessors "knew" that sugar pills did all sorts of wonderful things for patients, and thus they could prescribe them with considerable success. Double-blind studies give the final confirmation of this. In these experimental situations, even today's physician can prescribe an inactive medication and have it produce symptom relief, precisely because he does not know the medication is inactive but rather believes it to be at least possibly therapeutic. Again we can turn to Evans' outstanding work (1974b) for elucidation of this point. He writes: "The placebo's effectiveness is directly proportional to the apparent effectiveness of the active analgesic agent that doctor and patient think they are using. When the physician assumes he is using a powerful pain-killer, such as morphine, the result is a strong placebo effect. If, however, the physician assumes that the analgesic is mild, the result is a much smaller placebo effect, even though it is still proportionately about half as effective as the actual drug."

The positive placebo effect is brought about, then, by a patient and a doctor who together expect a particular medication (active or inert) to produce relief of symptoms. The question remains to perplex us: How does this positive placebo effect operate? By what mysterious mechanism is this beneficial effect caused? We have no satisfactory answers for this, but then, we know precious little about how or why many of the active medications in our therapeutic armamentarium work. The expeditious assumption is that the placebo effect is brought about by "suggestion," and that placebo responders are suggestible people. This idea has not been confirmed in various experimental investigations, however. The best description that we are then left with is that the hope and confidence of a physician can be instilled into a patient in such a way as to relieve the anxiety which is a secondary component of pain and of virtually every form of medical symptom. "It appears that the drug-giving ritual, and all of the associated nonspecific variables of trust and belief existing within the doctor-patient relationship, produce powerful curative effects" (Evans, 1974a).

THE NEGATIVE PLACEBO EFFECT

We have established that a doctor who is confident and hopeful about the medication he prescribes may convey that trust and belief to his patients and produce the positive placebo effect in about one third of them. Now we need to look for a bit at the other side of the coin. What about the patient who does not have confidence in the prescription he is given and who does not start off with the anticipation that the medication may well be helpful? Similarly, what about the physician who prescribes a medication whose efficacy he doubts, and who proffers a prescription to his patient with little or no expectation that it is going to do the slightest bit of good? Clearly, with such a patient and such a doctor, there can be no positive placebo effect. Moreover, it is quite possible that what will be produced is a *negative placebo effect* which detracts substantially from the effectiveness of the medication given, even when that medication is an active substance that may possess very real pharmacologic powers for relieving the patient's complaints. If the positive placebo effect works by minimizing or relieving anxiety through trust and belief, then the negative placebo effect works by augmenting and aggravating anxiety through distrust and disbelief. Nowhere is this more important than in the prescribing of mind-influencing drugs; whatever the intrinsic merits of the medication, it may well be the placebo effect—positive or negative—that determines the success or failure of therapy with antidepressants, major tranquilizers, anxiolytics, sedatives, and hypnotics.

What this all adds up to is that the prescribing physician should not be at all embarrassed or hesitant about considering and manipulating the placebo effect to the best advantage of his patients. That means that the physician will want, whenever possible, to have a positive placebo effect, as well as the physiologic effects of the medication, operating for the patient. Additionally, the physician will wish to avoid the negative placebo effect, which can only detract from therapeutic results. I would make the following suggestions toward achieving these ends:

1. Whenever possible, prescribe medications that you are quite familiar with and with which you have seen beneficial therapeutic results. Of course, we all have to prescribe "new" medications at times in order to test out their efficacy. However, it is clinically wisest to prescribe the tried-and-true medicine that you know well first; if and when this should fail, then you can turn to newer remedies.

2. Share with your patient some or all of your reasons for prescribing a particular medication. When you write for a trusted old-standby remedy, tell the patient that is what you are doing: "I'm ordering some medicine for your nervousness that seems to be really effective. I've used it with many people, and it seems to do the trick!" If, on the other hand, you have to prescribe a medicine that is relatively new to you, you still base your choice of prescription on something: what you have heard from other clinicians or what you have read in the medical literature. Share this reasoning with your patient also: "This medicine is relatively new on the market, but a lot of doctors are reporting great success with it," or "Let's try something different for your headaches, since the previous drugs haven't helped you. There's a good bit of evidence that this medicine I'm going to order for you helps headaches when other drugs fail."

3. Never write a prescription for a medication that you firmly believe is ineffective or that you are convinced will be useless for your patient. Usually you are writing a prescription because there is *some* chance of it being helpful, no matter how slim the chance is. Total pessimism on your part pretty much indicates that a particular prescription should not be written. Patients are quite adept at detecting the physician's skepticism or pessimism, just as they are adept at sensing his confidence or optimism.

4. Utilize your own personality type and your own style in conveying hope and reassurance with your prescription. Some doctors have the kind of bluff, hearty, authoritarian personality that enables them to say "Now you get this prescription filled and take it just like I say, and I'm sure you'll feel better," and to say this in a convincing, genuine, effective manner. For others of us, such an approach would sound phony or contrived. We may be better able to convey our confidence and reassurance by gently, calmly, and definitely prescribing the medication and by indicating with a few words or gestures that we expect it will be helpful. Whatever your personal style, bring it to play in offering your patient some relief from the anxiety that inevitably accompanies his other medical complaints.

5. If you are firmly convinced that there is *no* medication that will help a particular patient's complaint, then do not prescribe any drug. As we all know, the sick patient has a need for the doctor to give him something, but there are things we can give other than medications. Consider prescribing something you feel *will* be helpful: a diet change, a change of life-style, some hygienic advice. Or, give the patient something that may be more helpful than any prescription: your best counsel and wisdom, expressed in a sympathetic manner.

ABOUT OVERPRESCRIBING

From both popular and scientific circles we frequently hear the accusation that people in general today are "over-medicated" and that physicians overprescribe wildly. This charge is frequently levelled primarily at American doctors, even though statistical studies show that people in many other countries use substantially greater amounts of medications than do the inhabitants of the United States. We should consider this question of overmedication and overprescribing, however. Certainly, it seems true that a great many Americans are overmedicated. A large percentage of these people, however, are overmedicated because of their use of over-the-counter, nonprescription drugs. Even a greater number—in fact, a vast majority of overmedicated Americans—are ingesting drugs that are not used for medicinal purposes at all: drugs such as alcohol, caffeine, and nicotine.

In terms of prescribed medications, the situation is more complex. We may well be overprescribing for some maladies. For example, as is noted elsewhere in this book, there is a tendency to overprescribe various sedative and anxiolytic agents, such as the barbiturates, meprobamate, and the benzodiazepines (Valium, Librium, etc). Amphetamines were overprescribed in the recent past, but fortunately this is abating. On the other hand, various medications may well be underprescribed. A recent study (Raft et al, 1975) confirms the fact that antidepressant drugs are underprescribed—a fact that many experienced clinicians have suspected for some time.

The issue is also complex on the patient's side. Much attention is paid to people who are drug abusers and overusers, and certainly there are many of them. But we should also concern ourselves with those people who, for one reason or another, will never use a drug even when one is clearly needed; or with those patients (not at all uncommon) who consistently underuse prescribed medication. These people take too little of their medicine, skip prescribed doses, or discontinue needed medication because of exaggerated fears of drugs or because of some sort of "moral" conviction that it is better to do without any medicine at all. This conviction has deep roots in many people and often leads to much unnecessary suffering and to deterioration and disease that could well have been checked by proper medication.

I believe we must arrive at the conclusion, then, that generalizations about the prescribing and the taking of drugs are very misleading and inaccurate. Both patients and physicians might be best guided by the rule: When you need a medicine, it is wise to take one, and when you don't need medicine, then by all means shun it. Physicians should be alert against prescribing medicines or amounts of medicines that are unnecessary or excessive. Hopefully, they will be equally alert to the danger of not prescribing those remedies that are indicated, or of prescribing them in insufficient, inadequate dosages. The ideal amount of medicine to use is neither a lot nor none at all; the ideal amount is the least amount that will cure or alleviate suffering, pain, or disease.

REFERENCES

Dorland's Illustrated Medical Dictionary, 25th ed., s.v. "placebo."
Evans, F.J. and McGlashan, T.H.: Work and effort during pain. In *Perceptual and Motor Skills,* edited by Carol Ammons. Missoula, Mont: Southern Universities Press, 1967.

Evans, F.J.: The power of a sugar pill. *Psychol Today* 9:54–60, 1974a.

Evans, F.J.: The placebo response in pain reduction. In *Advances in Neurology*, Vol. 4, edited by J.J. Bonica. New York: Raven Press, 1974b.

Kabat, H.F.: Making sure the drug is used. Read before the Hennepin County Medical Society, Minneapolis, Minn., January 14, 1976.

McGlashan, T.H., Evans, F.J., and Orne, M.T.: The nature of hypnotic analgesia and placebo response to experimental pain. *Psychosom Med.* 31:227–246, 1969.

Orne, M.T.: Pain suppression by hypnosis and related phenomena. In *Advances in Neurology*, Vol. 4, edited by J.J. Bonica. New York: Raven Press, 1974.

Raft, D., Davidson, J., Toomey, T.C. et al: Inpatient and outpatient patterns of psychotropic drug prescribing by nonpsychiatric physicians. *Am J Psychiatr.* 132:1309, 1975.

Shapiro, A.K.: A contribution to a history of the placebo effect. *Behav Sci.* 5:109–135, 1960.

Stewart, W.K.: The dysplacebo effect. *Mod Med.* 44:98–101, 1976.

17 Michigan Department of Mental Health Guidelines for the Use of Psychotropic Drugs

Raymond W. Waggoner, M.D.

INTRODUCTION

That there was an important need for guidelines in the use of psychotropic drugs became apparent in the course of reviewing approximately 1500 treatment summaries submitted by community-based and mental hospital psychiatrists requesting prior certification for Medicare and Medicaid extension of psychiatric hospitalization. These reviews indicated a therapeutically inconsistent use of psychotropic drugs that was of such magnitude as to seriously interfere with the optimal psychiatric care of the patients receiving these medications.

It was therefore decided that the Department of Mental Health should develop guidelines concerning the appropriate use of psychotropic drugs to help the psychiatrists avoid some of the more prevalent errors found in the review of their certification requests. Dr. Raymond W. Waggoner[1] and Dr. Homer F.

[1]Senior Clinical Consultant, Michigan Department of Mental Health

Weir[2] undertook the development of these guidelines. The preliminary copy was completed, and it was sent to the directors of all (Michigan) state facilities for comment. When these comments were returned, they were incorporated into the draft, which was then submitted to Dr. Edward Domino[3] for his comments. These were incorporated into the final draft to be sent to the various facilities under the control of the Department of Mental Health.

The original guidelines were based on clinical experience with drugs and on reports from current literature, which were coordinated with the material. An attempt was made to follow the orientation of the AMA *Drug Evaluations,* the *Physicians' Desk Reference*, and the *American Hospital Formulary Service.* It is interesting to note that Dr. Aaron Mason[4] had arrived at essentially the same conclusions as had we in reviewing prescriptions written by psychiatrists practicing in mental hospitals.

It should be emphasized that the guidelines were intended primarily for the use of the physicians in state facilities, and that they might be of value to other psychiatrists in their individual practices. It should also be noted that all guidelines, as such, are subject to modification, revision, and/or deletion as continuing research and new clinical data may indicate. We feel that when guidelines are established with this kind of flexibility in mind, they become a document valuable not only in helping the physician to provide optimal services but also in establishing a baseline for assessing treatment accountability.

Purpose

These standards were compiled to establish a set of guidelines for treatment with psychotropic drugs.

Application

All facilities and hospitals operated by the State of Michigan Department of Mental Health and all county community mental health programs shall adhere to these standards.

---

[2]Senior Advisor on Medical Care Services, Michigan Department of Mental Health
[3]Professor of Pharmacology, University of Michigan
[4]Chief Psychiatrist, Medical Center, University of Kentucky

References

Public and Local Acts   52 Stat. 1040 et seq. (1938), as amended; 21 U.S.C. 301 et seq., as amended; Act 151, Public Acts of 1962, Michigan Pharmacy Act (338.1106); Act 149, Public Acts of 1967, Nursing Practice Act (338.1151); Act 196, Public Acts of 1971, Michigan Controlled Substances Act (335.301); Act 185, Public Acts of 1973, Medical Practice Act (338.1801).

Administrative and Emergency Rules   Emergency Rules, Department of Mental Health, August 15, 1975; General Rules Relating to the Practice of Nursing, Department of Licensing and Regulation; Interim Rules Relating to the Practice of Medicine, Department of Licensing and Regulation; State Board of Pharmacy, Department of Licensing and Regulation, June, 1974, Supplement October 28, 1974, Supplement July 9, 1975; Controlled Substances, State Board of Pharmacy, Department of Licensing and Regulation, May 31, 1974, Supplement October 28, 1974; Joint Commission, Accreditation of Hospital Standards, *Accreditation Manual for Psychiatric Facilities*, 1972.

Policy and Legal Authority: Emergency Administrative Rules

The Michigan Department of Mental Health's guidelines to psychotropic drug use outline the following rules to promote a **safe, sanitary, and humane living environment** for the inpatient:

1. A facility shall have a pharmacy, or shall contract for pharmaceutical services within a pharmacy, licensed and subject to and conducted in accordance with existing statutes, rules, and procedures.
2. Residents shall receive prompt and adequate medical treatment, for physical ailments and for the prevention of illness or disability, which meets standards of the medical community.

Guideline rules governing the policies and procedures of administration of **medication** specify:

1. Medication shall be administered only at the order of a physician. (*Note*: Emergency phone orders may be used

providing the physician countersigns the order within 24 hours.)

2. Medication shall not exceed United States Food and Drug Administration standards (as defined in current *Physicians' Desk Reference*; AMA *Drug Evaluations* [Second Edition]; and/or *American Hospital Formulary Service* [current issues]) unless the medical rationale is documented in the patient's clinical record in accordance with written review procedures established by the hospital staff. (See "Use of Potentially Toxic Dosages," later in this chapter.)

3. Medication shall not be used as punishment, for the convenience of staff, or as a substitute for other appropriate treatment. (*Note*: Department of Mental Health policy is to interpret this rule as, "Medication shall not be used as a punishment or for the convenience of staff.")

4. Administration of a psychotropic medication shall be reviewed not less frequently than every 30 days to determine the appropriateness of continued use.

5. Medications shall be administered by qualified and trained facility personnel in accordance with the Medical Practice Act and the Nursing Practice Act.

6. Administration of medication shall be recorded in the resident's medical record. (*Note*: Department of Mental Health policy is to interpret this rule as, "All medication shall be recorded, including aspirin.")

7. Medication cards or other approved systems shall be used in the preparation and administration of medication.

8. Nursing units shall be equipped with adequate medication areas which provide appropriate and sufficient spaces for dosage preparation and set-up. Administration shall be in accordance with existing statutes and rules of the Michigan Pharmacy Act and the Michigan Controlled Substances Act.

9. Medication errors and adverse drug reactions shall be immediately reported to a physician and the facility director and shall be recorded in the resident's clinical record. (*Note*: Department of Mental Health policy interprets this rule as, "Medication errors and adverse drug reactions shall be immediately reported to

a physician, who will promptly deal with the problem. The facility director shall record the incident in the resident's clinical record.")

10. Medications given to residents upon leave or discharge shall be only on written authorization of a physician.
11. Medications given to residents upon leave or discharge shall comply with state rules and federal regulations pertaining to labelling and packaging.

The guidelines define the following policies in respect to **medical diagnostic service**:

1. Medical diagnostic services shall be provided only on the request of a physician.
2. A facility shall have provision of promptly and conveniently obtaining required clinical, laboratory, x-ray, and other diagnostic services.
3. Results of clinical tests shall be immediately brought to the attention of the physician and incorporated in the clinical record.

Use of psychotropic **chemotherapy** shall be subject to restriction as follows:

1. Unless the individual consents, or unless administration of chemotherapy is necessary to prevent physical injury (as described below) to the individual or to others, psychotropic chemotherapy shall *not* be administered to:
   a) A resident who has been admitted by medical certification or by petition until after a final adjudication;
   b) A defendant undergoing examination at the center for forensic psychiatry or at another certified facility to determine competency to stand trial;
   c) A person acquitted of a criminal charge by reason of insanity who is undergoing examination and evaluation at the center for forensic psychiatry.
2. Consent shall meet the requirements of an informed consent.
3. Chemotherapy may be administered to prevent physical injury after signed documentation of the physician is placed in the record of the resident and when

acts of a resident, or other objective criteria, clearly demonstrate to a physician that a resident is presently dangerous to self or others.

4. Initial administration of psychotropic chemotherapy may not be extended beyond 48 hours unless there is consent. The initial period of treatment shall be as short as possible, shall be terminated as soon as there is little likelihood that the resident will quickly return to an actively dangerous state, and shall utilize the smallest dosage necessary.

5. Additional chemotherapy may be administered if a resident again becomes dangerous to self or to others following termination of a period of medication, whether prior to final adjudication or whether during a period of examination or evaluation ordered by a criminal court.

6. A governing body shall adopt policies and procedures regarding psychotropic chemotherapy which:
   a) Define psychotropic chemotherapy;
   b) Establish objective criteria for determining present dangerousness;
   c) Provide for the medical staff to develop agreement on the minimum duration of treatment for different disorders;
   d) Establish when and how documentation is placed in records of residents.

Prior to final adjudication, or during a period of examination or evaluation ordered by a criminal court, the medical staff of a facility may provide essential emergency physical treatment as requested or consented to by the resident or the individual empowered to give consent. When the life of a resident is in danger and consent cannot be obtained, essential emergency physical treatment may be performed after the medical necessity has been documented and entered into the record of the resident.

DEFINITION OF PSYCHOTROPIC DRUGS

Psychotropic drugs are defined as those agents which exercise direct effects upon the central nervous system and which are capable of influencing and modifying behavior. Drugs included in this category and to which the guidelines apply are:

Antipsychotics (eg, chlorpromazine)
Antidepressants (eg, imipramine)
Agents for control of mania and depression (eg, lithium)
Antianxiety agents (eg, diazepam)
Sedatives and hypnotics to promote sleep (eg, flurazepam hydrochloride)
Psychomotor stimulants (eg, methylphenidate hydrochloride)

STANDARDS OF PROCEDURE

Establishment of Dosage

A comprehensive drug history should be obtained, if possible, before treatment is initiated. A detailed account should include a consideration of the use of other drugs by the patient as well as any history of cardiac, liver, renal, central nervous system, or other disease. Communication between the physician treating the behavioral disorder and any physicians who may be treating other disease entities in the same patient is essential if serious drug interactions are to be avoided.

The target symptoms and behaviors to be treated should be entered in the clinical record. These signs and symptoms constitute a baseline against which the patient's clinical condition is evaluated, and they also permit evaluation of the effectiveness of treatment. Effects of medication on the target symptoms and on patient behavior should be recorded weekly in the patient's progress notes.

Adequate initial dosages should be used to obtain desired results. Concern over exceeding recommended maximum dosages or over the possibility of producing side effects tends to lead doctors to prescribe dosages too low to achieve optimum results. The adequacy of initial dosage has to be cautiously and individually determined. Experts should be consulted when there is any doubt about dosage effectiveness and amount. (The exception to this high initial dosage practice is the occasional drug which should be started on a low dosage and gradually built up to an adequate amount. This procedure is especially indicated in elderly or debilitated patients and in those patients who have exhibited reactions to other psychotropic drugs.)

Initially, very large dosages should not be given for longer than a week. Sometimes a brief medication review after 2 or 3 days of drug treatment may be helpful in quickly evaluating the appropriateness of dosage amount. The initial period of administration of a prescription should never exceed 30 days without an evaluation of patient response. Dosage should be gradually reduced to a minimum maintenance level after the desired clinical result is obtained and the patient's condition has stabilized.

In each case, a psychotropic drug should be administered for a period sufficient to determine its clinical effectiveness. Frequently patients have been shifted from one drug to another after only very short trials. In general, a period of from three to six weeks may be required before significant improvement in psychotic symptoms is observed. In acute cases, the patient's management problems may be so severe that a change in drug within a shorter period (less than three to six weeks) may be necessary. And occasionally, even longer periods of treatment may be needed before a change in medication is indicated.

In adults, a single daily dose of some psychotropic drugs may be used, especially antipsychotic and antidepressant agents, which have a long half-life in the body. Either a morning or an evening schedule may be used. There is evidence that large, single daily doses of some psychotropic drugs, such as antidepressants, given to children may result in undue toxicity and therefore should not be used. With single evening doses, complaints of side effects are frequently reduced, and sedative properties may aid in sleep. Morning doses may be used in patients who show fewer side effects during the daytime. It is recognized that small dosages of even long-acting drugs tend to cause less fluctuation in plasma levels and may be of clinical value.

Drug Holidays

Drug holidays may be established as part of the drug schedule for some patients. Prolonged daily doses are required by very few patients, and the minimum required dosage should be individually determined. In the use of antipsychotic and antidepressant drugs, a drug-free day each week, a drug-free weekend, an every-other-day dosage schedule, or a drug-free week per month may be established where possible.

The chronic use of antianxiety agents (eg, chlordiazepoxide and diazepam) is not generally justified. The effectiveness of antianxiety agents is short-lived (a matter of a few days to a few weeks); prolonged use may increase the likelihood of drug dependence and/or a therapeutic paradox. The maxim for use of antianxiety agents might well be that only that anxiety which markedly interferes with human performance should be treated with drugs—and then only with drugs that are not tolerance or dependence forming.

Use of Potentially Toxic Dosages

If dosage levels significantly in excess of the maximums listed in the AMA *Drug Evaluations,* the *Physicians' Desk Reference*, or an *American Hospital Formulary Service* are used, the medical rationale should be documented in the patient's clinical record in accordance with written review procedures established by the hospital staff.

Nonpsychotic (as diagnosed by a psychiatrist) residents of centers for the retarded shall not receive dosages in excess of maximum amounts as defined by the sources above. Thioridazine should not be given in amounts exceeding 800 mg daily in either hospitals for the mentally ill (MI hospitals) or in Regional Human Development (MR) Centers, because dosages in excess of this can cause retinopathy.

The use of psychotropic drugs in children is under continuing study. Generally, because long-term toxicity studies pertinent to the growing child are unavailable, most drug manufacturers and the Food and Drug Administration are not recommending use of certain psychotropic drugs, such as haloperidol, Prolixin, or the antidepressants (used to treat either depression or enuresis), in children. Nevertheless, there are a number of therapeutic situations where the use of these psychotropic drugs in children is clearly indicated. These include the use of haloperidol in the treatment of Gille de la Tourette's syndrome not responsive to approved medications, and of antipsychotic agents in the treatment of psychoses which are resistant to approved medications at approved dosage levels. There are other examples; it is to be understood that in those situations where the manufacturer and/or the Food and Drug Administration do not recommend a higher dosage level, or where a specific medication is not approved for children in spite of its apparent clinical effectiveness, the physician should seek a second opinion (in writing) from a qualified child psychiatrist or psychopharmacologist. Written, informed consent should also be secured from the parents or guardians.

Use of Psychotropic Drug Combinations

Generally, only one psychotropic drug should be prescribed at a time. There is little evidence to support the use of psychotropic drug combinations under most circumstances. Such a practice has the disadvantage of not permitting identification of the offending drug if side effects occur. Drug consultations may be indicated when combined medications are used. There are important exceptions to the suggestion of prescribing only one drug at a time, and some of these are described below.

1. Combinations (Etrafon, Triavil) of an antidepressant such as amitriptyline with an antipsychotic such as perphenazine may have therapeutic value in affective illness.

2. The prophylactic use of an antiparkinsonism agent with an antipsychotic is held by some drug experts to be justified. Even so, such routine use should be discouraged because of the side effects (anticholinergic psychosis) which can result with high dosages of antiparkinsonism drugs. Hence, the use of antiparkinsonism drugs usually is indicated only when extrapyramidal side effects appear. Antiparkinsonism drugs are not effective in preventing extrapyramidal side effects, and their routine use increases the severity of lethargy and dizziness and may produce a toxic psychosis with memory loss. Such a disturbance of the cholinergic system with the atropine-like antiparkinsonism drugs may be treated temporarily with a cholinergic agonist like physostigmine. However, reduction in the dosage of the anticholinergic is the long-term solution.

3. If the maximum dosage of a psychotropic drug is accompanied by toxic symptoms, then treatment may be helped by lowering the dosage of the first drug and adding an appropriate second drug to the regimen.

4. Severe mania may benefit from the combination of lithium carbonate with an antipsychotic drug.

Although this combination has been said to result in enhanced toxicity on some occasions, there is not good evidence that this is the case.

PRN Dosage Regimens

The use of psychotropic drugs on a PRN (as needed) basis is not indicated after the first two or three weeks of treatment with a significant dosage of medication. PRN dosage of a psychotropic is frequently used to control acutely disturbed behavior or other symptoms. The need for such use usually indicates that the patient has not yet been stabilized on a clinically effective dosage. One exception might be the PRN usage of chlorpromazine for the treatment of LSD flashback, even though the patient may be generally stabilized for his anxiety on a clinically effective dosage.

Precautions in the Use of Lithium

Because of potential, serious toxicity, lithium should be used only after a complete history, physical examination, and laboratory assessment of the patient have been done. The standards we mention are being actively studied and may change, but the following are the current essential parts of the work-up done before lithium use:

1. A history of previous use of lithium is solicited, with particular attention to evidence of lithium sensitivity.
2. A medical history must probe for any evidence of heart, kidney, or thyroid disease. Tests should be made in verification:
   a) An electrocardiogram should be done;
   b) Laboratory tests should be performed to determine adequate kidney functioning;
   c) Thyroid assessments should consist of a physical examination, and T-3 and T-4 determinations as indicated by history and physical.

Once treatment with lithium has been instituted, various monitoring procedures must be maintained. The American Psychiatric Association's guidelines for laboratory work are as follows:

1. Serum lithium levels and sodium chloride blood levels should be determined according to the following schedule (*Note*: The morning dose should be held until blood is drawn for lithium study):
   a) Two to three times weekly until the patient is stabilized;
   b) Then weekly for one month;
   c) Then monthly for one year;
   d) After one year, both levels should be determined at three- to six-month intervals as long as the patient is on the medication;
   e) Every three to six months, maintenance surveillance for thyroid, cardiac (blood pressure and electrocardiogram), and renal functions should be implemented.
2. Serum lithium levels should not exceed 2.0 mEq/liter in initial therapy or 1.5 mEq/liter during maintenance therapy.

Adjunctive therapeutic requirements include:

1. A daily fluid intake of 2500 to 3000 cc;
2. Dietary sodium chloride to be adjusted as indicated by laboratory findings; and
3. Avoidance of tricyclic antidepressants for treating slight or moderate depressions that occur during lithium therapy.

Choice of Drugs and Treatment Review

A general guideline might be to select the psychotropic drug which in the physician's clinical judgment offers the most effective treatment for the target symptoms exhibited by the patient. Better results will be obtained if the physician becomes quite familiar with one or two of the different classes of antipsychotics (the phenothiazines, the thioxanthenes, a butyrophenone, a dibenzoxazepine, and an indole) than if he relies on minimal experience with many drugs.

Semiannually, annually, or at other times as appropriate, there should be a formal review of each patient's drug treatment plan. Direct care personnel and the clinical pharmacist, as well as the physician, should be involved in the therapy review. The

---

RESPONSE TO CHEMOTHERAPY: ANNUAL OR BIANNUAL REVIEW IN INPATIENTS AND OUTPATIENTS

Name: _____ Case No.: _____ Date: _____

Diagnosis: _____

_____

Medication: _____

Date First Administered: _____

Duration of Chemotherapy: _____

Symptomatology and Course of Illness
Degree of Impairment and Nature of Improvement

Annual or biannual review of the effects of chemotherapy along with other treatment regimens involves:

  a. Estimation of initial degree of impairment (symptomatology) and of nature of improvement with application of drugs

  b. Evaluation of nature of adjustment without chemotherapy: medication is discontinued for two- to four-week intervals

---

Exhibit A. Form used by the Fairlawn Center at Clinton Valley Center (a Department of Mental Health psychiatric hospital in Pontiac, Michigan) in the review and evaluation of inpatient and outpatient response to chemotherapy.

Symptomatology	With Chemotherapy From: _____ To: _____					Without Chemotherapy From: _____ To: _____	
	Degree of Impairment			Nature of Improvement		Nature of Adjustment	
	Severe	Moderate	Mild	Improved	Not Improved	Moderate Change	Mild or No Change
Thought Disorder							
Impaired Affect							
Impaired Motivation							
Regressive-Bizarre Behavior							
Aggressive-Assaultive Behavior							
Impaired Work Habits & Daily Activity							
Depression							
Suicidal Behavior							
Mania or Hypomania							
Other Symptoms							
Overall Evaluation							

Recommended Course of Treatment:_____

_____

_____

_____

Chemotherapy:_____

_____

_____

Reviewed by: _____ M.D. Date:_____

results of these reviews, and new treatment recommendations, should be recorded in the patient's record. A simple format, similar to the sample devised by the Fairlawn Center of Clinton Valley Center, should be used (see Exhibit A).

Each individual institution (MI hospital or MR center) should develop inhouse training/retraining seminars at which consultants in the use of antipsychotic and other behavioral drugs can discuss chemotherapy with the hospital or center medical staff, including those responsible for outpatient care. Clinical psychopharmacology consultants should be designated for the purpose of helping inhouse staff with ongoing therapeutic problems (dosages, new drugs, new reactions, drug interactions, etc) as needed. If additional funding is needed to support such consultative services, the individual institution should designate its need for such funds in its budget request. The Michigan Department of Mental Health is currently studying the feasibility of retaining a centrally supported Office of Psychopharmacology Consultation, Education, and Research.

When psychotropic drugs have been prescribed, laboratory surveillance of hemoglobin levels, of white blood cell count (with differential as indicated), and of liver and renal functions (through SMA, eg) should be maintained.

GLOSSARY

Table 1
Mind-Influencing Drugs by Trade Name

Trade Name	Generic Name	Type of Drug
Adapin	Doxepin hydrochloride	Tricyclic antidepressant
Akineton	Biperiden	Antiparkinsonism agent
Amphedroxyn	Methamphetamine	Stimulant
Antitrem	Trihexyphenidyl hydrochloride	Antiparkinsonism agent
Artane	Trihexyphenidyl hydrochloride	Antiparkinsonism agent
Atarax	Hydroxyzine	Antianxiety agent
Aventyl	Nortriptyline hydrochloride	Tricyclic antidepressant
Bendopa	Levodopa	Antiparkinsonism agent
Benzedrine	Amphetamine	Stimulant
Chlor-PZ	Chlorpromazine	Antipsychotic (aliphatic phenothiazine)
Cogentin	Benztropine mesylate	Antiparkinsonism agent
Compazine	Prochlorperazine	Antipsychotic (piperazine phenothiazine)
Dalmane	Flurazepam hydrochloride	Antianxiety agent (benzodiazepine)
Dartal	Thiopropazate	Antipsychotic (piperazine phenothiazine)
Daxolin	Loxapine succinate	Antipsychotic
Deaner	Deanol	Stimulant
Deprol	Meprobamate plus benactyzine hydrochloride	Antianxiety agent; antidepressant (???)
Desoxyn	Methamphetamine	Stimulant
Dexedrine	Dextroamphetamine	Stimulant
Dilantin	Diphenylhydantoin	Anticonvulsant
Disipal	Orphenadrine hydrochloride	Antiparkinsonism agent
Dopar	Levodopa	Antiparkinsonism agent
Elavil	Amitriptyline hydrochloride	Tricyclic antidepressant
Equanil	Meprobamate	Antianxiety agent
Eskalith	Lithium carbonate	Miscellaneous
Etrafon	Amitriptyline hydrochloride plus perphenazine	Combination tricyclic antidepressant and antipsychotic
Haldol	Haloperidol	Antipsychotic (butyrophenone)
Imavate	Imipramine hydrochloride	Tricyclic antidepressant
Inapsine	Droperidol	Used for I.V. and I.M. tranquilizing (butyrophenone)
Inderal	Propranolol hydrochloride	Beta-adrenergic blocking agent
Janimine	Imipramine hydrochloride	Tricyclic antidepressant
Kemadrin	Procyclidine hydrochloride	Antiparkinsonism agent

Table 1 *(continued)*

Trade Name	Generic Name	Type of Drug
Larodopa	Levodopa	Antiparkinsonism agent
Levsin	L-hyoscyamine sulfate	Antiparkinsonism agent
Levsinex	L-hyoscyamine sulfate	Antiparkinsonism agent
Librium	Chlordiazepoxide	Antianxiety agent (benzodiazepine)
Lithane	Lithium carbonate	Miscellaneous
Lithonate	Lithium carbonate	Miscellaneous
Lithotabs	Lithium carbonate	Miscellaneous
Loxitane	Loxapine succinate	Antipsychotic
Marplan	Isocarboxazid	MAO inhibitor; antidepressant
Mellaril	Thioridazine	Antipsychotic (piperidine phenothiazine)
Miltown	Meprobamate	Antianxiety agent
Moban	Molindone	Antipsychotic (oxoindole)
Nardil	Phenelzine sulfate	MAO inhibitor; antidepressant
Navane	Thiothixene	Antipsychotic (thioxanthene)
Norpramin	Desipramine hydrochloride	Tricyclic antidepressant
Pagitane	Cycrimine hydrochloride	Antiparkinsonism agent
Parnate	Tranylcypromine	MAO inhibitor; antidepressant
Permitil	Fluphenazine	Antipsychotic (piperazine phenothiazine)
Pertofrane	Desipramine hydrochloride	Tricyclic antidepressant
Pipanol	Trihexyphenidyl hydrochloride	Antiparkinsonism agent
Presamine	Imipramine hydrochloride	Tricyclic antidepressant
Prolixin	Fluphenazine	Antipsychotic (piperazine phenothiazine)
Proketazine	Carphenazine	Antipsychotic (piperazine phenothiazine)
Quide	Piperacetazine	Antipsychotic (piperidine phenothiazine)
Rau-Sed	Reserpine	Antipsychotic (rauwolfia alkaloid)
Repoise	Butaperazine	Antipsychotic (piperazine phenothiazine)
Ritalin	Methylphenidate	Stimulant
Sandril	Reserpine	Antipsychotic (rauwolfia alkaloid)
Serax	Oxazepam	Antianxiety (benzodiazepine) agent
Serentil	Mesoridazine	Antipsychotic (piperidine phenothiazine)
Serpasil	Reserpine	Antipsychotic (rauwolfia alkaloid)
Sinemet	Carbidopa plus levodopa	Antiparkinsonism agent
Sinequan	Doxepin hydrochloride	Tricyclic antidepressant
SK-Bamate	Meprobamate	Antianxiety agent
SK-Pramine	Imipramine hydrochloride	Tricyclic antidepressant
Solacen	Tybamate	Antianxiety agent

Table 1 *(continued)*

Trade Name	Generic Name	Type of Drug
Sparine	Promazine	Antipsychotic (aliphatic phenothiazine)
Stelazine	Trifluoperazine	Antipsychotic (piperazine phenothiazine)
Symmetrel	Amantadine hydrochloride	Antiparkinsonism agent
Taractan	Chlorprothixene	Antipsychotic (thioxanthene)
Thorazine	Chlorpromazine	Antipsychotic (aliphatic phenothiazine)
Tindal	Acetophenazine	Antipsychotic (piperazine phenothiazine)
Tofranil	Imipramine hydrochloride	Tricyclic antidepressant
Tofranil-PM	Imipramine pamoate	Tricyclic antidepressant
Tranxene	Clorazepate dipotassium	Antianxiety agent (benzodiazepine)
Tremin	Trihexyphenidyl hydrochloride	Antiparkinsonism agent
Triavil	Amitriptyline plus perphenazine	Combination tricyclic antidepressant plus antipsychotic
Trilafon	Perphenazine	Antipsychotic (piperazine phenothiazine)
Tybatran	Tybamate	Antianxiety agent
Valium	Diazepam	Antianxiety agent (benzodiazepine)
Vesprin	Triflupromazine hydrochloride	Antipsychotic (aliphatic phenothiazine)
Vistaril	Hydroxyzine	Antianxiety agent
Vivactil	Protriptyline hydrochloride	Tricyclic antidepressant (stimulant)

Table 2
Mind-Influencing Drugs by Drug Type

Type of Drug	Generic Name	Trade Name
Antianxiety Drugs or Minor Tranquilizers		
Benzodiazepines	Chlordiazepoxide	Librium
	Clorazepate dipotassium	Tranxene
	Diazepam	Valium
	Flurazepam hydrochloride (promoted as hypnotic)	Dalmane
	Oxazepam	Serax
Glycerol derivatives	Meprobamate	Milton
		Equanil
		SK-Bamate
Diphenylmethane derivatives	Hydroxyzine	Atarax
		Vistaril
Antipsychotic Drugs		
Aliphatic phenothiazines	Chlorpromazine	Thorazine
		Chlor-PZ
	Promazine	Sparine
	Triflupromazine	Vesprin
Piperazine phenothiazines	Acetophenazine	Tindal
	Butaperazine	Repoise
	Carphenazine	Proketazine
	Fluphenazine	Permitil
		Prolixin
	Perphenazine	Trilafon
	Prochlorperazine	Compazine
	Thiopropazate	Dartal
	Trifluoperazine	Stelazine
Piperidine phenothiazines	Mesoridazine	Serentil
	Piperacetazine	Quide
	Thioridazine	Mellaril
Butyrophenones	Droperidol	Inapsine (used for I.V. and I.M. tranquilizing)
	Haloperidol	Haldol
Thioxanthenes	Thiothixene	Navane
	Chlorprothixene	Taractan
Dibenzoxazepines	Loxapine succinate	Daxolin
		Loxitane
Oxoindoles	Molindone	Moban
Rauwolfia alkaloids	Reserpine	Rau-Sed
		Sandril
		Serpasil
Antidepressants		
Tricyclic antidepressants	Amitriptyline	Elavil
	Desipramine	Norpramin
		Pertofrane
	Doxepin	Adapin
		Sinequan

Table 2 *(continued)*

Type of Drug	Generic Name	Trade Name
Tricyclic antidepressants (*cont'd*)	Imipramine	Imavate
		Presamine
		SK-Pramine
		Tofranil
	Nortriptyline	Aventyl
	Protriptyline	Vivactil
MAO inhibitors	Isocarboxazid	Marplan
	Phenelzine	Nardil
	Tranylcypromine	Parnate
Antiparkinsonism Drugs	Amantadine hydrochloride	Symmetrel
	Biperiden	Akineton
	Benztropine mesylate	Cogentin
	Carpidopa plus levodopa	Sinemet
	Cycrimine hydrochloride	Pagitane Hydrochloride
	L-hyoscyamine sulfate	Levsin
		Levsinex
	Levodopa	Bendopa
		Larodopa
		Dopar
	Orphenadine hydrochloride	Disipal
	Procyclidine hydrochloride	Kemadrin
	Trihexyphenidyl hydrochloride	Antitrem
		Artane
		Pipanol Hydrochloride
		Fremin
Stimulants	Amphetamine	Benzedrine
	Dextroamphetamine	Dexedrine
	Deanol	Deaner
	Methamphetamine	Desoxyn
		Amphedroxyn
	Methylphenidate	Ritalin
Miscellaneous		
Beta-adrenergic blocking agent	Propranolol hydrochloride	Inderal
Anticonvulsant	Diphenylhydantoin (phenytoin sodium)	Dilantin
Drugs used in manic-depressive disease	Lithium carbonate	Eskalith
		Lithane
		Lithonate
		Lithotabs
Combination drugs (anxiety plus depression)	Amitriptyline hydrochloride plus perphenazine	Etrafon
		Triavil
	Meprobamate plus benactyzine hydrochloride*	Deprol

*Antidepressant activity highly questionable